# THERAPEUTIC APPROACHES TO
# MYOCARDIAL INFARCT SIZE LIMITATION

# Therapeutic Approaches to Myocardial Infarct Size Limitation

Editors

## David J. Hearse, B.Sc., Ph.D., D.Sc., F.A.C.C.
*Head of Research*
*Honourary Senior Lecturer in Biochemistry*

## Derek M. Yellon, Dip. Pharm., Ph.D.
*Senior Investigator*
*Honourary Lecturer in Biochemistry*

*The Heart Research Unit*
*The Rayne Institute*
*St. Thomas' Hospital*
*London, England*

Raven Press ■ New York

**Raven Press, 1140 Avenue of the Americas, New York, New York 10036**

Made in the United States of America

**Library of Congress Cataloging in Publication Data**
Main entry under title:

Therapeutic approaches to myocardial infarct size limitation.

    Includes bibliographies and index.
    1. Heart—Infarction. 2. Heart—Infarction—
Treatment. I. Hearse, David J. II. Yellon, Derek M.
[DNLM: 1. Myocardial Infarction—Therapy.
WG 300 T398]
RC685.I6T48   1984         616.1′237       84-13430
ISBN 0-88167-035-9

# Preface

It is paradoxical that, at a time when "infarct size reduction" is appearing in textbooks of cardiology and is becoming accepted by some as a routine clinical procedure, more and more experimental cardiologists are asking: "Is infarct size reduction really possible?" This book, the first devoted solely to the principles, problems, and possibilities of infarct size reduction, presents personal viewpoints on this major medical problem from a group of internationally acknowledged experts. Consideration of the arguments presented is likely to lead to a radical reappraisal of current concepts of the natural history and therapy of acute myocardial infarction.

A review of the literature over the last 15 years reveals many hundreds of experimental and clinical studies in which a wide variety of agents, as diverse as β-blockers, hyaluronidase, and cobra venom have all been claimed to reduce substantially the ultimate size of an evolving infarct. *Despite these encouraging studies with perhaps as many as 50 different agents, we must accept the fact that no single intervention has been adopted for widespread and sustained clinical use as an antiinfarct agent.*

After a decade of enthusiasm over the concept of the pharmacological protection of the regionally ischemic myocardium, a wave of caution and pessimism has engulfed many experimental and clinical cardiologists. *This is unfortunate since myocardial protection is undoubtedly possible.* One need go no further than the operating theater to see how the rational application of antiischemic procedures has revolutionized cardiac surgery. In the decade that cardiologists have begun to question the clinical value of antiinfarct agents, cardiac surgeons have used chemical cardioplegia to increase the duration of tolerable ischemic arrest by at least sixfold. Despite ever-increasing durations of ischemia, cardiac surgeons have exploited myocardial protection to achieve major increases in surgical safety and success.

Why is the protection of the ischemic myocardium becoming such a controversial issue, and why can we not apply successful surgical principles to evolving myocardial infarction? Although part of the answer can be attributed to the greater requirements and difficulties of treating myocardial infarction, we believe that much of the problem lies in failings of experimentation and interpretation. We now know, for example, that in the dog heart, the model upon which most concepts and clinical studies have been based, there is no lateral "border zone" of intermediate flow and injury. However, it was this border zone that was supposed to act as the target for therapeutic interventions. We now know that many widely used indices of tissue injury and protection are inadequate and cannot necessarily prove that we have prevented tissue death let alone returned cells to contractile function. We now realize that the term "protection" has been used far too loosely such that cardiologists have rarely made the critical distinction between slowing the rate of development of injury and achieving an absolute reduction in the extent of injury. This latter problem has stemmed from a general failure to acknowledge the overwhelming importance of the coronary artery anatomy and its collateral flow in determining patterns of cell death and survival.

It is now abundantly clear that without the "early" restoration of "substantial" coronary flow, ischemic tissue will die. It now remains for us to define the limits of "early" and "substantial" and then develop therapeutic methods to extend these limits. The advent of thrombolytic and angioplastic procedures will do much to stimulate these developments.

If infarct size reduction is to become a clinical reality, as we believe it can, there will have to be more and better studies; and this can only be achieved on the basis of a fuller understanding of: the natural history of ischemic injury, its spatial and temporal characteristics in various disease states in man and appropriate experimental models, and, finally, the pharmacology of injury modification and the manipulation of collateral flow.

Stimulated by our own confusion, we asked a small group of internationally acknowledged experts each to write a personal and speculative essay stating their view on various aspects of infarct size reduction. Not only has this allowed us to compile up-to-date and authoritative views on well established facets of the problem (for example, the anatomy and control of the coronary microcirculation and the vital role of the collateral supply), but we have also been able to introduce new and exciting concepts such as the likelihood that oxygen-derived free radicals and leukocytes may play a role in the evolution of tissue injury. In this integrated collection of essays, we have italicized certain sections of the text in order to highlight some of the important or provocative views held by our contributors. These opinions, together with the essays themselves, range from the pure clinical to the applied experimental. As a result, we believe that this book provides invaluable guidance (and, it is hoped, encouragement) to the practicing clinician, while also providing the experimentalist with the relevant clinical questions and the conceptual framework in which to devise those urgently needed investigations.

David J. Hearse
Derek M. Yellon

# Acknowledgments

Our most sincere thanks must go to our distinguished contributors who, despite the enormous pressures permanently placed upon them, all readily agreed to participate and who tolerated our bullying reminders which have allowed this book to go from inception to publication in less than 12 months. It is also appropriate to offer our gratitude to Andrew Henderson who, in addition to acting as a contributor, helped us to devise the content and essay format of the book. We would like to acknowledge our colleagues Vivien Baeza and Gillian Perrett, both of whom have committed much of their time and care to the preparation of the texts, and John Lovegrove, who skillfully prepared all art work. Our thanks go to Michael Oliver for writing the foreword and expressing so forcefully the clinicians' reservations about infarct size reduction; such reservations were of course the stimulus for this book.

# Contents

# Contributors

**Robert J. Bache, M.D.**
*Professor of Medicine*
*Department of Medicine*
*Cardiovascular Section*
*University of Minnesota Medical School*
*Minneapolis, Minnesota 55455*

**Sanford P. Bishop, D.V.M., Ph.D.**
*Professor of Pathology*
*Department of Pathology*
*University of Alabama in Birmingham*
*Birmingham, Alabama 35294*

**James M. Downey, Ph.D.**
*Professor of Physiology*
*Department of Physiology*
*University of South Alabama*
*College of Medicine*
*Mobile, Alabama 36688*

**David J. Hearse, B.Sc., Ph.D.,
    D.Sc., F.A.C.C.**
*Head of Research*
*Honourary Senior Lecturer in*
    *Biochemistry*
*The Heart Research Unit*
*The Rayne Institute*
*St. Thomas' Hospital*
*London SE1 7EH, England*

**Andrew H. Henderson, M.B.,
    F.R.C.P.**
*Chairman and Professor of Cardiology*
*British Heart Foundation Sir Thomas*
    *Lewis Chair of Cardiology*
*Honorary Consultant Cardiologist*
*Department of Cardiology*
*Welsh National School of Medicine*
*Heath Park*
*Cardiff CF4 4XN, South Wales*

**Michiel J. Janse, M.D.**
*Chief, Laboratory of Experimental*
    *Cardiology*
*Department of Cardiology and*
    *Experimental Cardiology*
*Academisch Medisch Centrum*
*Meibergdreef g*
*1105 AZ Amsterdam, Netherlands*

**Robert B. Jennings, M.D.**
*James B. Duke Professor and Chairman*
*Department of Pathology, Box 3712*
*Duke University Medical Center*
*Durham, North Carolina 27710*

**Stanley R. Jolly, Ph.D.**
*Research Associate*
*Department of Pharmacology*
*Medical College of Georgia*
*Augusta, Georgia 30912*

**Wolfgang Kübler, M.D.**
*Medizinische Universitatsklinik*
    *Heidelberg*
*Abt Innere Medizin III*
*(Kardiology)*
*Bergheimer Str 58*
*6900 Heidelberg 1, West Germany*

**Benedict R. Lucchesi, M.D., Ph.D.**
*Professor of Pharmacology*
*Department of Pharmacology*
*University of Michigan Medical School*
*Ann Arbor, Michigan 48109*

**Melvin L. Marcus, M.D.**
*Professor of Medicine*
*Department of Internal Medicine*
*Cardiovascular Division*
*University of Iowa*
*Iowa City, Iowa 52242*

**Joe M. McCord, Ph.D.**
*Chairman and Professor of Biochemistry*
*Department of Biochemistry*
*University of South Alabama*
*Mobile, Alabama 36688*


**Michael Oliver, M.D., F.R.C.P.**
*Professor of Cardiology*
*Cardiovascular Research Department*
*University of Edinburgh*
*Hugh Robson Building*
*George Square*
*Edinburgh, Scotland*


**Philip A. Poole-Wilson, M.D., F.R.C.P.**
*Professor of Cardiology*
*National Heart Hospital*
*Cardiothoracic Institute*
*2 Beaumont Street*
*London WIN 2DX, England*


**Keith A. Reimer, M.D., Ph.D.**
*Associate Professor of Pathology*
*Department of Pathology, Box 3712*
*Duke University Medical Center*
*Durham, North Carolina 27710*


**Joseph L. Romson, Ph.D.**
*Postdoctoral Fellow*
*Department of Surgery*
*Division of Cardiothoracic Surgery, RF25*
*University of Washington*
*Seattle, Washington 98195*


**Wolfgang Schaper, M.D., Ph.D.**
*Chairman and Professor of Cardiology*
*Department of Cardiology*
*Max-Planck-Institut*
*Parkstrasse 1*
*D-6350 Bad Nauheim, West Germany*


**Harald Tillmanns, M.D.**
*Senior Cardiologist*
*Medizinische Universitatsklinik*
  *Heidelberg*
*Abt Innere Medizin III*
*(Kardiology)*
*Bergheimer Str 58*
*6900 Heidelberg 1, West Germany*


**Derek M. Yellon, Dip. Pharm., Ph.D.**
*Senior Investigator*
*Honourary Lecturer in Biochemistry*
*The Heart Research Unit*
*The Rayne Institute*
*St. Thomas' Hospital*
*London SE1 7EH, England*

# Foreword

## Has the Study of Infarct Size Limitation
## Done Any Good?

While attending a recent conference on infarct size limitation, I observed that views more than facts were being exchanged, and that in the last 10 years, there has been little progress towards the clinical objective of reducing infarct size. This failure may be due partly to the lack of definition of objectives, partly to a lack of understanding of the limitations of clinical intervention, and partly to too much optimism. I must confess that I was disheartened to hear yet more discussions about "border zones," microcirculatory flow, and myocardial energy consumption, and to learn that there is still no firm definition of irreversible cell injury. It seems that many investigators find it difficult, or do not try, to relate their findings to humans and that many clinicians either suspect that infarct size reduction may be irrelevant, or do not realize its potential.

There should be two main objectives for the enthusiasm, research, and investment that has been directed into reducing the size of a myocardial infarct: *the first is the hope that there will be fewer deaths, and the second is that there should be an improvement of ventricular function such that survivors will have a better exercise tolerance and an improved capacity to return to and sustain a normal life.* Are either of these objectives well-founded?

The chief cause of early death is reentry ventricular arrhythmias. These develop during the time when local areas of myocardial ischemia vary, regress, or become confluent and lead rapidly to the development of infarction and necrosis. Later, lethal ventricular arrhythmias resulting from heterogeneous alterations in ions and substrates consequent upon reperfusion must contribute considerably and, still later, and to a lesser extent, arrhythmias arise from Purkinje tissue.

Ventricular arrhythmias are also the chief cause of death during the days, weeks, and months following recovery from myocardial infarction. However, only when the area of infarction is very large is there a strong correlation between the extent of tissue damage and the prevalence of either early or late ventricular arrhythmias. In those with moderate or small infarcts, lethal arrhythmias are common and not predictable. *If the primary objective of reducing infarct size is to decrease death rate, then it follows that it is only with interventions in patients with very large infarcts that success is likely to be achieved. Yet it is exactly this category of infarct, both experimentally and in man, where least success appears to have been achieved.* In general, arrhythmic deaths are likely to occur before intervention can be implemented.

Ventricular function is usually only seriously and noticeably impaired when a large infarct is present, varying widely in those with mild or moderate infarcts and measurement is unreliable in the acute phase. As far as ultimate left ventricular function is concerned, it may be irrelevant to show that it is possible to achieve a 10% reduction in the size of a moderate infarct.

Should we conclude, therefore, that the only worthwhile yield to the community is likely to come from attempts to reduce the size of large infarcts? If this is true, then the whole enterprise relates to a small minority.

We know that one-third of all patients with acute heart attacks die within the first 3 weeks, and that one-half of these are dead within two hours of the onset of the heart attack. Unless there is a great change in attitudes toward early resuscitation and faster transfer to intensive care areas, treatment to reduce infarct size cannot be instituted in this 15%. Of the remaining 15% reaching hospital, two-thirds probably die from ventricular arrhythmias and not from large infarcts. This leaves only about 5% likely to benefit from intervention. To them might be added another 10% of immediate survivors with large infarcts. *Thus, at the most, approximately 20% of patients might benefit, but we have no idea how much reduction of infarct size would be necessary to achieve either of the primary aims. It may be realistic to estimate that no more than a quarter of these might be helped, in other words, about 5 in every 100 patients.*

There is little evidence to suppose that the normal processes of healing are impaired in the majority of patients with infarcts whereas there is evidence to suggest that some interventions designed to reduce infarct size might also change the normal processes of healing adversely. For example, is it really wise to consider suppressing white cell invasion of damaged tissue because these cells might release leukotrienes and so cause greater damage? Why are they there in the first place? If the means used to reduce infarct size delay healing and seriously impede the development of the collagen-fibrosis reaction, then it could be argued that the moderately good left ventricular function, which exists in the majority of patients recovering from infarction, might actually be reduced by the intervention.

My next concern, expressed more eloquently by others, is the unrealistic laboratory conditions under which so many studies have been, and are being, conducted. Although I am the first to admit that there is no satisfactory experimental model for testing whether it is possible to reduce infarct size, we should have learned certain lessons by now. These should include recognizing that the administration of a "protective substance" prior to ligation or experimental occlusion of a coronary artery bears no relation to any current clinical management of infarction in man. Nor is there much relevance to the acute situation in man when the "protective substance" is given into the coronary arterial system. And it is not helpful to show that a given "protective substance" appears to reduce infarct size in one species but not in another, particularly when the studies use pharmacological doses which, because of other effects, would preclude the use of the substance in humans. Ought we not by now to have made more attempts to limit infarct size in chronically ischemic conscious animals with the intention of reproducing something of the situation that is present in a middle-aged adult human? Partial occlusion of two arteries weeks before major occlusion of the third might represent the human situation. Why is this not done? Why is the effect of intervention not studied in hearts with previously induced damage or infarction? Surely this is more relevant to the situation in man, whose first major event is often preceded by other unrecognized ones.

The methods used for coronary occlusion are often strikingly different, some sudden and some slow. This is also true of reperfusion, with some investigators using constant pressure then variable pressure, and others using pulsatile or constant flow. Additionally, there is still a lack of observance of the now widely accepted discipline adopted in clinical trials of "intention to treat;" studies are still reported where animals are excluded because they died or the experiment was judged to be "unsatisfactory."

Fortunately our methods of measuring infarct size are now on more solid ground, and much is being made of, for example, a maintained or slowly decreasing R:Q ratio, or of improvement in ST vector and QRS (40 or 100) vectors, combined with various methods of expressing creatine kinase isoenzyme release or left ventricular ejection fraction. *When all of these indices of infarct size appear to be improved, it might be justified to conclude that some impact has been made. However, I would still maintain that it is not justified to conclude that this will be useful to a middle-aged patient with acute myocardial infarction.* There are two recurring and outstanding deficiencies in the quest for reduction of myocardial infarct size. The first is the dearth of information concerning the effects of intervention in man, as compared with an appropriate control group, on the incidence of cardiac death at, say, 6 and 12 weeks after the heart attack. The second is the lack of information concerning ventricular function and exercise tolerance several weeks after the acute heart attack is over.

Unfortunately, accounts of change in either of these critical endpoints, whether they appear to have been improved, remain unchanged, or are worsened, are either based on small numbers or are anecdotal. This is not good enough. Recently (*N. Engl. J. Med.*, 310:9–15, 1984), there has been at least one serious attempt to meet this deficiency with the demonstration that intravenous timolol appears to reduce infarct size and also reduce sudden cardiac death. *Not that this means cause and effect and that reduction of sudden death is due to infarct size. More likely, both may be ascribed to early and continuous modulation of myocardial catecholamine activity.*

Until death and functional capacity are measured at three and six months after the administration of "antiinfarct agents" in a large number of patients within a formal clinical trial design, suspicion will continue to exist that little has really been achieved. Such a clinical trial, or preferably trials, should be established and conducted within the discipline and experience that has been so hard learned during the last 15 years. This requires that the trials will have to be large because of the heterogeneous nature of myocardial infarction, they will have to be double-blind and randomized, and the statistical aims will have to be identified prospectively.

I am bound to conclude that the area of investigation that I feel would be most worthwhile is preinfarct intervention. Modification of acute ischemia and its arrhythmic and thrombotic consequences would seem a far better bet in terms of reducing mortality and maintaining ventricular function than proceeding much further with attempts to modify infarct size, when, as I commented earlier, successful modification may help only 5 in every 100 of the infarct population.

Despite my personal view, I have no doubt that experimental and clinical studies of infarct size limitation will continue. If this is the case, then they should consider past and present failings and enter a new investigative era that will take into account the natural history of myocardial infarction, the relevance of experimental design, the limitations of interpretation and extrapolation, and the need for clinical trial to prove benefit. This volume, under the editorship of David Hearse and Derek Yellon, is the first to take a cold, critical, and detailed look at these and other problems, which should do much to make these long overdue improvements possible.

Michael Oliver
*Cardiovascular Research Unit*
*University of Edinburgh*
*Edinburgh, Scotland*

*Therapeutic Approaches to Myocardial Infarct
Size Limitation*, edited by D. J. Hearse and
D. M. Yellon. Raven Press, New York © 1984.

# 1

# The Problem and the Question: A Clinician's Viewpoint

### Andrew H. Henderson

*Department of Cardiology, Welsh National School of Medicine,
Cardiff CF4 4XN, South Wales*

## INFARCT SIZE LIMITATION

### The Concept

The concept of infarct size limitation is built on the idea that an intervention, after the onset of the acute process leading to myocardial infarction, can result in the ultimate size of that infarct being smaller than it would otherwise have been.

It is, of course, the clinical setting which gives the concept its potential importance, and it is in the clinical arena that its contribution has to be put to the test. Given the responsibilities of clinical care and the costs (in all senses of the word) of intervention, *the onus of proof rests on the advocates of intervention. Most conservative clinicians have yet to be convinced that infarct size limitation is a practical proposition.*

## Clinical Practice as Practiced

Clinical practice depends on a judicious mix of: (a) empirical evidence drawn from exclusive clinical trials and extrapolated from specific animal trials, (b) an understanding of underlying mechanisms, (c) the collective influence of clinical fashion (the swings of which are commonly underdamped), and (d) anecdotal experience. The difficulties of obtaining evidence from clinical trials have been well illustrated by the history of secondary prevention trials with β blockers; the problem of applying the hard-won evidence from such trials to individual patients remains with us as a source of everyday debate. The dangers of equating animal experiments with the human situation are well recognized. Likewise the inadequacy of our understanding of underlying mechanisms, despite the bewildering rate of progress in this field, needs no elaboration; yet rational practice must be based on a synthesis, unique to each patient, constructed from our limited knowledge of the underlying pathophysiology. Fashion reflects consensus judgment borne of such inadequate sources.

## The Background

*The difficulty with the concept of infarct size limitation is that we have had no accepted precise means of measuring infarct size in man, and we have had no adequate animal model of the overall clinical problem.* Add to this the natural history of the metaphor which degenerates into jargon (what of "myocardial salvage" and the "border zone," or even "infarct size limitation" itself?) and the reasons for the present clinical uncertainty begin to become apparent.

Infarct size limitation is inescapably linked in most people's minds with the series of experimental studies reported in the early 1970s (27,28). A wide variety of agents was found to be capable of reducing the ultimate extent of an infarct caused by acute coronary artery occlusion, generally in dogs. Recognition of deficiencies in the experimental design of some of these studies has led to some modification of the conclusions but they remain generally valid within their terms of reference, i.e., a number of agents given within, say, an hour of acute occlusion in previously healthy animals can limit infarct size. The "time for testing" of the concept in clinical practice was said to have come (5).

The time for testing may have come but it never really took off. It lost momentum. *Translated into the realities of the coronary care unit, such limited trials as have been conducted have been disappointing or ironically contrary, as with early β-blocker treatment where there is growing evidence of benefit in clinical trials (21) but little benefit in the more carefully controlled experimental studies (23).* In truth, the disappointments of negative results may be due to the difficulties of demonstrating benefit with the limited means available and against the background of biological scatter in the uncontrolled clinical setting. Very large numbers are needed: For example, some 3,000 patients would be needed to demonstrate a 15% difference in the extent of the infarct, and more if the endpoint was mortality (43); the number, of course, would be larger if a given intervention were to be effective only in an unidentified subgroup of patients. *The onus of proof remains with the interventionists. The responsible clinician is not easily persuaded into giving drugs by percentage points of statistical benefit.*

Meanwhile, the concept of infarct size limitation has been unnecessarily limited in most clinicians' minds to the type of experimental circumstances which gave it birth. Myocardial infarction in man differs in many important respects. Rarely is it amenable to therapeutic intervention as early as one hour after the onset of the acute process. Rarely is it likely to be the result of acute coronary artery occlusion without previous coronary artery disease and preexisting collaterals. And it would be naive to assume that every clinical myocardial infarct occurs as a result of a single acute irrevocable coronary occlusion.

*This difference between the clinical situation and the experimental model of acute coronary artery occlusion probably has two main explanations: (a) the complex pathogenesis and dynamic behavior of clinical coronary occlusion, and (b) the extent of preexisting collaterals capable of maintaining some flow in the proximally occluded system.*

## Is It Worth It?

The first point to establish is that the clinical goal of infarct size limitation is worth pursuing. *Of this there can be no real doubt (16).* There appear to be three main determinants of prognosis following a myocardial infarct, reflecting what are probably three different contributory causes of death: (a) the amount of myocardium lost, (b) the residual presence of myocardium still vulnerable to ischemia, and (c) an associated or separate liability to ventricular arrhythmias. The extremes of the relationship between prognosis and infarct size can be seen as the development of cardiogenic shock with its near 90% mortality if the infarcted area exceeds 40% of the myocardium (34), and the self-evident benefits of preventing infarction at all if the causal process can be reversed in time.

## Is It Practicable?

The next question is whether any therapeutic intervention to limit infarct size can be given to the patient in time. To some extent this question feeds on itself: *If major benefit could be established from early intervention, impetus would be given to the provision of mobile coronary care with which to deliver early intervention—*or to take another view, the widespread provision of mobile coronary care should provide the platform from which to test and provide such treatment. The practicability of infarct size limitation rests, at present, on the view that it may not be too late to intervene when the patient is seen some 4 hr after the clinical onset, despite the evidence from experimental coronary artery occlusion studies. For this, there is growing circumstantial evidence from many sources, though the potential for benefit clearly fast diminishes with time, and the scope for limiting infarct size is probably rather small by this time in most cases.

## CLINICAL SPECTRUM

### Simple Coronary Occlusion: A Simple View of Myocardial Infarction

Myocardial infarction at its simplest presents with the unheralded onset of chest pain, electrocardiographic evidence of regional ischemia progressing to infarction, and enzyme leakage from dying myocardium—attributed equally simply to the acute occlusion of a large coronary artery occurring at the site of a preexisting atheromatous stenosis often not severe enough to have limited perfusion to the point of symptomatic angina. With good fortune, arrhythmias and other complications do not ensue and the patient recovers to resume normal life, the loss of myocardium and cardiac reserve being too small for him to notice, the residual myocardium having compensated for any resultant conformational changes and increase in wall stress. In the less fortunate 50% of patients, ventricular fibrillation is the first manifestation of the ischemia, or it occurs before the patient reaches coronary care, so precluding any possibility of intervening to limit infarct size.

### Dynamic Coronary Occlusion: A Not-So-Simple View

*More careful evaluation suggests that the myocardial infarct frequently is not a single isolated event.* Over half the patients carefully questioned will recall unrecognized episodes of similar pain, or of nonspecific tiredness in the hours or days leading up to the infarct. This vague but clinically well recognized harbinger remains unexplained: We now know that episodes of ECG-documented myocardial ischemia are very commonly painless and also that complete functional recovery following ischemia may be long delayed; it may, therefore, conceivably reflect symptoms of intermittent pump failure following "silent" episodes of ischemia. The relatively high incidence of acute infarction following unstable angina with rest pain is also well known; and intracoronary thrombosis appears to play a pathogenetic role in unstable angina as well as in myocardial infarction (26). Aspirin has recently been reported to reduce the occurrence of myocardial infarction in unstable angina, suggesting a role for platelet aggregation (25). Unstable angina usually occurs with severe effort angina on a background of severe stenosis. Rarely it can be due to true "variant angina" (without effort angina or stenosis), where it appears that a temporary abnormality predisposes the artery to episodes of nonspecifically induced coronary constriction or "spasm." The occurrence of myocardial infarction with thrombus in some such patients illustrates, in an extreme way, the role that vasomotor tone can sometimes play in its pathogenesis (29). Anecdotal evidence of extreme stress at the onset of such a period of variant angina in some patients should perhaps not be dismissed as irrelevant to its initiating pathogenesis. Angina of effort, on the other hand, is generally a very stable situation which can persist for many years without infarction. After an acute myocardial infarct, further episodes of myocardial infarction (so-called "infarct extension"), usually in the same territory as the first, are not rare during the succeeding days (36). The impact of infarct size on mortality and the benefits of secondary prevention also appear to be more marked in the early than in the later months after infarction.

This circumstantial evidence all suggests that many clinical myocardial infarcts occur during a period of primary instability of coronary flow sufficient to cause a series of episodes of myocardial ischemia, any one of which might be the one which persists to cause myocardial infarction or triggers arrhythmic complications. *In many but not all cases the manifestation of this underlying coronary instability will be tidily terminated as the coronary artery occludes, or the vulnerable region of myocardium infarcts, or its owner succumbs.* The scenario is reminiscent of variant angina, where the susceptibility to coronary spasm seems to run a naturally self-limiting time course (which is not to imply that vasomotor tone is anything more than one possible mechanism for the coronary instability). On a shorter time scale, too, the possibility of spontaneous reperfusion and the "stuttering" nature of the development of many myocardial infarcts are becoming recognized clinically, and as documented by secondary humps in the time course of the ST-segment shifts or in the myoglobin or creatine kinase release curves (24,36). Whether this short-term variability is fundamentally different from the longer-term variability or is part of the same spectrum of pathogenetic events is unknown. *In any event, the clinical evidence is accumulating that at least a substantial proportion of myocardial infarcts do not occur as a consequence simply of a single, once-and-for-all coronary artery occlusion. The occlusive process may be gradual or intermittent.*

In some patients there seems little doubt that infarction is initiated by severe exertion or emotional stress, as if a particularly severe episode of angina were to get stuck. In these cases the ischemia may be demand-led and not the consequence of a primary constriction or occlusion of a large coronary artery.

In other cases, patchy, diffuse subendocardial necrosis is found at autopsy, generally on a background of severe, three-vessel coronary stenosis and with a history of recurrent angina without infarction, or with hemodynamic overload as with severe aortic valve disease. By definition this is here regarded as distinct from the gross regional lesion of an infarct occurring within the territory of a single major coronary artery, although the final pathway of necrosis is similar.

## Sudden Death *Sine* Infarct

"Sudden death syndrome" (the diagnostic pigeon hole for those who drop down dead) is attributable to the arrhythmic complications of ischemia occurring too soon for an infarct to have ensued. There is no reason to regard the situation as pathogenetically different from the early stage of myocardial infarction in some, whereas in others it may represent an episode of what would otherwise have been reversible angina. Successful resuscitation finds clinical evidence of an infarct in only about one-third of patients. Autopsy in those who are not so rescued finds almost invariably a critical stenosis but thrombotic occlusion in only about a third of patients (8).

### Occlusion or Not?

Complete occlusion of a coronary artery is the usual angiographic finding in acute myocardial infarction (10); early intracoronary thrombolysis is frequently successful; and the weight of pathological evidence appears to have swung back to the view that thrombotic occlusion is the rule rather than the exception, since it has been found, usually at the site of an intimal erosion (7), at subsequent autopsy in over 90% of cases in recent careful studies. Angiography of patients surviving an infarct, however, has shown a decreasing proportion with occluded vessels, though critical stenosis remains (10). This implies that the coronary artery occlusion presumed to have caused the myocardial infarct is often not permanent, but it tells us little about the duration of the occlusion or its behavior during the development of the infarct. Spontaneous reversal of some of the processes responsible for the occlusion must be presumed. *Coronary occlusion thus appears to be a feature of acute myocardial infarction but, commonly, it is not permanent.*

Conversely, it is not rare to find a complete occlusion at autopsy in the absence of any myocardial infarct (2). This is further discussed in relation to collaterals (see below).

### PATHOGENESIS OF REDUCED CORONARY FLOW

#### A Multifactorial Phenomenon

The pathogenesis of myocardial infarcts (see Fig. 1) is probably multifactorial. At the level of the large coronary arteries it involves plaque rupture, platelet aggregation and activation, changes in coronary vasomotor tone, and thrombosis. Platelet aggregation or emboli may impair the microcirculation. Hemodynamic factors will affect perfusion pressure. Collaterals will supply residual flow. The mechanical effects of myocardial contracture and the metabolic effects of myocardial ischemia will alter resistance downstream and, thus, the flow upstream. The scope for variety is wide, the possible permutations multiple, the interactions at all levels complex.

These multiple contributory causes need to be understood and, ideally, to be identified in any given patient and at any given stage. *Different interventions may be beneficial in different circumstances, though this remains a matter for speculation*, as would then be the practical question of the relative rarity of these different states. It may well be that occlusion in the majority of cases is due to one or other of very few possible main chains of events—with structural intimal lesions initiating platelet aggregation and thrombosis, for example, or perhaps with functional en-

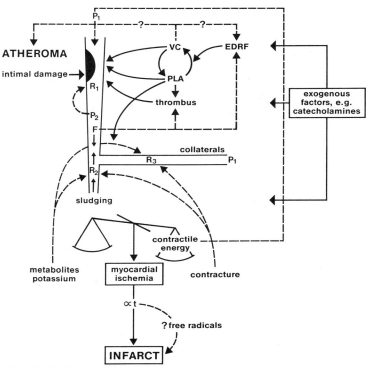

**FIG. 1.** Possible Pathogenetic Mechanisms in Myocardial Infarction. $P_1$ = perfusion pressure; $P_2$ = pressure downstream; $R_1$, $R_2$, $R_3$ = resistance at different sites; F = flow; t = time; VC = vasoconstriction; PLA = platelet activation/aggregation; EDRF = endothelium-derived relaxant factor.

dothelial disturbance initiating vasoconstriction, either of which may then converge to thrombotic occlusion as the final common path.

## Contributory Mechanisms

### *To State the Obvious*

Where flow is good, component control mechanisms leave much room for maneuver without detriment to perfusion. Where flow is absent, these controls are irrelevant. Where flow is critically reduced their contribution and interaction become vitally important.

### *Coronary Occlusion*

In respect of the dynamic processes responsible for coronary occlusion, consideration must be given to changes in vasomotor tone of the large coronary arteries at the site of a stenosis (where even minor superimposed changes in caliber may critically affect flow); to humoral and mechanical factors which promote or inhibit platelet activation; to platelet aggregation, which may cause intermittent occlusion of flow at the site of a stenosis (12) or in the microcirculation; to the effect of vasoactive metabolites released from platelets activated during passage through critically narrowed arteries; to the contribution of endothelium-dependent vasodilatation (14,17), which may be flow-related and increased by endothelial shear stress (20); to the mechanical effect whereby decreased resistance to run-off downstream can increase resistance at the site of a proximal stenosis (41,45); and to thrombosis.

## Demand-Led Ischemia

Consideration must be given to the direct effect on small vessel flow of contraction and of contracture of ischemic myocardium (19); to the influence of myocardial metabolites and potassium leakage on local coronary resistance vessels, still poorly understood (3); and to the effects of reduced flow on sludging and closure of microcirculatory channels. These factors may contribute also to the reduction in flow following coronary occlusion or from collateral supply.

## Collaterals

### Life Lines

The territory of one coronary arterial system appears to be clearly demarcated peripherally from that of another, without capillary interchange. Proximal collateral communications between one system and another exist naturally, though to widely varying extent in different species; these can allow intersystem flow if pressure gradients develop. New collateral channels develop slowly over a time course of days and weeks following infarction. Although important questions remain about what controls the development of these new collaterals, it would appear that recurrent episodes of ischemia can also cause them to develop. Preexisting good collaterals are the usual finding in patients with myocardial infarction, which generally occurs on a background of coronary stenosis. It is generally recognized that the consequences of coronary occlusion can be catastrophic in the absence of previous coronary artery disease; conversely, complete occlusion may be found at autopsy without infarction (2). Without some collateral flow, the irreversible changes of total ischemia would ensue within 30 min (22), yet all models show considerable myocardial preservation towards the periphery and epicardial layers of the territory of the occluded artery for some hours as the infarction slowly progresses. Collateral communication between one arterial system and another is therefore a life line which enables the maintenance of flow, albeit at a low rate, to a system that becomes occluded proximally. *The extent of the collateral flow is of major importance in determining the outcome of coronary occlusion. It will critically determine the amount of residual flow to the jeopardized territory and thus the rate of decline in energy and ultimately the amount of myocardium that will survive* (as modulated by other influences).

## Wavefronts and Beachheads

A major portion of jeopardized myocardium within the territory of a proximally occluded artery is preserved beyond 30 min by low-flow perfusion contributed to that arterial system by collaterals, yet with more prolonged occlusion it succumbs to infarct, presumably with little or no residual flow to the infarcted region. This implies that *the wavefront of the relatively slowly progressive infarction is associated with a receding beachhead of flow from the collaterals.* An important objective may therefore be to prevent this recession of flow. There is evidence that collaterals to an ischemic region can be pharmacologically dilated, which may help (13). Potentially more important may be the microcirculation, as influenced by the mechanical and metabolic effects of ischemic myocardium, by the effects of ischemia on small vessel tone, and by the effects of white cells, platelets, and stasis within the vascular compartment.

### Clinical Implications

On the clinical front, it is to be expected that there may be difficulty in demonstrating benefit from clinical trials of an interaction aimed at one component of a complex train of events. This is especially so when each is likely to be represented to a differing extent throughout the clinical spectrum of patients with developing myocardial infarcts. We may, however, be lucky if a given intervention turns out to have a major effect on a major link in the chain in a major proportion of patients.

## DELAYING TACTICS

### Rationale

Returning to the more pedestrian purpose of "myocardial preservation" by reducing the consequences of inadequate perfusion, considered in isolation this has always seemed of rather limited potential. *The primary insult is the reduction of coronary flow and it is to the maintenance and restoration of flow that our main efforts should be urgently directed. The rationale for any other intervention is dependent on:* (a) *delaying the consequences of ischemia until some reperfusion occurs (see below), and* (b) *preventing the fatal consequences of ischemia to the myocardial cells (see below).*

### Delaying the Decline in the Economy

#### Time Factor

Considering, first, the simple truth that cell necrosis is ultimately related to energy lack within the cell, *time may obviously be bought by altering the rate at which the energy levels decline.* As discussed in Chapter 5, this can be achieved either on the supply side or on the demand side. The practical question then remains whether there is ultimately anything to gain simply by delaying the decline in energy levels. Does this achieve anything more than a postponement of cell death? From experimental evidence of acute coronary occlusion in previously healthy animals, the rate of development of new collaterals would, at first sight, seem too slow to rescue myocardium subjected to total ischemia. Experimental evidence from dogs indicates that new collaterals begin to develop in about 24 hr (40), whereas cell necrosis in totally ischemic tissue begins within 30 min. The gap is formidably wide!

Preexisting collaterals are clearly all important. First, naturally existing collaterals maintain some flow. Second, for reasons which are not yet clear, there is evidence that perfusion spontaneously increases over the 24 hr following acute coronary occlusion. Third, the additional potential of highly developed preexisting collaterals is considerable: witness the well-endowed guinea pig whose natural collaterals protect it against infarction following coronary occlusion; witness also the fortunate people whose subsequent autopsies showed them to have been protected from myocardial infarct by collaterals when their coronary arteries occluded. The spectrum is clearly wide enough to embrace the possibility of complete protection in some cases without further intervention. It thus gives hope that there is much to fight for within the presenting population of patients with myocardial infarction. *We must conclude that residual flow often slows the decline in energy enough to bring energy-saving measures within temporal range and worthwhile purpose.*

Add to this the newer techniques of therapeutic thrombolysis and instrumental recanalization (see below) and it is clear that the time which needs to be bought by such delaying tactics may be greatly shortened. *The gap can clearly be narrowed.*

## Supply Side

The supply side we have considered is determined by flow through the coronary artery in question (sometimes only intermittently blocked), flow through collaterals (a critical determinant), and flow through the microcirculation. It should not be forgotten that perfusion pressure and diastolic duration become important under conditions of limited flow.

## Demand Side

The demand side appears amenable to moderation in several ways (though, as discussed in Chapter 2, it must be remembered that the heart must keep the circulation going and maintain coronary perfusion pressure, unlike the situation with cardiopulmonary bypass surgery and cardioplegia, so that a compromise may need to be struck). The determinants of myocardial energy consumption are well known. There is good experimental evidence that the setting of these determinants at the time of coronary occlusion influences ultimate infarct size though the setting 45 min later is without effect (32). This poses questions about the duration of effect of these factors, given also that the completely ischemic cell very rapidly turns its contractile performance off in an act of self-preservation. Clinical evidence that the cell's economy can still be influenced after the early minutes of ischemia would lead again to the conclusion that much of the jeopardized myocardium is in a balanced, though probably deteriorating, state of low-flow ischemia for some hours.

### Endocardial Versus Epicardial Vulnerability

As discussed in detail in Chapter 8, the endocardium is more vulnerable to infarction. Infarction may thus be restricted to the endocardium in less severe or less prolonged ischemia. The "wavefront" of experimental infarction progresses with time and severity from the subendocardial layers (where systolic wall stress and energy consumption are highest) outwards eventually to become transmural (37).

### Catecholamines

The role of catecholamines is of particular interest. They are known to induce myocardial necrosis in experimental animals and in clinical situations of high catecholamine drive. They are released locally by ischemic myocardium and systemically (often to very high levels) in clinical myocardial infarction. Catecholamines undoubtedly exert strong positive inotropic effects even when contractile performance is declining from lack of energy, as can be elegantly demonstrated in isolated preparations of heart muscle where the inotropic effect is clearly at the cost of myocardial survival (4). Catecholamine-induced myocardial necrosis probably reflects simply the imbalance between known determinants of energy supply and consumption, even in the absence of coronary artery disease.

### Clinical Pointers

Clinically, there is considerable circumstantial evidence to suggest that there is benefit to be had from energy conservation. Therapeutic lowering of high blood pressure following the onset of acute myocardial infarction is beneficial. Nitrite infusion may be helpful if blood pressure is maintained (9,11), though the data and the possible mechanisms are confusing. The adverse effects of tachycardia find convincing corroboration in respect of serious ventricular arrhythmias. The prophylactic use of antiarrhythmic drugs has proved disappointing. There can be no doubt though that tachycardias and particulary ventricular tachycardias seriously upset the energy balance and merit urgent treatment. The immediate treatment of ventricular arrhythmias when they occur probably accounts for the lower incidence of cardiogenic shock where mobile coronary care units that can deliver this sort of care are available. *We should perhaps learn from the diving seal which gets away with it by the most extreme slowing of heart rate. The most recent evidence of benefit from early β-blocker treatment started within 4 hr (21) is persuasive, despite purist reservations about the validity of the methods used to estimate infarct size.* The paradoxical lack of benefit from β blockers in the more recent animal studies (23) may be due to a low level of sympathetic drive in these animals. Experimental evidence that calcium antagonists preferentially depress ischemic myocardium (42) offers another approach which invites exploitation and where the results of clinical trials are awaited.

Occult myocardial ischemia can lead to cell necrosis in a number of conditions with normal coronary arteries, such as aortic valve disease, myocardial hypertrophy, cardiomyopathy, and hyperthyroidism. This emphasizes the importance of noncoronary factors.

*Delaying tactics on the demand side would thus seem to come into their own to the extent that collateral perfusion and time permit.* Recent evidence from early β-blocker treatment provides encouraging support for this approach.

## PREVENTING THE CONSEQUENCES OF ISCHEMIA

Recognition that energy lack may only indirectly cause cell death offers scope for intervention at the level of the coupling links. As discussed in Chapters 12 and 13, recent evidence about the damaging effects of free radicals derived from myocardial cells (31) or released from activated leukocytes (39) excitingly extends this possibility. It seems likely that this previously unrecognized phenomenon contributes to the ultimate size of the infarct and that it may be amenable to therapeutic moderation.

## CORONARY DEOCCLUSION

Open heart surgery with coronary vein grafting early in the course of myocardial infarction is possible (35) but it carries hazards and takes some time to set up when minutes matter. Its advantages appear to be outweighed by its disadvantages, though conceivably its day might yet come. Instrumental angioplasty (18) clearly has great potential but it is too recent a development to have been evaluated thoroughly for the relief of coronary occlusion in this context. Intracoronary infusion of vasodilators has also been reported to reestablish flow in a proportion of patients during the early hours of infarction (33), though more studies have found that in most cases flow is restored only after (additional) thrombolysis. Earlier trials of pharmacological thrombolysis by intravenously administered streptokinase suggested some statistical benefit but were not beyond criticism. The more targeted administration of thrombolytic agents has subsequently found more favor. Intracoronary infusion of streptokinase is now at the stage of rigorous evaluation; the evidence from a number of good and careful studies (1,15,30,38) suggests increasingly that it can be effective—if given within 4 hr and followed by surgery to prevent reocclusion at the site of the underlying critical (? unstable) stenosis. The advent of new tissue plasminogen activators which can be effective in lysing coronary thrombus when given intravenously and which avoid the bleeding dangers of systemic fibrinolysis (as with streptokinase) promises to bring exciting possibilities within range (44). If and when these agents become available, they should circumvent the difficulties and delays inherent in instituting thrombolysis by the intracoronary route. This would have a dramatic impact. The major practical problem would then shift to the logistic one of very early recognition and immediate treatment on site, together with an even greater demand for subsequent surgical or instrumental relief of the underlying stenosis.

## REPERFUSION DAMAGE

Spontaneous reperfusion occurs with increasing collateral flow and "stuttering" infarction as well as with therapeutic recanalization. It is a necessary step of recovery, yet it is associated with arrhythmias and can be shown in isolated preparations to be associated with an exacerbation of ischemic injury and an overwhelming influx of cations. Whether this paradoxical phenomenon is an irrevocable consequence of the preceding ischemia, or whether it is at least in part amenable to therapeutic intervention, remains a matter of dispute. *I am persuaded that it is independently amenable to treatment*, as by preventing the influx of calcium, and I believe that some of the "calcium antagonist" drugs may be capable of achieving this by nonspecific effects (6). The gross and obvious adverse effects of reperfusion (arrhythmias and hemorrhage into the infarct) appear in practice to be uncommon complications of clinical recanalization and are probably related critically to the timing of the reperfusion; with growing experience they seem unlikely to pose an insuperable problem.

## CONCLUDING COMMENTS

The variety of pathogenetic mechanisms contributing to coronary occlusion and the common preexistence of stenosis with well developed collaterals distinguish clinical infarcts from the usual animal models of coronary occlusion. *Residual low-flow perfusion slows energy depletion and the temporal and spatial progression of the infarct. The rate of energy decline can be somewhat further slowed by reduction of myocardial energy consumption.* Slowing the decline is only useful, however, if rescue is at hand. *Vasodilatation, disaggregation of platelets, and anticoagulation should favor reperfusion and discourage further impairment of flow, both through native vessels and through collaterals.* Maintaining the microcirculation into ischemic myocardium could be important. Minimizing the adverse effects of reperfusion could bring further benefit. An attack on free radical-mediated damage, whether the free radicals are derived from myocardial cells or activated leukocytes, offers a novel and potentially rewarding approach to infarct size limitation, yet to be evaluated.

*Therapy directed towards maintaining flow, reducing energy consumption, and minimizing the consequences of ischemia may, in combination, buy more time than expected. Trials of multiple intervention seem indicated:* they are probably no dirtier than trials of single drugs with multiple effects. *Something more than marginal benefit needs to be demonstrated if infarct size limitation is to become widely accepted as a practical proposition.*

*Therapeutic thrombolysis has brought a new dimension to the concept.* It promises to increase the reward for time bought, though it is difficult to envisage it as ever being available by the intracoronary route for more than a fortunate few. *The potential for infarct size limitation by any means diminishes rapidly with time; it is probably very limited after 4 hr except to prevent further episodes.* The advent of tissue plasminogen activators that can be given intravenously could overcome this major problem and transform the situation. *This is for the future, but the time may be ripe for the more widespread provision of mobile coronary care to provide a platform for the developments in view.*

## REFERENCES

1. Anderson, J. L., Marshall, H. W., Bray, B. E., Lutz, J. R., Frederick, P. R., Yanowitz, F. G., Datz, F. L., Klausner, S. C., and Hagan, A. D. (1983): A randomized trial of intracoronary streptokinase in the treatment of acute myocardial infarction. *N. Engl. J. Med.*, 308:1312–1319.
2. Baroldi, G., and Scomazzoni, G. (1967): Coronary circulation in the normal and the pathogenic heart. *U.S. Government Printing Office*, Washington, D.C.
3. Belloni, F. L. (1979): The local control of coronary blood flow. *Cardiovasc. Res.*, 13:63–85.
4. Bing, O. H. L., Brooks, W. W., and Messer, J. V. (1972): Effects of isoproterenol on heart muscle performance during myocardial hypoxia. *J. Mol. Cell. Cardiol.*, 4:319–328.
5. Braunwald, E., and Maroko, P. R. (1974): The reduction of infarct size—an idea whose time (for testing) has come. *Circulation*, 50:206.
6. Chappell, S. P., Lewis, M. J., and Henderson, A. H. (1983): Myocardial reoxygenation damage can be circumvented. *J. Mol. Cell. Cardiol.*, 15:329.
7. Davies, M. J., Futton, W. F. M., and Robertson, W. B. (1979): The relation of coronary thrombosis to ischaemia myocardial necrosis. *J. Pathol.*, 127:99–110.
8. Davies, M. J. (1981): Pathological view of sudden death. *Br. Heart J.*, 45:88–96.
9. Derrida, J. P., Sal, R., and Chiche, P. (1977): Nitroglycerin infusion in acute myocardial infarction. *N. Engl. J. Med.*, 297:336.
10. De Wood, M. A., Spores, J., Hensley, G. R., Simpson, C. S., Eugster, G. S., Sutherland, K. I., Grunwald, R. P., and Shields, J. P. (1983): Coronary arteriographic findings in acute transmural myocardial infarction. *Circulation*, 68(Suppl. 1):39–49.
11. Flaherty, J. T., Becker, L. C., Bulkley, B. H., Weiss, J. L., Gerstenblith, G., Kallman, C. H., Silverman, K. J., Wei, J. Y., Pitt, B., and Weisfeldt, M. L. (1983): A randomized prospective trial of intravenous nitroglycerin in patients with acute myocardial infarction. *Circulation*, 68:576–588.
12. Folts, J. D., Gallagher, K., and Rowe, G. G. (1982): Blood flow reductions in stenosed canine coronary arteries: vasospasm or platelet aggregation. *Circulation*, 65:248–259.
13. Forman, R., Eng, C., and Kirk, E. S. (1983): Comparative effect of verapamil and nitroglycerin on collateral blood flow. *Circulation*, 67:1200–1204.
14. Furchgott, R. F. (1983): Role of endothelium in responses of vascular smooth muscle. *Circ. Res.*, 53:557–573.
15. Ganz, W., Buchbinder, N., Marcus, H., Mondkar, A., Maddaahi, J., Charuzi, Y., O'Connor, L., Shell, W., Fishbein, M. C., Kass, R., Miyamoto, A., and Swan, H. J. C. (1981): Intracoronary thrombolysis in evolving myocardial infarction. *Am. Heart J.*, 101:4–13.
16. Geltman, E. M., Ehsani, A. A., Campbell, M. K., Schetman, K., Roberts, R., and Sobel, B. E. (1979): The influence of location and extent of myocardial infarction on longterm ventricular dysrhythmias and mortality. *Circulation*, 60:805.
17. Griffith, T. M., Edwards, D. H., Lewis, M. J., Newby, A. C., and Henderson, A. H. (1984): The nature of endothelium-derived vascular relaxant factor. *Nature*, 308:645–647.
18. Gruntzig, A. R., Senning, A., and Siegenthaler, W. E. (1979): Non-operative dilatation of coronary-artery stenosis: percutaneous transluminal coronary angioplasty. *N. Engl. J. Med.*, 301:61–68.

19. Harris, P. (1975): A theory concerning the course of events in angina and myocardial infarction. *Eur. J. Cardiol.*, 3/2:1157–1163.
20. Holts, J., Busse, R., and Giesler, M. (1983): Flow-dependent dilation of canine epicardial coronary arteries *in vivo* and *in vitro*: Mediated by the endothelium. *Naunyn-Schmiedebergs Arch. Pharmacol.*, 322:R44.
21. International Collaborative Study Group (1984): Reduction of infarct size with the early use of timolol in acute myocardial infarction. *N. Engl. J. Med.*, 310:9–15.
22. Jennings, R. B., Sommers, H. M., Smyth, G. A., Flack, H. A., and Linn, H. (1960): Myocardial necrosis induced by temporary occlusion of the coronary artery in the dog. *Arch. Pathol.*, 70:68–78.
23. Jennings, R. B., and Reimer, K. A. (1979): Effect of beta-adrenergic blockade on acute myocardial ischemic injury. In: *Modulation of Sympathetic Tone in the Treatment of Cardiovascular Diseases*, edited by F. Gross, pp. 103–114. Hans Huber, Berne.
24. Kagen, L., Scheidt, S., and Butt, A. (1977): Serum myoglobin in myocardial infarction: The "staccato phenomenon." Is acute myocardial infarction in man an intermittent event? *Am. J. Med.*, 62:86–92.
25. Lewis, H. D., Davis, J. W., Archibald, D. G., Steinke, W. E., Smitherman, T. C., Doherty, J. E., Schnaper, H. W., LeWinter, M. M., Linares, E., Pouget, J. M., Sabharwal, S. C., Chesler, E., and DeMots, H. (1983): Protective effects of aspirin against acute myocardial infarction and death in men with unstable angina. *N. Engl. J. Med.*, 209:396–403.
26. Mandelkorn, J. B., Nelson, M., Wolf, M. D., Sing, S., Schechter, J. A., Kersh, R. I., Rodgers, D. M., Workman, M. B., Bentivoglio, L. G., LaPorte, S. M., Meister, S. G., and Tucker, B. (1983): Intracoronary thrombus in nontransmural myocardial infarction and in unstable angina pectoris. *Am. J. Cardiol.*, 52:1–7.
27. Maroko, P. R., Kjeksus, J. K., Sobel, B. E., Watanabe, T., Covell, J. W., Ross, J., Jr., and Braunwald, E. (1971): Factors influencing infarct size following experimental coronary artery occlusions. *Circulation*, 43:67–82.
28. Maroko, P. R., and Braunwald, E. (1973): Modification of myocardial infarction size after coronary occlusion. *Ann. Int. Med.*, 79:720–733.
29. Maseri, A., L'Abbate, A., Baroldi, G., Chierchia, S., Marzilli, M., Ballestra, M., Severi, S., Parodi, O., Biagini, A., Distante, A., and Pesola, A. (1978): Coronary vasospasm as a possible cause of myocardial infarction. A conclusion derived from the study of "preinfarction" angina. *N. Engl. J. Med.*, 299:1271–1277.
30. Mathey, D. G., Kuck, K. H., Tilsner, V., Krebber, H. J., and Bleifeld, W. (1981): Non-surgical coronary artery recanalisation after acute transluminal infarction. *Circulation*, 67:489–497.
31. McCord, J. M., and Roy, R. S. (1982): The pathophysiology of superoxide: Roles in inflammation and ischaemia. *Can. J. Physiol. Pharmacol.*, 60:1346–1352.
32. Muller, K. D., Lein, H., and Schaper, W. (1980): Changes in myocardial oxygen consumption 45 minutes after experimental coronary occlusion do not alter infarct size. *Cardiovasc. Res.*, 14:710–718.
33. Oliva, P. B., and Breckenridge, J. C. (1977): Arteriographic evidence of coronary arterial spasm in acute myocardial infarction. *Circulation*, 56:366–374.
34. Page, D. L., Caulfield, J. B., Kastor, J. A., DeSanctis, R. W., and Sanders, C. A. (1971): Myocardial changes associated with cardiogenic shock. *N. Engl. J. Med.*, 285:133.
35. Phillips, S. J., Zeff, R. H., Kongtahworn, C., Skinner, J. R., Iannone, L., Brown, T. M., Wickemyer, W., and Gordon, D. F. (1982): Surgery for evolving myocardial infarction. *JAMA*, 248:1325–1328.
36. Reid, P. R., Taylor, D. R., Kelly, D. T., Weisfeldt, M. L., O'Neal Humphries, J., Ross, R. S., and Pitt, B. (1974): Myocardial infarct extension detected by precordial ST-segment mapping. *N. Engl. J. Med.*, 290:123–128.
37. Reimer, K. A., Lowe, J. E., Rasmussen, M. M., and Jennings, R. B. (1977): The wavefront phenomenon of ischemic cell death. Myocardial infarct size versus duration of coronary occlusion in dogs. *Circulation*, 56:786–794.
38. Rentrop, K. P., Blanke, H., Karsch, K. R., Kaiser, H., Kosotering, H., and Leitz, K. (1981): Selective intracoronary thrombolysis in acute myocardial infarction and unstable angina pectoris. *Circulation*, 63:307–317.
39. Romson, J. L., Hook, B. G., Kunkel, S. L., Abrams, G. D., Schork, A., and Lucchesi, B. R.

(1983): Reduction of the extent of ischemic myocardial injury by neutrophil depletion in the dog. *Circulation*, 67:1016.

40. Schaper, W. (1982): Collateral anatomy and blood flow: its potential role in sudden coronary death. *Ann. NY Acad. Sci.*, 382:69–75.
41. Schwartz, J. S., Carlyle, P. F., and Cohn, J. N. (1980): Effect of coronary arterial pressure on coronary stenosis resistance. *Circulation*, 61:70–76.
42. Smith, H. J., Goldstein, R. A., Griffith, J. M., Kent, K. M., and Epstein, S. E. (1976): Regional contractility: selective depression of ischemic myocardium by verapamil. *Circulation*, 54:629–635.
43. Sobel, B. E., and Braunwald, E. (1980): The management of acute myocardial infarction. In: *Heart Disease*, edited by E. Braunwald, p. 1373. Saunders, Philadelphia.
44. Van de Werf, S., Ludbrook, P. A., Bergmann, S. R., Tiefenbrunn, A. J., Fox, K. A. A. DeGeest, H., Versteraete, M., Collen, D., and Sobel, B. E. (1984): Coronary thrombolysis with tissue-type plasminogen activator in patients with evolving myocardial infarction. *N. Engl. J. Med.*, 310:609–614.
45. Walinsky, P., Santamore, W. P., Wiener, L., and Brest, A. N. (1979): Dynamic changes in the haemodynamic severity of coronary artery stenosis in a canine model. *Cardiovasc. Res.*, 13:113–118.

*Therapeutic Approaches to Myocardial Infarct Size Limitation*, edited by D. J. Hearse and D. M. Yellon. Raven Press, New York © 1984.

# 2

# Why Are We Still in Doubt About Infarct Size Limitation? The Experimentalist's Viewpoint

### David J. Hearse and Derek M. Yellon

*The Heart Research Unit, The Rayne Institute, St. Thomas' Hospital, London SE1 7EH, United Kingdom*

During the last decade we have witnessed the development and establishment of the major cardiological concept that with appropriate interventions it is possible to reduce the size of an evolving myocardial infarct (21,22). Since there is a direct relationship between mortality and infarct size, this concept has become highly attractive and from the early 1970s numerous experimental studies with at least 50 agents, as diverse as hyaluronidase, β blockers, glucose, steroids, pyruvate, cobra venom, and rutosides have provided encouraging results. With good justification Braunwald and colleagues in 1974 stated: "Just because myocardial tissue lies within the distribution of a recently occluded coronary artery does not mean that it is necessarily condemned to death" (2), and "abundant experimental evidence indicates that this (limitation of necrosis) is now possible. Pilot studies support its clinical feasibility and a careful, rigorously conducted prospective trial is likely to provide useful results and would be timely" (3).

*Despite numerous experimental and clinical studies, most of which have reported encouraging results, we must accept the fact that no single intervention has been adopted for widespread and sustained clinical use as an "antiinfarct" agent.* In 1980, in a major review of the effect of drugs upon evolving myocardial infarction, Opie (26) cautiously concluded "the time has not yet come to introduce antiinfarct agents into general cardiological practice," and in the 1984 edition of Dr. Braunwald's *A Text Book of Cardiovascular Medicine*, Sobel and Braunwald (32) state: "It must be acknowledged that *definitive* proof that substantial quantities of tissue can be salvaged and that prognosis can thereby be improved is not yet available, despite (a) the inherent logic in attempting to reduce infarct size; (b) the availability of a wide variety of interventions that are effective in experimental animals; (c) the ability to apply these techniques with reasonable safety in patients; and (d) the results of an increasing number of trials in patients with encouraging results." Contributing to the current sense of caution and uncertainty about the feasibility of infarct size reduction are a growing number of experimental reports (5,13,15,23,33) questioning whether traditional antiinfarct agents such as β blockers (19,20,27,30) are really able to reduce infarct size. Increasingly the question is being asked: *Is infarct size reduction really possible?*

The objective of this chapter is to discuss various factors which, in our opinion (12,13), have contributed to the current state of controversy and confusion over the vital issue of infarct size reduction. These factors include the adequacy of various models of myocardial infarction; the limitation of various indices of injury and protection; the confusion which has arisen over "border zones" of injury; and the failure of most studies to distinguish between the ability of interventions to reduce, as opposed to delay, injury. In a number of instances it becomes apparent that much of the confusion has arisen from the inappropriate use of terminology. In discussing this we conclude by proposing a series of definitions of key terms frequently used in the study of infarct size limitation.

## MYOCARDIAL PROTECTION: IS IT REALLY POSSIBLE?

### Nature of Ischemic Injury

Myocardial ischemia initiates (Fig. 1) a sequence of progressively more severe cellular changes. Initially these changes are reversible such that reperfusion results

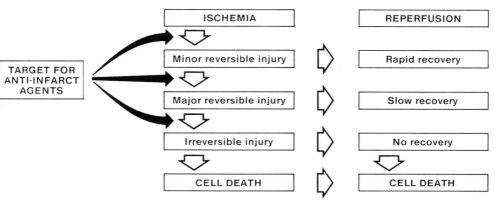

**FIG. 1.** The Progression of Ischemic Injury and Targets for Therapeutic Interventions. Myocardial ischemia initiates a sequence of progressively more severe cellular changes which, unless halted by early reperfusion or some suitable antiinfarct agent, will culminate in cell death and tissue necrosis. Effective protection demands that the intervention be applied before the critical transition from reversible to irreversible cellular injury.

in a rapid and complete return to contractile function and a normalization of any metabolic impairment. As the duration or severity of ischemia increases, then cellular injury becomes more severe and reperfusion may not result in an immediate return of function. However, if injury is still reversible, then a full recovery should eventually occur although this may take some time. For example, after even brief periods of ischemia, tissue energy stores may not return to normal for several hours or days (29). With more prolonged ischemia, injury eventually becomes irreversible and here, by definition, reperfusion cannot lead to recovery and cell death is inevitable.

*The concept of myocardial protection is based on the argument that pharmacological or biochemical manipulation of cellular activity (for example, the use of a β blocker to reduce energy demand, or the provision of glucose as an anaerobic energy supply) during the reversible phase of injury may halt or, in the case of mild ischemia, even reverse the progression of ischemic injury.*

## Surgical Success Versus Clinical Failure?

The general failure of antiinfarct agents to be adopted for clinical usage has led some to question whether myocardial protection is really possible. *There is, however, no doubt that the modification of ischemic injury is possible and that it can find major clinical application.* Evidence for this proposition is the widespread and highly successful application of cold chemical cardioplegia during cardiac surgery (11). Many cardiac surgical procedures necessitate cardiopulmonary bypass and the deliberate induction of whole heart ischemia. Although offering the surgical advantage of a bloodless, still, and relaxed heart on which to operate, ischemic cardiac arrest induces major and sometimes irreversible (17) injury in the human heart. Because of this, a decade ago the limit for the tolerable duration of unmodified ischemic arrest was generally considered to be less than 1 hr. Cardioplegia (the infusion of cold protective solutions into the coronary network at the onset of, and intermittently throughout, a period of global ischemia) has now extended the limits of tolerable ischemia to several hours. Despite the associated increase in duration of ischemic arrest, the use of cardioplegic protection has also resulted in improved postischemic recovery and reduced mortality. The mechanisms underlying this form of myocardial protection are well defined and include the conservation of cellular energy through the use of agents (such as potassium) to induce rapidly total cardiac arrest, the slowing of degradative and deleterious cellular reactions by hypothermia, and the combating of unfavorable ischemia-induced changes by the inclusion of various protective agents such as magnesium and procaine in cardioplegic solutions. Is it perhaps reasonable to ask: *Why then, if cardioplegia is so successful, cannot its principles be applied to evolving myocardial infarction?* The answer to this question lies in a number of key differences between surgically induced global ischemia and regional ischemia with evolving myocardial infarction.

### Global Versus Regional Ischemia: Critical Differences for Protection

A comparison of the conditions during surgical ischemia and evolving myocardial infarction not only provides an answer to the above question, but also serves to highlight a number of investigative inadequacies in the study of infarct size limitation. Important features of surgically induced ischemia (see Fig. 2) are that it can be anticipated and it is of a fixed, relatively short duration; reperfusion can be initiated at will; and protective agents can be administered at the moment of, or before, the induction of ischemia. In contrast, with myocardial infarction the duration of ischemia is not finite and cannot necessarily be reversed; the time of onset may be unknown and rarely is it possible to administer drugs before or during early ischemia. An additional important factor is that with surgical ischemia contractile activity is not required (its active suppression is an important component of the protection process), whereas in the case of infarction, the maintenance of pump function is essential. Finally, under surgical conditions the heart is far more accessible, the highly protective procedure of hypothermia can be applied, and the ischemia is relatively uniform throughout the myocardium, a factor which may be of considerable importance in preventing various secondary problems arising from the heterogeneity of regional ischemia.

In concluding this section *it is clear that myocardial protection is indeed possible if by "protection" we mean delaying the onset of irreversible injury beyond such a time as reperfusion can be assured.* This point serves to introduce a major contributor to the controversy over infarct size reduction, namely, the failure of most investigations to distinguish between altering the *rate* as opposed to the *extent* of injury.

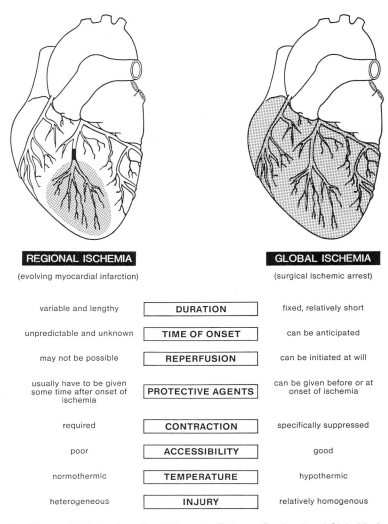

| | | |
|---|---|---|
| **REGIONAL ISCHEMIA** | | **GLOBAL ISCHEMIA** |
| (evolving myocardial infarction) | | (surgical ischemic arrest) |
| variable and lengthy | DURATION | fixed, relatively short |
| unpredictable and unknown | TIME OF ONSET | can be anticipated |
| may not be possible | REPERFUSION | can be initiated at will |
| usually have to be given some time after onset of ischemia | PROTECTIVE AGENTS | can be given before or at onset of ischemia |
| required | CONTRACTION | specifically suppressed |
| poor | ACCESSIBILITY | good |
| normothermic | TEMPERATURE | hypothermic |
| heterogeneous | INJURY | relatively homogenous |

**FIG. 2.** Myocardial Protection: Key Differences Between Regional and Global Ischemia. Regional ischemia arises in the myocardium during evolving myocardial infarction and global ischemia arises as a consequence of surgically induced ischemic cardiac arrest. In both cases tissue injury can result and this may lead to cell death and tissue necrosis. However, a variety of endogenous and exogenous factors combine to dramatically alter the prospects for sustained tissue protection in each condition.

## DISTINCTION BETWEEN REDUCING AND DELAYING ISCHEMIC INJURY

### Changes in Rate or Extent of Injury?

The action of cardioplegia in a globally ischemic heart with little or no coronary flow is to *slow* the rate of development of injury and, hence, *delay* the onset of irreversible damage (eventually inevitable in this low or zero flow condition) beyond the time of reperfusion. Thus, *in the context of surgical ischemia a delay of injury can find great practical application.* By contrast, during regional ischemia and evolving myocardial infarction, slowing injury is of relatively little value if cell death is eventually going to occur. In regional ischemia, the ultimate aim must be to achieve an absolute reduction in the extent of injury (or an extremely long delay such that natural collateral growth can occur). *This is far more difficult to achieve and in the case of severe flow impairment it might be argued (13) that it is impossible unless the intervention achieves a near normalization of coronary flow.*

## Difficulties of Interpretation

Early studies of infarct size limitation are characterized by their *failure to distinguish between the ability of antiinfarct agents to reduce and to delay injury.* Many studies were either of too short a duration (4 hr or less, some being as short as 30 or 45 min) or reperfusion was introduced too early to allow definitive proof of absolute tissue salvage. By way of illustration the authors have recently undertaken a study (5) in which the ability of the nonsteroidal antiinflammatory agent, flurbiprofen, to reduce infarct size was assessed in a dog model with relatively short and relatively long durations of ischemia. This study was prompted by the report (6) (now retracted) that this agent achieved a major reduction of infarct size after 6 hr of regional ischemia in the dog. As Fig. 3 shows, our studies confirmed the finding that the area of necrosis, as assessed by tetrazolium staining, was much smaller in the drug-treated hearts 6 hr after the onset of coronary occlusion; *however, after 24 hr of elapsed ischemia the infarct size was almost identical in both groups.* This result suggested that, at best, the drug was only delaying injury but was having no effect upon the final extent of injury.

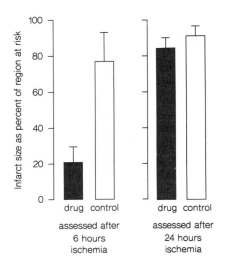

**FIG. 3.** The Distinction Between Reducing and Delaying Tissue Injury. Dog studies (35) showed that flurbiprofen reduced the size of an infarct when the assessment was made 6 hr after the onset of ischemia. However, by 24 hr the size of the infarct was almost identical in drug-treated and control groups indicating the absence of a sustained effect.

We went on to question this conclusion by undertaking a study in which we (35) used reperfusion to ascertain if the observed delay in the detection of necrosis was a true delay in its development or if it was merely an artifact arising from some ability of the drug to alter the sensitivity of the tetrazolium staining procedure. The results of this study suggested that this delay may have indeed been artifactual since the entire mass of "early" drug-salvaged tissue progressed to necrosis in spite of a restored perfusion. This study, like those of Kirlin et al. (18) and Factor et al. (8), appears to question the widespread use of tetrazolium staining for the gross detection of acute myocardial infarction. This problem is further discussed in Chapter 10.

## Objectives for Protection

In concluding this section we stress that *protection of the regionally ischemic myocardium should ideally involve an absolute reduction in the extent, as opposed to merely a delay in the onset, of irreversible injury.* However, as is discussed in Chapter 3 and in the next section, it is not always easy to determine whether an agent delays or reduces injury. This is because certain ischemia-induced reversible changes, which may be used as markers of injury, may not normalize for days or even weeks after the onset of reperfusion.

Finally, although we have stressed the importance of designing interventions which cause a sustained reduction of injury, we would concede that *achieving a substantial delay is not without value* since it might act to buy time for natural collateral growth or for the application of secondary procedures such as thrombolysis or balloon angioplasty.

## ADEQUACY OF INDICES OF INJURY AND PROTECTION

A major criticism of many studies of infarct size reduction relates to incorrect interpretation and inadequacy of many indices of tissue injury and protection. We would contend that this has often resulted in *the inappropriate use of the term "tissue protection."*

## Meaning of "Protection"

Many early, influential studies of infarct size reduction used electrocardiographic or enzymatic assessments of tissue injury and infarct size. Although these were the best procedures available at the time, it is now widely accepted that indices such as ST-segment elevation or cumulative creatine kinase leakage are often imprecise and prone to serious artifact. It is quite possible, for example, to use drugs such as steroids (10) or calcium antagonists (1) to reduce substantially the extent of enzyme leakage from severely injured tissue. If, however, sufficient injury remains such that there is no improvement in functional recovery, then *the applicability of the term "protection" seems questionable.* However, even when used carefully and correctly, there is a further problem relating to indices of protection which could be called *"the limitation of association" and this problem has contributed greatly to the current confusion over infarct size limitation.*

## Limitation of Association

Although a drug may reduce some index of injury such as ST-segment elevation or enzyme leakage, *this cannot necessarily be equated with an increase in tissue viability. The authors would propose (13) that true tissue protection should involve not only preventing the critical transition from reversible to irreversible injury, but also promoting the return of the physiological role of the organ, i.e., pump function.* Often in experimental studies, changes in staining or metabolism have been equated with a return of physiological as well as biological function. Such associations may be quite unjustified as, indeed, are other often-made associations such as those between "intermediate" staining, "intermediate" metabolite depletion, and "intermediate" or reversible injury. It seems to us that *there are few studies where drug treatment has achieved an unquestioned and sustained reduction of the infarct size, while at the same time promoting the return of previously ischemic cells to normal or near normal contractile function.*

## "BORDER ZONE" CONTROVERSY

Most early experimental studies, and some recent studies of infarct size reduction have been based on the assumption that gradients of flow, metabolism, and injury characterize the transition from normal to ischemic tissue in a zone of regional ischemia. Specifically it was *assumed* (see Fig. 4) that encapsulating the severely ischemic core of an area of regional ischemia, and separating it from the surrounding normal tissue, was a lateral "border zone" of intermediate flow and injury. It was this border zone that was supposed to act as the target for therapeutic interventions, and it was the salvage of this border zone which was supposed to account for the reduction of the physical dimensions of an evolving infarct. *We believe that this, more than any other factor, has contributed to the confusion over the feasibility of infarct size limitation.*

## Is There a Lateral Border Zone?

The traditional view of the lateral border zone is illustrated in Fig. 5A. For many years it was assumed that intramural anastomoses, and an element of interdigitation between adjacent coronary beds, gave rise to a quantitatively significant border zone of intermediate perfusion at the interface between an area of ischemia and adjoining normally perfused tissue. As is discussed more fully in Chapters 5 and 6, *this view failed to take adequate account of our knowledge of coronary artery anatomy, of the nature of collateral vessels, and of the characteristics of the distribution of the collateral blood.*

It is now well recognized in a number of species (24), particularly the pig and the dog, that individual coronary arteries serve discrete beds of tissue such that in the pig, for example, the occlusion of one artery will result in an almost complete loss of flow in the affected bed with little or no collateral supply entering the tissue

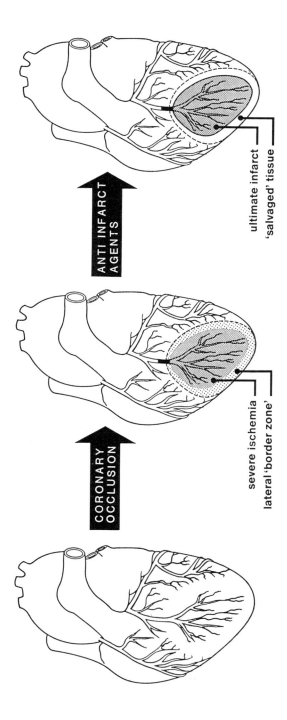

**FIG. 4.** Myocardial Infarct Size Reduction: The Disputed View. The concept became established that following the occlusion of a coronary artery an area of regional ischemia developed which was heterogeneous in terms of severity of injury. It was thought that a core of severely ischemic tissue existed and that encapsulating this, and separating it from the surrounding normal tissue, was a "border zone" of intermediate flow, metabolism, and injury. Thus, the transition from ischemic and normal tissue was characterized by a progressive gradient of flow. This spatially identifiable lateral border zone was presumed to act as the target for therapeutic agents designed to salvage tissue and thereby reduce the ultimate size of the evolving infarct. *This view of a lateral border zone of salvable tissue is now disputed in a number of models.*

**A** Lateral border zone of intermediate perfusion

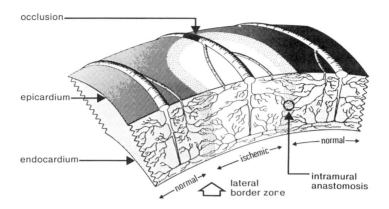

**B** No lateral border zone : sharp but irregular interface

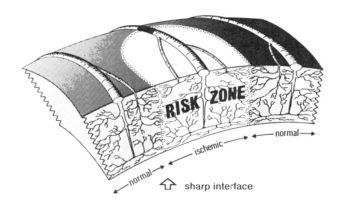

**FIG. 5.** The Border Zone Controversy: Vascular Arrangements That Might Give Rise to Differing Interfaces of Injury. The model depicts three adjacent coronary arteries, each supplying a distinct tissue bed. The middle vessel is occluded and this renders its perfusion bed ischemic. **A:** *A lateral border zone* might arise if there were intramural anastomoses between small vessels from adjacent coronary beds together with a complex pattern of interdigitation between beds. In this way, collateral flow and diffusion at the interface might generate a qualitatively significant border zone of intermediate injury *(dotted area). In many models and species this view is now disputed.* **B:** *No lateral border zone* will exist if there are no interconnections between adjacent perfusion beds. In this model, occlusion of the middle coronary artery will result in an abolition of flow throughout its perfusion bed without there being any great effect upon adjoining perfusion beds. Under these conditions the transition between normal and ischemic tissue would be characterized by a sharp interface of flow and injury and not by a progressive gradient. No spatially identifiable border zone would arise. This condition may occur in the pig heart and possibly young human hearts.

**C** No border zone : uniform distribution of collateral flow

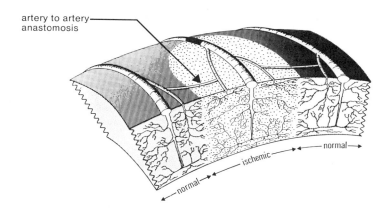

**D** Transmural border zone : nonuniform distribution of collateral flow

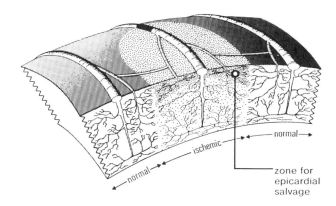

**FIG. 5. Cont.** **C:** *Some collateral flow* is delivered to the ischemic zone from adjacent perfusion beds in some models and species. In the dog, for example, artery-to-artery connections often result in collateral flow values on the order of 20% of control. Once delivered to the ischemic bed this collateral flow endeavors to distribute itself in the manner of normal arterial blood, i.e., it is uniformly distributed across the ischemic zone and would not be expected to be preferentially delivered to the margins of the ischemic mass, and as such would not be expected to generate any lateral border zones. **D:** *Transmural border zones* may possibly be generated in models such as the dog by a combination of a number of factors. Firstly, collateral flow arising from artery-to-artery connections, although being distributed uniformly in the lateral plane of the infarct is not delivered uniformly in the transmural plane. This results in the preferential delivery of collateral flow to the subepicardial tissue at the expense of subendocardial tissue. This gradient of flow and injury is exacerbated by a greater energy requirement in the endocardial tissue and a greater vulnerability to ischemic injury in the endocardial tissue. These factors may combine to generate a transmural border zone where epicardial tissue is more susceptible to natural salvage and to protective interventions. This model most likely represents the situation pertaining in the dog heart.

from other beds (see Fig. 5B). Such an anatomical arrangement makes it very difficult to envisage how border zones of flow could arise in the pig heart, and, as such, it would seem reasonable to speculate *that without reperfusion, sustained tissue salvage and infarct size reduction is a remote possibility in the pig.*

In the dog, there is a substantial degree of collateral supply between adjacent coronary beds such that even with the total occlusion of the artery serving one bed, residual flows of 10 to 20% may occur. However, as discussed in Chapter 8, *this collateral flow is delivered by artery-to-artery connections and, once delivered to the ischemic bed, it distributes itself in the manner of normal arterial blood.* Such a situation should not give rise to preferential flow at the lateral borders of an ischemic zone but would be expected to distribute itself across the infarct, giving rise to the situation depicted in Fig. 5C.

Thus, *purely on the basis of vascular anatomical considerations, the superficially attractive concept of a lateral border zone must be questioned.* This doubt has been confirmed by a variety of definitive studies (7,9,34) which have shown in a number of models (including the dog, which has formed the cornerstone of most antiinfarct studies) *that no lateral border zone of intermediate flow exists and that the interface between normal and ischemic tissue is characterized by a sharp (but irregular) interface with severely ischemic tissue lying adjacent to normal, well perfused tissue (see Fig. 6A),* any lateral border zone being supported only by diffusion and being quantitatively insignificant.

### Is There a Transmural Border Zone?

Before dismissing infarct size limitation on the basis of lateral border zone studies it is important to appreciate that natural tissue salvage often occurs, usually in the epicardium, and that it may well be possible to promote tissue salvage in this zone. As is discussed fully in Chapter 8, *epicardial salvage tends to occur because of a variety of factors including a transmural gradient of energy require-*

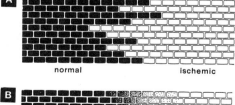

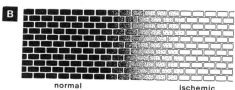

**FIG. 6.** Lateral Interfaces of Injury at a Cellular Level. In a number of models such as the dog the lateral transition between normal and ischemic tissue is thought to be characterized by a sharp (but irregular) interface of flow and injury such that essentially normal cells lie adjacent, or very close to, severely ischemic cells. This model is illustrated in **A**. Progressive gradients of flow and injury such as are illustrated in **B** are no longer thought to characterize the lateral boundaries of an ischemic bed; however, such gradients may possibly arise in the transmural plane thus accounting for natural salvage in the subepicardium, the wavefront phenomenon of cell death and the possible susceptibility of the subepicardial tissue to protective interventions.

*ment and vulnerability to ischemia, coupled with (in models receiving some collateral supply) an uneven transmural distribution of residual flow. Thus, a situation exists where there is a gradient of increasing energy demand and decreasing energy supply as one moves from the epicardium to the endocardium.* This means that, in the case of the dog, the illustration in Fig. 5D is probably the most correct in the series. Such a model can then be used to readily explain the occurrence of significant, variable, natural salvage in models such as the dog; the reported "wavefront" phenomenon of cell death (28); and recent reports (36,37) that some agents, e.g., verapamil and nifedipine, can afford substantial and sustained salvage in the dog, but that this salvage is predominantly in the transmural plane with salvage occurring preferentially in the epicardial zone.

## What Relevance to the Human Heart?

What does the conclusion that the possibility of infarct size limitation in the transmural plane in the dog tell us about the human? *How relevant is the dog, the pig, or the rat to man?* The difficulty of extrapolating from the dog or any other species to the human heart needs no elaboration. Undoubtedly, differences in basal metabolism, pharmacological responsiveness, and vulnerability to ischemic injury exist. As highlighted in Chapter 5, vital differences in collateral supply exist between different models, and it is still debated whether the dog is the best model for the human heart. It is certainly true that in the dog heart with coronary artery ligation, a sharply demarcated area of severe ischemia is created in an otherwise healthy mass of myocardial tissue; this differs considerably from diffuse forms of ischemia seen in the human, and it may also bear little resemblance to the situation arising with only a partial occlusion of a coronary artery. Add to this the complications arising from the major surgery and trauma associated with most large animal studies, the presence of anesthesia, and the fact that coexisting diseases frequently seen in the human (e.g., diabetes) are rarely simulated in experimental studies, then it takes a major leap of faith to extrapolate current animal studies to the human heart. *Animal studies are, however, essential, and we feel that leaps of faith are necessary, placing a high priority on today's investigators to devise better models and apply more cautious and well considered interpretations.*

## FEASIBILITY OF INFARCT SIZE LIMITATION

*Coronary flow, and its degree of impairment, is the ultimate determinant of tissue injury, and the speed and extent to which flow can be restored must be the most important factor in any consideration of tissue salvage.* Although the relationship is neither linear nor simple, the greater the reduction of coronary flow in a zone of regional ischemia then the less time there is before the onset of irreversible injury, the less time there is for the successful application of protective agents, and the less chance there is that a true functional recovery can be achieved. *The extent of flow impairment in both clinical and experimental ischemia can be highly variable as can be the degree of ischemic injury within a single zone of injury.*

## Three States of Flow Deprivation?

Recently we have speculated (14) that three distinct states of flow reduction and ischemic injury may exist and that these may determine the practicability of tissue salvage (see Fig. 7). On the basis of dog heart studies in which the three variables flow deprivation, duration of ischemia, and cellular energy metabolism were interrelated, *we developed the hypothesis that ischemia might be designated as either "tolerable," "critical," or "lethal."*

### *"Tolerable" Ischemia*

*In our dog study (14), coronary flow reductions of up to approximately 50% were found to have relatively little effect on tissue energy stores, even if the reduction was maintained for 2 hr.* In this state of "tolerable" ischemia, tissue energy balance was probably maintained by a combination of increased oxygen consumption per unit flow, reduced contractile performance, and more efficient substrate utilization (for example, switching from fatty acid to glucose utilization). Thus, in this state, although contractility may be reduced, the tissue should remain free of major metabolic or morphological injury for long or indefinite periods. Such tissue might not be expected to undergo infarction (unless subject to excessive stimulation such as catecholamine overload) and might represent a tolerable but chronically ischemic mass which may respond well to metabolic or pharmacological interventions designed to maximize the energy supply: demand status. *In this tissue, drugs, such*

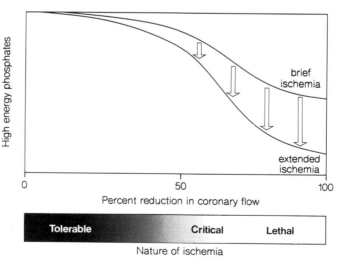

**FIG. 7.** States of Coronary Flow and the Evolution of Tissue Injury. A speculative diagram in which tissue injury (represented by depletion of tissue high energy phosphates) is related to the degree of deprivation of coronary flow. The injury may be designated as "tolerable," "critical," or "lethal" ischemia. Each has different characteristics and may respond differently to pharmacological modification. (For details see text.)

*as coronary vasodilators, might reasonably be expected to afford real protection with a sustained improvement or even a normalization of contractile performance.*

### "Critical" Ischemia

In our second proposed state of ischemic injury, with flow reductions of about 60 to 80%, tissue energy levels were seen to decline. The greater the flow reduction, or the greater the duration of ischemia, then the greater was the energy imbalance. In this phase, which we designated as "critical" ischemia, *small changes in flow or duration could result in large changes in tissue energy status.* It is possible that this tissue could be appropriately identified as "jeopardized" (12,31) since a small improvement in flow might halt the time-dependent decline of energy reserves and possibly convert the tissue to the time-independent state of tolerable ischemia. It may well be that in this relatively narrow range of flow deprivation, metabolic and pharmacological salvage, or very considerable delays in the onset of irreversible injury, may be feasible. However, *the time-dependency of this phase would necessitate that interventions be made as soon after the onset of ischemia as possible,* perhaps within 1 to 2 hr with 80% reduction of flow, and 6 to 12 hr with 60% reduction of flow.

### "Lethal" Ischemia

The third state of injury we designated as "lethal" ischemia and here flow reductions of greater than 80% were proposed to occur. In this phase, injury was suggested to develop very rapidly and have a complex time-dependency such that tissue energy stores fell rapidly with time up to about 45 min. With increasing durations of ischemia, residual energy supplies were found to decline more slowly, the tissue probably being in a state of irreversible injury. *Thus, with flow deprivations of 80% or more (a condition usually observed in a dog or pig heart with coronary artery ligation), it is probably more appropriate to call the tissue "condemned" (12) rather than "jeopardized" since without reflow there is little likelihood of tissue salvage by any metabolic or pharmacological agent.*

### Relation to Transmural Salvage

If transmural gradients of flow deprivation exist, and if (as discussed in Chapter 8) the resulting gradient of vulnerability to ischemic injury is amplified by a gradient of energy requirement and one of inherent metabolic vulnerability, then under some conditions the transition from epicardium to endocardium may encompass the full spectrum of tolerable, critical, and lethal ischemia. *Under these conditions, it is highly likely that an intramural interface of injury may exist, the position of which might be modified by appropriate interventions so as to affect tissue salvage* (see Fig. 8 and later discussion).

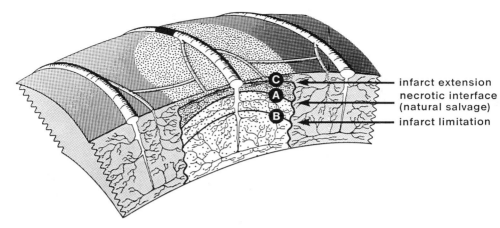

infarct extension
necrotic interface
(natural salvage)
infarct limitation

**FIG. 8.** Infarct Size Manipulation. In the dog heart with significant collateral flow an element of natural salvage often occurs such that a subepicardial band of tissue (perhaps 25% of the original risk zone) does not deteriorate to necrosis. It is envisaged that a transmural wavefront of irreversible injury migrates from the endocardial surface towards the epicardial surface and may stabilize at position **A**. Under certain circumstances such as where vasoconstriction may reduce the blood supply or catecholamines induce increases in heart rate and energy demand, it is conceivable that the interface of necrosis may migrate further towards, or completely to, the epicardium, perhaps stabilizing at position **C**. This we would call infarct size extension and it may well be that infarct size reduction could be achieved by using agents such as β blockers to counter endogenous or exogenous factors which act to extend the infarct. Thus, infarct size limitation could be construed as a limitation of extension. The therapeutic principles behind such an effect might perhaps be different to the situation where vasodilators or agents which increase collateral supply act to attenuate the migration of the wavefront of irreversible injury such that it stabilizes in position **B**. Thus, the term infarct size reduction might be applied where the intervention results in the ultimate volume of the evolving infarct being smaller than it would have been had the intervention not been used.

## DEFINITIONS AND CONCEPTS

At the beginning of this chapter we identified the inappropriate use of terminology as a major factor contributing to the confusion over infarct size modification. Words such as "jeopardized myocardium," "border zones," "wavefronts of cell death" are highly attractive and are equally as dangerous. We believe that their liberal use, often prior to the establishment of their existence or relevance, has done much towards the present state of affairs where in many departments of cardiology infarct size reduction is viewed as an established clinical procedure.

In concluding our chapter we would like to present a series of definitions and criteria which we feel should be applied in any discussion of myocardial protection. These definitions have been evolved in light of some of the problems discussed in previous sections and we hope that they may aid in the interpretation of other chapters in this book.

### States of Oxygen Deprivation

It is important to distinguish between various forms of oxygen deprivation that can be completely different in both origin and consequence. Terms such as ischemia, hypoxia, and anoxia have often been used inappropriately and interchangeably, particularly in the surgical literature.

### Ischemia

Ischemia represents an imbalance between the myocardial demand for, and the vascular supply of, coronary blood. *This condition not only creates a deficit of oxygen, substrates, and energy in the tissue, but also results in an insufficient capacity for the removal of potentially toxic metabolites* such as lactate, carbon dioxide, and protons. *The cessation of coronary flow is not a prerequisite of myocardial ischemia*, in fact, it rarely occurs clinically, and even under experimental conditions (with multiple coronary artery ligations) the collateral circulation may provide substantial perfusion in the ischemic zone. In assessing energy metabolism and tissue injury under conditions of ischemia with residual coronary flow, it is important to appreciate a point stressed by Opie (25). This is that glycolytic adenosine triphosphate (ATP) production represents the only source of ATP under *totally* anaerobic conditions and, as such, the promotion of anaerobic metabolism during ischemia has received much emphasis (probably too much). However, it only requires a very low level of collateral flow for residual oxidative metabolism to become the quantitatively dominant source of ATP.

### "Stuttering" Ischemia and "Stunned" Myocardium

*Another important characteristic of ischemia that is often overlooked is its dynamic nature.* Ischemic crises may come and go giving rise to *"stuttering ischemia."* Transient ischemia of this nature may arise from a number of factors, for example, as a consequence of changing patterns of flow distribution, from the occurrence and relief of coronary spasm, and as a result of the spontaneous lysis of thrombotic occlusions.

Spontaneous or induced reperfusion of ischemic tissue during the phase of reversible injury results in the eventual recovery of the metabolic and contractile capabilities of the tissue. However, as stressed several times in this and other chapters, this recovery may take some time. Thus, the resynthesis of adenine nucleotides lost during as little as 15 min of ischemia, may take days or weeks (29), and the restoration of normal contractile function may take a similar period of time (16). Tissue suffering such an ischemic "hangover" has been appropriately designated by Braunwald and Kloner as *"stunned"* myocardium (4). *Tissue in this partially recovered state would, of course, be particularly vulnerable to subsequent ischemic insults. The combination of stunned myocardium and stuttering ischemia may well create a scenario for the initiation of a sequence of progressively more severe self-inflicted injury which could easily culminate in irreversible injury and cell necrosis.*

### Anoxia and Hypoxia

The conditions of anoxia and hypoxia are quite distinct from ischemia in both their origins and consequences. In anoxia or hypoxia, the oxygen delivery to the myocardium is reduced by the removal of all or some of the oxygen in the coronary supply. Thus, while the partial pressure of oxygen is reduced, coronary flow may be normal or even elevated, and substrate delivery and metabolite removal may also be normal. In contrast to ischemia with residual flow, in anoxia anaerobic glycolysis is the dominant source of ATP. In hypoxia, depending on the extent of oxygen availability, there will be a variable balance between aerobic and anaerobic ATP production.

### Myocardial Infarction

Unless checked, the continuum of increasingly severe tissue injury initiated by myocardial ischemia will eventually lead to cell death and the generation of a mass of necrotic tissue (the myocardial infarct). The entire process represents myocardial infarction, the critical event being the transition from reversible to irreversible cell injury. *Before this time myocardial infarction is not an obligatory consequence of ischemia but beyond this point infarction becomes inevitable.*

## States of Ischemic Injury

Tissue injury conventionally has been divided into "reversible" and "irreversible," however, exactly what these terms qualify is not always clear.

### Reversible Injury

The time-related condition of reversible injury requires that the degree of tissue injury be such that restoration of adequate coronary flow results in "recovery." Recovery of what? Tissue ATP levels, mitochondrial function, ion pumping ability, and morphological integrity have often been used as markers of tissue recovery. We would maintain (as discussed in the section dealing with the inadequacy of indices of injury and protection) that this is inadequate and that the loosely used term "recovery" should take account of the physiological role of the organ as well as selected aspects of its biological function, i.e., *the ability to return eventually to a state of contractile function should be a mandatory component of the definition of reversible injury.* We say this, because at this time we cannot discount the possibility that a state of "chronic cell injury" may exist.

### Chronic Cell Injury: Does It Exist?

*The interesting and as yet unresolved possibility arises that tissue injury may be such that a cell is biologically alive in the sense that many of its metabolic characteristics, e.g., mitochondrial function, are normal but it is physiologically "dead" in that it remains acontractile.* It does not seem inconceivable that protective interventions might prevent the process of necrosis while not evoking a return of contraction. Under such conditions, cells might exhibit misleadingly normal profiles for some indices of injury, e.g., tissue ATP content. *If* such a condition exists, it underscores the importance of contractile assessments of injury and protection, or at least the use of multiple independent indices of injury and protection.

Some investigators (see Chapter 3) question the existence of chronic injury, arguing that such a condition could not exist in a steady state indefinitely and that eventually it would either deteriorate to necrosis or progress to recovery. If this turns out to be the case then the term stunned myocardium can be used instead of chronic injury.

### Irreversible Injury

In the light of the preceding two sections we would propose that *for tissue to be designated as irreversibly damaged, it should have permanently lost the ability to contract, irrespective of the duration of reperfusion.*

## Potential for Tissue Salvage

If tissue is to recover then it must still be in a state of reversible injury. However, reversible injury may arise as a consequence of a very brief period of severe ischemia or a longer period of mild ischemia. In the context of therapeutic protection where (at least in the first instance) attempts are being made to prevent cell death by methods which do not involve reperfusion, we believe it is necessary to consider the practicality of salvage. To do this we would divide reversibly injured tissue into "jeopardized" and "condemned."

### Jeopardized or Salvable Tissue

Jeopardized or salvable tissue exist in a situation in which cell injury is reversible primarily because the degree of ischemia is not very severe. Thus, these cells may be receiving suboptimal flow but although their mechanical function may be severely impaired they are able to remain in a viable condition for some time. In other words, *tissue salvage is a practical consideration.* This condition would contrast with one in which the ischemia is severe and the injury is reversible only because the duration of elapsed ischemia is short; to this latter condition we would apply the term "condemned."

### Condemned Tissue

Condemned tissue cells are also reversibly damaged but flow is greatly impaired and ischemia is very severe. In practical terms, without early reperfusion, salvage is not possible and *deterioration to irreversible injury and cell death is inevitable.* The term condemned tissue should probably be applied to the subendocardial portion of a zone of regional ischemia.

## Spatial Characterization of Interfaces of Injury

In any consideration of tissue salvage and infarct size reduction it *is essential that there be a geographically identifiable zone of tissue to act as a target for the therapeutic intervention.* The term "border zone" was thus coined, but in many instances (13) this was confused with an analytical transition zone.

### Transition Zone: An Analytical Entity

The transition zone is that zone of tissue in which the change from predominantly normal to predominantly abnormal flow, metabolism, and electrophysiology is *analytically detected.* It is *within* this zone that sharp interfaces, or border zones, if they exist, are *located.* However, two important limitations must always be considered. First, the width of the zone is a reflection of the resolving power of the detection procedure (for example, the distance between biopsy or electrocardiographic recording sites) rather than the width of the biological gradient. Second, analytically generated border zones might arise in a situation where there was a sharp but highly irregular interface between an ischemic and normal tissue bed (see Fig. 6A). Tissue biopsies taken from such an interface might retrieve an admix of normal and ischemic cells which upon homogenization and analysis might incorrectly indicate intermediate levels of flow or metabolism.

### True Border Zone

*The true border zone must be a spatially identifiable zone of reversibly injured tissue in which the cells are jeopardized, and where the fate of the tissue lies in the balance, and where the progression to functional recovery or the regression to cell death can be influenced by several endogenous or exogenous factors.* Condemned tissue, although reversibly injured, would not necessarily qualify for designation as border zone.

### Risk Zone

The risk zone is the perfusion field of an occluded coronary artery. It is within this field, in the absence of reflow or an appropriate protective intervention, that a myocardial infarction will develop. It is also within this zone that any spatial border zone of potentially salvable cells must be located.

## Infarct Size Manipulation

In the past considerable confusion has arisen over the terms infarct size reduction or limitation and infarct size extension. This has arisen primarily because of a failure to consider the events within the framework of the risk zone.

### Infarct Size Reduction

*Infarct size reduction is the application of interventions which result in the ultimate volume of the evolving infarct being smaller than it would have been had the intervention not been used. A requirement of the definition is that the protection is sustained,* i.e., the effect is not just a delay in the development of necrosis. We would argue that the definition should also require that the salvable tissue eventually return to normal contractile function. *Few, if any, experimental studies claiming successful infarct size reduction fulfill this last requirement.*

Infarct size reduction would normally be expected to occur *within* the original risk zone and on the basis of our current knowledge *we would expect that in the dog for example, it would result in the movement of a critical transmural interface of injury towards the endocardium,* i.e., epicardial salvage. Alternatively, if the transmural wavefront of death hypothesis (28) is accepted, then infarct size reduction would necessitate that *the protective agent attenuates the migration of this wavefront towards the epicardium.*

### Infarct Size Limitation

The terms infarct size limitation and reduction are used interchangeably by most authors and any distinction may only be a matter of semantics. Some investigators would however argue for a difference in that agents which limit infarct size might act by combating factors which might act to extend the infarct *within* the original zone of risk. This distinction is illustrated in Fig. 8, where under "normal" circumstances with a transmural risk zone the final interface of necrosis might be expected to stabilize in position A, i.e., 75% of the risk zone ultimately becoming necrotic. It may well be that the application of an appropriate intervention (e.g., an agent which increases epicardial collateral flow) might result in less cell death such that the interface of necrosis eventually stabilizes in position B—this we would call infarct size reduction. It might, however, be that in some instances endogenous factors such as heart rate, circulating catecholamine levels, or substrate availability act to increase energy demand or reduce flow in the epicardial zone such that the position of the interface of injury eventually stabilizes closer than expected to the epicardial surface—say, in position C. If this were the case then it is possible that agents such as β-adrenergic agonists might counter such a naturally occurring extension, i.e., salvage is accomplished by *limiting extension.*

*Although this distinction between reducing the size of the infarct below that expected and limiting the spread of the infarct beyond that expected might seem trivial, it could be argued that different therapeutic principles might be involved.*

### Infarct Size Extension

A number of early studies suggested that certain factors, e.g., increasing heart rate, vasoconstrictors, or excessive catecholamines might result in the extension of the dimensions of an evolving infarction. Some investigators suggested that such extensions could be substantial and arise at the lateral interfaces of the ischemic zone. This led some to conclude that infarct size extension involved the development of an infarct *beyond the limits of the risk zone* of the occluded coronary artery. In uncomplicated models, with single or multiple occlusions of coronary arteries in otherwise normal hearts, *we do not accept that such an event can occur. In our view, infarct size extension in such models can only involve extension within the confines of the existing risk zone*, i.e., as discussed in the previous section, a movement of the position of the ultimate interface of necrosis towards the epicardium into the zone which would normally exhibit natural salvage. *Thus, in a simple occlusion model we would argue that the maximum extent of infarct size extension would be when all natural salvage is prevented and a full transmural infarct develops.*

Development of an infarct in other perfusion beds, beyond the risk zone of the original bed, might occur under a number of circumstances. For example, a thrombus might extend in a retrograde manner and subsequently occlude the perfusion bed of an adjacent coronary artery. This could lead to the development of a second area of infarction; *however, it would be more appropriate to designate this as reinfarction rather than infarct extension since it would not be a progressive spread of injury from the existing infarct, but the independent development of a new infarct.* It should of course be possible to use therapeutic agents, e.g., anticoagulants, to prevent such an event. Another situation which might arise is the existence of various degrees of ischemia within the heart as a result of various degrees of occlusion in different coronary arteries. One artery might, for example, be diseased to such an extent that flow in its bed is reduced by 60%, thus putting the entire bed at risk of infarction. At the same time another artery may be less severely damaged and may only limit flow to its bed by, say, 40% and, as such, this tissue may not be at high risk of infarction. If the more severely compromised tissue bed deteriorates to infarction then a number of factors including increased work load might act to exacerbate ischemic injury in the second bed which could then go on to infarct. Again we would argue that this is not an extension of the original infarct but an independent reinfarction. Such an event might however be responsive to appropriate therapeutic interventions.

## CONCLUDING COMMENTS

In this chapter we consider the question: "Is infarct size reduction possible?" from the experimentalist's viewpoint. We started by showing that *manipulation of ischemic injury is undoubtedly possible* since, in the context of cardiac surgery, relatively simple interventions are routinely used to protect the heart against ischemic periods of 4 hr or more. This observation led us to question what is really meant by the term protection. With surgically induced ischemia it is only required that the intervention delays the onset of irreversible injury beyond the time of reperfusion. However, whereas slowing the rate of injury development finds great application in the operating theater, it is of less value in the case of regional ischemia and evolving myocardial infarction where our ultimate aim must be to reduce the extent of tissue injury. As the last 10 years testify, this objective is far more elusive but we would maintain that it is not impossible. Although it is crucial that we distinguish between the ability of a drug to reduce rate and extent of injury, it is important to stress that injury-slowing procedures are not without value in the treatment of evolving infarction. We know, for example, that after 1 or 2 days of regional ischemia new collateral vessels can develop and eventually revascularize the ischemic mass. Unfortunately, this usually occurs after the onset of irreversible injury, too late to salvage any tissue. *In the coming years we should perhaps concentrate on developing interventions which delay serious injury for 24 or 48 hr and so allow natural repair and salvage to play a more important role.* The interest in long-term preservation for cardiac transplantation might provide an enormous stimulus for such developments. Further impetus to the development of really effective injury-slowing drugs will undoubtedly come from the growing use of fibrinolysis where, at the present time, application at an early stage of injury poses logistic problems.

We have stressed that the failure to distinguish between injury-slowing and injury-reducing has led to considerable misinterpretation with both experimental and clinical studies. Another important contributor has been the inadequacy of many of the classical indices of injury and protection. Reducing ST-segment elevation or creatine kinase leakage, while obviously a favorable indicator, cannot be equated automatically with preventing cell death or returning cells to contractile function. *In the future there will be a great need for better markers of injury and a better understanding of these markers, particularly in relation to the contractile capabilities of tissue.* Achieving this improvement will be limited considerably by the fact that reversibly injured tissue which is potentially capable of a full functional recovery may remain in a "stunned" state for days or even weeks after the onset of reperfusion. *As experimentalists we must prepare ourselves for more complex and much longer studies.*

Resolving the controversy over border zones of injury should help greatly in planning better experiments; at least now we know where to look for salvage. In the last 5 or 6 years it has become abundantly clear that the lateral margins of an area of ischemia are sharply demarcated with severely injured tissue lying adjacent to essentially normal cells. The absence of a lateral border zone, at least in the dog and the pig, raised considerable doubts about infarct size reduction. Investigators naturally asked: "If there is no spatially identifiable zone of intermediate injury then where is the target for antiinfarct agents? Is infarct size reduction really possible?" *A new wave of optimism is however developing* with the realization that in models with collateral flow, such as the dog, transmural gradients of flow, energy demand, and ischemic vulnerability combine to render subepicardial tissue considerably more resistant to the early onset of irreversible injury than the subendocardial tissue. *It therefore appears that in the transmural plane an epicardial border zone may exist and that the ultimate position of the necrotic interface can be influenced by a variety of factors such as natural collateral flow, agents enhancing this flow, and agents altering the energy demand or processes of cell death in the tissue.* As is evident from many chapters in this book, the extent of collateral flow and the nature of its distribution are critical to both natural and induced tissue salvage. Unfortunately, collateral flow is highly variable and, also, we still do not have a consensus on the collateral status of various human disease states. This last factor makes the design of adequate experimental models very difficult.

*So, is infarct size reduction possible? In the experimental laboratory we believe that it is; natural tissue salvage can often occur and we are confident that this can be made more predictable and more extensive.* Achieving it and demonstrating it will require better markers and models and much more emphasis on the promotion of early collateral flow in combination with the development of really effective injury-slowing interventions. *The answer to this question when applied to man is more difficult.* Existing results of clinical trials are extremely difficult to interpret. For example, there are many complex trials with β blockers which have claimed to demonstrate a reduction of infarct size. Unfortunately, these are dependent upon indirect indices such as creatine kinase leakage or mortality. The latter index is particularly problematic since agents such as β blockers can undoubtedly reduce lethal arrhythmias without necessarily reducing infarct size and protecting cardiac rhythm can improve various electrocardiographic and enzymatic profiles. *Despite these problems we are optimistic that antiinfarct agents will eventually achieve an undisputed role in the treatment of myocardial infarction.*

## REFERENCES

1. Baker, J. E., and Hearse, D. J. (1983): Slow calcium channel blockers and the calcium paradox: comparative studies in the rat with seven drugs. *J. Mol. Cell. Cardiol.*, 15:475–485.
2. Braunwald, E. (1974): Reduction of myocardial infarct size. *N. Engl. J. Med.*, 291:525–526.
3. Braunwald, E., and Maroko, P. R. (1974): The reduction of infarct size—an idea whose time (for testing) has come. *Circulation*, 50:206–209.
4. Braunwald, E., and Kloner, R. A. (1982): The stunned myocardium: prolonged postischemic ventricular dysfunction. *Circulation*, 66:1146–1149.
5. Chambers, D. E., Yellon, D. M., Hearse, D. J., and Downey, J. M. (1983): Effects of flurbiprofen in altering the size of myocardial infarcts in dogs: reduction or delay? *Am. J. Cardiol.*, 51:884–894.
6. Darsee, J. R., Kloner, R. A., and Braunwald, E. (1981): Demonstration of lateral and epicardial border zone salvage by flurbiprofen using an *in vivo* method for assessing myocardium at risk. *Circulation*, 63:29–35 (retracted).
7. Factor, S. M., Sonnenblick, E. H., and Kirk, E. S. (1978): The histological border zone of acute myocardial infarction—islands or peninsulas? *Am. J. Pathol.*, 92:111–120.
8. Factor, S. M., Cho, S., and Kirk, E. S. (1982): Non-specificity of triphenyl tetrazolium chloride (TTC) for the gross diagnosis of acute myocardial infarction. *Circulation*, (Suppl. II)66:84.
9. Harken, A. H., Barlow, C. H., Harden, W. R., and Chance, B. (1978): Two and three dimensional display of myocardial ischemic "border zone" in dogs. *Am. J. Cardiol.*, 42:954–959.
10. Hearse, D. J., and Humphrey, S. M. (1975): Enzyme release during myocardial anoxia: a study of metabolic protection. *J. Mol. Cell. Cardiol.*, 7:463–482.
11. Hearse, D. J., Braimbridge, M. V., and Jynge, P. (1981): *Protection of the Ischemic Myocardium: Cardioplegia.* Raven Press, New York.
12. Hearse, D. J., and Yellon, D. M. (1981): The border zone in evolving myocardial infarction: controversy or confusion? *Am. J. Cardiol.*, 47:1321–1334.
13. Hearse, D. J. (1983): Critical distinctions in the modification of myocardial cell injury. In: *Calcium Antagonists and Cardiovascular Disease*, edited by L. H. Opie, pp. 129–145. Raven Press, New York.
14. Hearse, D. J., Crome, R., Yellon, D. M., and Wyse, R. K. H. (1983): Metabolic and flow correlates of myocardial ischemia. *Cardiovasc. Res.*, 17:452–458.
15. Heng, M. K., Noris, R. M., Peter, T., Nisbet, H. D., and Singh, B. N. (1978): The effects of glucose-insulin-potassium on experimental myocardial infarction in the dog. *Cardiovasc. Res.*, 12:429–435.
16. Heyndrickx, G. R., Millard, R. W., McRitcie, R. J., Maroko, P. R., and Vatner, S. E. (1975):

Regional myocardial function and electrophysiological alterations after brief coronary artery occlusion in conscious dogs. *J. Clin. Invest.*, 56:978–984.

17. Katz, A. M., and Tada, M. (1977): The "Stone Heart" and other challenges to the biochemist. *Am. J. Cardiol.*, 39:1073–1077.

18. Kirlin, P. C., Romson, J. L., Pitt, B., Abrams, G. D., Schork, M. A., and Lucchesi, B. R. (1982): Ibuprofen-mediated infarct size reduction: effects of regional myocardial function in canine myocardial infarction. *Am. J. Cardiol.*, 50:849–856.

19. Kudoh, Y., Maxwell, M. P., Hearse, D. J., Downey, J. M., and Yellon, D. M. (1984): Failure of metoprolol to limit infarct size during 24 hours of coronary artery occlusion in a closed chest dog. *J. Cardiovasc. Pharmacol. (in press).*

20. Lange, R., Nieminen, M., and Kloner, R. A. (1984): Failure of pindolol and metoprolol to reduce the size of non-reperfused infarcts in dogs using area at risk techniques. *Cardiovasc. Res.*, 18:37–43.

21. Maroko, P. R., Kjekshus, J. K., Sobel, B. E., Watanabe, T., Ross, J., Jr., Covell, J. W., and Braunwald, E. (1971): Factors influencing infarct size following experimental coronary artery occlusion. *Circulation*, 43:67–82.

22. Maroko, P. R., and Braunwald, E. (1973): Modification of myocardial infarction size after coronary occlusion. *Ann. Int. Med.*, 79:720–733.

23. Most, A. S., Capone, R. J., and Mastrofrancesco, P. A. (1976): Failure of hyaluronidase to alter the early course of acute myocardial infarction in pigs. *Am. J. Cardiol.*, 38:28–33.

24. Newman, P. E. (1981): The coronary collateral circulation: determinants and functional significance in ischemic heart disease. *Am. Heart J.*, 102:431–445.

25. Opie, L. H. (1976): Metabolic regulation in ischemia and hypoxia. *Circ. Res.*, (Suppl. I)38:I-52–I-74.

26. Opie, L. H. (1980): Myocardial infarct size. Part II. Comparison of anti-infarct effects of beta-blockade, glucose-insulin-potassium, nitrates and hyaluronidase. *Am. Heart J.*, 100:531–552.

27. Peter, T., Heng, M. K., Singh, B. N., Ambler, P., Nisbett, H., Elliot, R., and Noris, R. (1978): Failure of high doses of propranolol to reduce experimental myocardial ischemic damage. *Circulation*, 57:534–540.

28. Reimer, K. A., and Jennings, R. B. (1979): The "wavefront phenomenon" of myocardial ischemic cell death. II. Transmural progression of necrosis within the framework of ischemic bed size (myocardium at risk) and collateral flow. *Lab. Invest.*, 40:633–644.

29. Reimer, K. A., Hill, M. L., and Jennings, R. B. (1981): Prolonged depletion of ATP and of the adenine nucleotide pool due to delayed resynthesis of adenine nucleotides following reversible myocardial ischemic injury in dogs. *J. Mol. Cell. Cardiol.*, 13:229–239.

30. Reimer, K. A., and Jennings, R. B. (1982): Decreasing myocardial energy utilization. In: *Myocardial Infarction: Measurement and Intervention*, edited by G. S. Wagner, pp. 397–414. Martinus Nyhoff, London.

31. Sobel, B. E., and Shell, W. E. (1973): Jeopardized, blighted and necrotic myocardium. *Circulation*, 47:215–216.

32. Sobel, B. E., and Braunwald, E. (1984): The management of acute myocardial infarction. In: *Heart Disease: A Text Book of Cardiovascular Medicine*, edited by E. Braunwald, p. 1326. Saunders, Philadelphia.

33. Vogel, V. M., Zannoni, V. G., Abrams, G. D., and Lucchesi, B. R. (1977): Inability of methylprednisolone sodium succinate to decrease infarct size or preserve enzyme activity measured 24 hours after coronary occlusion in the dog. *Circulation*, 55:588–595.

34. Yellon, D. M., Hearse, D. J., Crome, R., Grannell, J., and Wyse, R. K. H. (1981): Characterization of the lateral interface between normal and ischemic tissue in the canine heart during evolving myocardial infarction. *Am. J. Cardiol.*, 47:1233–1239.

35. Yellon, D. M., Maxwell, M. P., Hearse, D. J., Yoshida, S., Eddy, L., and Downey, J. M. (1984): Flurbiprofen causes an apparent but not real delay of necrosis in the dog. *Advances in Myocardiology,* Vol. 6, edited by N. S. Dhalla and D. J. Hearse. Plenum, New York. *(in press).*

36. Yellon, D. M., Hearse, D. J., Maxwell, M. P., Chambers, D. E., and Downey, J. M. (1983): Sustained limitation of myocardial necrosis 24 hours after coronary artery occlusion: verapamil infusion in dogs with small myocardial infarcts. *Am. J. Cardiol.*, 15:1409–1413.

37. Yoshida, S., Downey, J. M., Chambers, D. E., Hearse, D. J., and Yellon, D. M. (1984): Nifedipine limits infarct size in closed chest coronary embolized dogs. *Basic Res. Cardiol. (in press).*

*Therapeutic Approaches to Myocardial Infarct Size Limitation*, edited by D. J. Hearse and D. M. Yellon. Raven Press, New York © 1984.

# 3

# What Causes Cell Death?

## Philip A. Poole-Wilson

*Cardiothoracic Institute, London W1N 2DX, England*

Over the last 20 years a large amount of research has been directed towards identifying biochemical events in ischemic heart muscle which characterize tissue which will subsequently recover from that which will eventually become necrotic. It has been argued that such knowledge might permit early diagnosis of myocardial infarction and lead to treatment designed to delay myocardial cell death until blood flow is restored. The now widespread use of cardioplegic solutions during cardiac surgery arose from these concepts. The subject has gained new impetus since the introduction of nonsurgical clinical techniques to improve blood flow to ischemic myocardium in patients with angina pectoris by dilatation of atheromatous lesions with angioplasty (37) and by dissolution of clot using thrombolytic techniques (32,76,104).

Myocardial ischemia is the end-result of several pathological processes in coronary arteries (7,20,95) and *a group of patients with myocardial infarction should not be regarded as homogeneous with regard to the etiology of infarction.* "Stuttering" ischemia in the context of myocardial infarction (95) may result from spontaneous thrombolysis, platelet emboli (27), progression of plaque rupture, or vasoconstriction. Repeated episodes of ischemia can precede acute myocardial infarction (75). If the key cellular events during ischemia could be identified then treatment might become more rational. At the present time there is no simple answer to the question of what is the cause(s) of cell death. I would argue that our increase in knowledge has led to a profusion of ideas rather than to the identification of any critical factor. In this chapter I discuss some of the concepts relating to cell injury, some factors that restrict our ability to study the phenomenon, and some important mechanisms that are currently under consideration as determinants of cell death or survival.

## MYOCARDIAL ISCHEMIA: CONCEPTS AND SEMANTICS

### Key Events

The consequences of myocardial ischemia are well known and are linked to the fact that the myocardium is highly dependent on the rate of blood flow for its supply of oxygen. The heart extracts almost 70% of oxygen from blood in the coronary arteries, and any increase of oxygen supply must therefore be achieved mainly by an increase of coronary blood flow. Under conditions of severe exercise, blood flow can increase as much as fivefold. Such is the oxygen demand of the myocardium that on cessation of blood flow, tissue and coronary sinus oxygen content fall almost immediately (109). The oxygen within the vasculature and that bound to myoglobin is only sufficient for two to six beats (57), and, in man, contractile function is reduced by the tenth beat after coronary occlusion (11). At this time the action potential is shortened (23) and in both animals (49,99,126) and man (123,124) an efflux of potassium can be detected. Acidosis also occurs within seconds (17), although some controversy exists as to its importance in relation to contractile failure (43,53). After a variable period of time (between 10–20 min) resting tension at constant muscle length rises, i.e., contracture develops (8,9,50,71). Early reperfusion partly reverses the mechanical changes and allows some degree of recovery, but *the timing and nature of events during both ischemia and reperfusion is dependent on many factors including species, temperature, and the preexisting oxygen consumption.*

### Ischemia: Problems of Removal and Supply of Metabolites

Ischemia has traditionally been regarded as an imbalance between oxygen supply and demand. If this is so, then the consequences of ischemia must depend solely on the availability of oxygen. But the heart does not only demand oxygen nor is the sole purpose of blood flow to supply oxygen. As discussed in Chapter 2, the removal of heat and metabolites are equally important functions and *I would contend that a more accurate definition might be that ischemia represents "an imbalance between the consumption of ATP and blood flow."* An important consequence of such a definition is that the emphasis is not solely on oxygen. Thus, for example, taking the argument that at least part of the early decline in developed tension is attributable to an intracellular acidosis (17,53), it should be noted that the acidosis itself is in part due to failure of blood flow to remove metabolites, particularly carbon dioxide. *Thus, acidosis in the initial seconds of ischemia may occur more as a consequence of low blood flow than oxygen lack.* Myocardial temperature is another factor which is determined by blood flow during early ischemia. *Later in ischemia the accumulation of many substances and the fall in pH are caused by the metabolic consequences of oxygen lack but the magnitude of these changes is determined by a failure to remove metabolites.*

### Terminology and Interpretation

Much innovative terminology has been used to emphasize particular aspects of myocardial ischemia or to stress favored concepts. Commonly encountered phrases are "reversible and irreversible cell injury," the "onset of necrosis," "infarct size," "border zone," "reperfusion damage," "stunned myocardium," and "oxygen paradox." *Not all these concepts need be correct. Like the clinical diagnosis of brain death, myocardial cell death is difficult to diagnose except under extreme conditions.* No one, for example, would believe that a cell whose membrane has been grossly disrupted, or whose intracellular organelles are totally disorganized could ever recover, but supposedly more subtle determinants of the inevitability of cell death, for example, staining with dyes, *are only valid until the exception is found. The incontrovertible diagnosis* of cell death can be made from the presence of fibrotic tissue many days after the ischemic insult. Despite these problems certain facts are now clear, for example: myocardial tissue made severely ischemic for periods greater than 3 hr is unlikely to recover at all, even 4 weeks (14,68) after reperfusion; the extent of necrosis increases rapidly after 15 min of ischemia and is greater than 70% after about 45 min (55,56,102); contractile function may partly recover after the myocardium has been ischemic for 1 hr but this recovery may take 4 weeks or more to be complete (14,68). *There is clearly a decreasing recovery of function with an increasing duration of ischemic period. The key question that must be asked is what determines the time-scale of those biochemical events which may lead to cell death?*

### Reperfusion: An Essential Event

It is a truism that permanent and total deprivation of blood flow to the myocardium must lead to cell death and likewise that reperfusion (depending on the duration of the ischemic period) is associated with recovery. Despite this basic consideration, there have been reports, in models of permanent coronary artery occlusion, that certain interventions can reduce infarct size, allegedly without a change of blood flow.

The phrase "reperfusion damage" (see Chapter 11) refers to the observation that reperfusion after a period of total or partial ischemia may lead to an increased enzyme release into the coronary effluent and that resting tension may transiently rise (42). "Reoxygenation damage" is a similar phenomenon (44). These phrases suggest that the observed damage was due to reperfusion or reoxygenation and could have been avoided by not reperfusing the tissue. *I would maintain that this is incorrect as failure to reperfuse will lead inevitably to cell death. The events at the time of reperfusion are merely an occurrence in the natural history of ischemia which may or may not be modified with a subsequent improvement in recovery.*

## EXPERIMENTAL COMPLICATIONS

The literature on the pathophysiology of myocardial ischemia is large and numerous experimental preparations have been used. Undoubtedly some of the discrepancies in results are due to differences in the design of experiments; a list of contributory factors is given in Table 1. *In vitro* preparations have been widely used and in many instances studies with partial and total ischemia have been compared to others which have been carried out with hypoxic and substrate-free perfusates. Although there are major metabolic differences between these two experimental conditions, the associated fall of developed tension, the rise of resting tension, the leakage of intracellular enzymes, and calcium exchange are remarkably similar (8,9,40,43,44). Two important considerations in ischemic preparations *in vitro* are the size of the extracellular space (94) and the extent of ionic redistribution (100). Since most isolated preparations lose potassium, gain sodium, and are edematous (100), the large extracellular space means that any consequence of ischemia which is dependent upon the distribution of a retained molecule *in vitro* will be diluted in a fluid volume substantially larger than *in vivo* (58). The alteration of tissue electrolytes *in vitro* may be important in two respects. First, a raised

TABLE 1. *Experimental factors that may complicate the study of myocardial ischemia*

Species: Differences in sensitivity to ischemia
Preexisting collaterals present or not?
Anesthetized or conscious preparations?
Mode of coronary occlusion. Sudden or slow? External or internal?
Mode of reperfusion. Sudden or slow? Constant pressure or flow?
Ischemia or hypoxia? With or without substrate?
Perfusion at constant pressure, pulsatile or constant flow?
Global or regional ischemia?
Total or partial ischemia?
Site and size of ischemic area
Duration of ischemia
Myocardial oxygen consumption at onset of ischemia
Method of measuring area of necrosis
Method of measuring predicted area of necrosis
Time of intervention. Before or after onset of ischemia?
Dose of drug and method of administration
*In vitro* perfusate. Blood, erythrocyte-enriched or crystalloid fluid?
Oxygen tension *in vitro* > 500 or = 100 mm Hg?
Edema in *in vitro* preparations
Altered intracellular ions in *in vitro* preparations
Randomized experiments
Concurrent controls
Blinded experimenters
Inclusion or exclusion of failed experiments or dying animals

intracellular sodium prior to any experimental procedure may exaggerate the role of sodium-calcium exchange in ischemia, and, second, a raised initial tissue calcium may influence the accumulation of calcium in diseased states. *In vitro* preparations are frequently perfused with physiological solutions with a calcium concentration of between 1.5 and 2.5 mmole/liter and have a high control calcium content (9,80,115,129). The calcium activity of blood is less than 1.0 mmole/liter and the calcium content of tissue *in vivo* (112,127) is less than that *in vitro* (80,115,129). The tissue calcium of heart muscle *in vitro* is directly related to the extracellular calcium concentration (115).

*It can be argued that a variety of changes under control conditions, such as those mentioned above for* in vitro *preparations, may substantially modify events during myocardial ischemia. If this is the case, then inappropriate experimental design may lead to misinterpretation of results from studies designed to identify critical metabolic changes leading to cell death.*

## POSSIBLE CAUSES OF CELL DEATH

Several theories (see Table 2) have been put forward to explain cell death. These can broadly be divided according to the supposed initiating factor. In the following sections I discuss some of the major theories which are currently receiving consideration. A major difficulty in assessing whether a proposed mechanism is of particular significance is that any variable which changes during ischemia will correlate with eventual cell necrosis and mechanical recovery on reperfusion. This is because the extent of necrosis increases with the duration of the ischemic period as does the change in the putative cause. In order to establish a causal link rather than an association, further evidence must be obtained. Common methods used to establish a causal link are either that with varying durations of ischemia the proposed relationship remains very close or that the relationship remains true when other factors, known to influence the severity of ischemia (such as temperature or heart rate), are varied. In addition to fulfilling the above requirements, I believe that any theory should always have a reasonable biological basis.

### Energy Hypothesis

Various modifications of this hypothesis have recently been advanced but the key feature is still that a lack of ATP is the cause of cell necrosis (55,56). *One of the problems I have in accepting this argument is that the mechanism by which a low ATP would lead to cell death is not satisfactorily explained.* Several possibilities have been proposed. These include the suggestion that ATP is essential for the preservation and repair of the cell membrane, for the phosphorylation of membrane channels in the sarcolemma or intracellular vesicles so as to maintain ionic homeostasis, for the energy required for ionic pumps, and for the maintenance of relaxation of the myofibrils (50,72,121). A correlation has been shown between tissue ATP content and cell necrosis after increasing periods of ischemia (55,56), and some authors have reported a threshold for ATP content below which necrosis

TABLE 2. *Possible mechanisms leading to myocardial cell death after ischemia*

| Primary mechanism | Secondary mechanism | Comments |
|---|---|---|
| Lack of energy | Low tissue ATP (42,56,57)<br>Loss of adenine nucleotides<br>(101)<br>Low tissue NAD (62)<br>Acidosis | Low ATP not a valid<br>mechanism in other<br>tissues. Precise<br>sequence of events<br>consequent to lack of<br>energy uncertain<br>? Membrane integrity<br>? Repair processes<br>? Cellular function<br>? Ionic homeostasis<br>? Energy for ion pumps<br>? Relaxation of<br>myofibrils |
| Mechanical effects | Cell tearing due to<br>contracture (28,29,31)<br>Myocardial cell swelling (93)<br>No-reflow phenomenon<br>(41,51,64,97,120) | Determined partly by<br>integrity of structure of<br>matrix |
| Membrane damage<br>Mitochondria (42,83)<br>Sarcolemma | Phospholipase activation<br>(125)<br>Protease activation (89)<br>Lysosomes (128)<br>Leukotrienes (118)<br>Acyl esters (59)<br>Lysophosphoglycerides<br>(18,119)<br>Oxygen radicals<br>(38,46,69,77,98,106,108)<br>Sodium-calcium exchange<br>(5,36,103)<br>Calcium (91)<br>$\alpha$ receptors (110) | A consequence is calcium<br>accumulation in the cell<br>which is a possible final<br>common pathway for cell<br>necrosis |

increases rapidly, although this is not a universal finding. On the other hand, substantial falls of ATP can occur without necessarily resulting in necrosis (39), and in other tissues, such as the brain or the liver, ATP content can approach zero while the tissue still has the potential for almost complete recovery (57,73). The fall in myocardial ATP content precedes the rise in the inulin diffusible space (58) suggesting that a low ATP is not the immediate cause of membrane disruption. It has also been shown that damage to the cell membrane, so great as to cause inevitable cell death, can occur in the absence of large changes in ATP (57). Drugs can greatly improve the postischemic recovery of mechanical function without affecting the tissue content of ATP (24). *These observations do not support a simple link between tissue ATP and cell death.*

For many years it has been believed that the initial fall of developed tension in myocardial ischemia is associated with only a small, or even no change in total tissue ATP content (39,53). The earliest mechanical changes arise as a consequence of the loss of turgor due to the collapse of the coronary arteries (2,122) in the absence of perfusion pressure. Intracellular pH then falls and this is followed by a decline in creatine phosphate (seen after approximately 20 sec) and ATP (seen from 1 min onwards). *It is my belief that it is impossible to relate changes in tissue ATP to the early contractile failure (53), but this view is not universally shared (43).* To account for the general lack of correlation between ATP content and contractile failure, it has been suggested that ATP is compartmentalized within the cell either physically, due to intracellular organelles, or functionally, due to the activity of local isoenzymes of creatine phosphokinase.

Ionic channels in myocardial cell membranes for potassium and calcium are sensitive to ATP-dependent phosphorylation (4,15,87), and their malfunction has been linked to ATP deficiency and the initiation of cell death (10,48,90). Evidence has been obtained suggesting that glycolytically derived ATP, which is presumed to be cytosolic, may be essential for the functional preservation of the cell membrane (78,79) and the prevention of contracture of the myofilaments (90). Changes in the cell membrane brought about by exogeneous phospholipases are also known to be dependent on the ATP content of the cell (48).

*In summary, despite the ubiquitous importance of ATP to cell function and cell survival, I do not believe that ATP deficiency has yet been shown to be the critical determinant for the onset of irreversible injury.*

## Mechanical Hypotheses

After 10 to 30 min of ischemia, resting tension begins to rise. Ganote and Kaltenbach (29) have proposed the concept that myofilaments contracting by different amounts in adjacent cells cause stresses sufficient to physically tear the membranes of cells apart. Such a process may be of importance not only during ischemia (28) but also during hypoxia (30) and the calcium paradox (31,131) when a similar rise of resting tension occurs. *Although such a mechanism may be critical under certain defined circumstances, I do not believe that it can have universal application.* I say this because cell necrosis can occur in the absence of contracture where sarcomeres are pulled apart rather than shortened. In addition, in some preparations contracture can be shown to occur without extracellular markers having access to the intracellular fluid (8,9,13,40), i.e., without gross physical disruption of the cell membrane.

Another mechanical effect which might possibly contribute to cell death is myocardial cell swelling (93). It could be argued that were such a process to occur against a rigid cell matrix then "blow-outs" might appear on the surface of the cell particularly at sites of "blebbing" observed during hypoxia.

The no-reflow phenomenon and its attendant consequences have been described in great detail (41,51,64,97,120). The observation is that reperfusion of ischemic tissue gives rise to an increased resistance to flow attributable primarily to endothelial cell swelling, contracture of the myocardium around the capillaries, and contraction of smooth muscle. Recent experiments (34) have shown that during partial regional ischemia there is a progressive increase in coronary resistance, which can be overcome by drugs. In the initial 45 min of ischemia this increase in resistance appears to be due primarily to contraction of smooth muscle. The cause of this effect may be the high extracellular potassium concentration which rapidly develops in ischemic myocardium (49,99,123,124,126). Vasoconstriction provides an additional mechanism for the efficacy of calcium antagonists during myocardial ischemia in some experimental preparations.

In summary, *although mechanical factors may contribute to cell death, and in some special cases (e.g., the calcium paradox) may be an important precipitating factor, it is my belief that they do not represent primary factors in the initiation of irreversible injury during myocardial ischemia.*

## Membrane Damage

Much recent work has been directed towards the hypothesis that early ischemia-induced changes in sarcolemmal (22) or mitochondrial membranes lead to a loss of ionic homeostasis and ultimately to cell death. Numerous causes for membrane damage have been proposed. One argument, for example, is that activation of phospholipase during ischemia, as a result of a decrease in pH or a rise in calcium, leads to a breakdown of phospholipids in the cell membrane. Another possibility is that the intracellular accumulation of acyl esters (59) or the formation of lyso-phosphoglycerides (18) can adversely alter cell membranes and their function through the ability of these compounds to act as nonspecific detergents (119). In addition, lysophosphoglycerides have been implicated in the genesis of arrhythmias (18). The leukotrienes might also contribute to membrane damage but recent studies show that they do not alter the contractile response to hypoxia (119). An additional possibility for the involvement of membranes in irreversible cell injury is that lipids in the cell membrane are acted on by oxygen radicals formed during ischemia and particularly during reperfusion (38,46,69,77,98,106,108). As discussed fully in Chapters 12 and 13, oxygen free radicals may be formed in mitochondria, in white cells (106), directly in membrane lipids (69), or from metabolites such as reduced nicotinamide adenine dinucleotide (NADH), flavoproteins, hypoxanthine (77), and catecholamines. In summary, *whatever the nature of the initial metabolic cause of ischemia-induced membrane derangement, the consequence is a severe disturbance of ionic homeostasis, and this I believe is a crucial factor in the genesis of irreversible cell injury.*

## Calcium Hypothesis

### Calcium in Cell Injury and Cell Function

Shen and Jennings (111,112) showed that reperfusion of ischemic muscle resulted in a large net gain of calcium and other changes of intracellular ions are also known to occur (55). *Fleckenstein (25,26) has emphasized the importance of calcium imbalance and has argued that calcium overload is a general cause of cell death.*

*Even if this is so, the hypothesis does not explain how the calcium gain came about in the first place.* Certainly, under many pathological conditions calcium accumulates in the heart (60), for example, in hypoxia (40,65,93), in ischemia (6,8,9,45,114), in the calcium paradox (44,131), in catecholamine-induced damage (107), and in various forms of heart failure (52,117) and cardiomyopathy (54,74).

One reason for the emphasis on calcium as a mediator of cell death is that no situation has yet been described in which massive calcium accumulation occurs and yet the cells survive. A second reason is that calcium is necessary for a multiplicity of cell functions. Thus, cytosolic calcium concentration affects contraction (105), the stability of cell membranes (33,91), the function of enzymes (21), and the mitochondrial production of ATP (70,92). Calcium is bound to (12,66) and closely associated with the myocardial cell membrane (6). The uptake of calcium by mitochondria dissipates the mitochondrial potential which is linked to ATP production (92,130), and calcium uptake into mitochondria can occur in preference to ATP production (70,92,130).

### Calcium Exchange in Ischemia and Reperfusion

Early experiments on ischemic myocardium clearly showed that an increase in tissue calcium occurs upon reperfusion (111,112). By contrast, calcium movements during ischemia or hypoxia were less clear and have only been reported recently. During total ischemia the quantity of unbound calcium in the extracellular and cystolic spaces is such that if equally distributed the concentration would be approximately $4 \times 10^{-5}$ mole/liter. Initial experiments on hypoxic substrate-free perfusion of the myocardium suggested that there was an accumulation of calcium during hypoxia (84). But these experiments were performed in a Langendorff preparation at a high heart rate and at 37°C. In later experiments, at a lower temperature (28, 32, and 35°C) and a lower heart rate, calcium efflux was shown to be unchanged and calcium influx decreased (40). This conclusion has now been substantiated by a number of groups (67,83,114). It seems that *a net gain of calcium during hypoxia is a late event* and is only evident in some Langendorff preparations because of the severity of the experimental conditions, but it should be stressed that even then calcium gain does not occur in the first 15 min of hypoxia (86). We have also shown that calcium gain does not occur during partial ischemia (9). *Thus, it can be concluded that calcium exchange between the vasculature and the myocardial cell is not greatly altered during hypoxia or ischemia even when there is a substantial rise of resting tension (8,9).* By contrast, on reoxygenation or reperfusion there is a sudden and large increase in calcium influx. The influx occurs within seconds suggesting that it is the reintroduction of oxygen that is the critical event. The increase of calcium influx is remarkably similar during reoxygenation and during reperfusion (8,9,40) and the calcium gain can be correlated with mechanical recovery (9) and with the fall of ATP (45).

## Mechanisms for Increased Calcium Influx

The net gain of calcium that occurs during reperfusion is attributable to an increased influx and not a decreased efflux (8,9,111). Although the precise mechanism causing the increased influx is not known, by exclusion it has been suggested that an increased calcium permeability permits the ion to move down the concentration gradient from the extracellular fluid to the intracellular space. The slow calcium channel appears not to be involved since calcium influx cannot be blocked by calcium antagonists or be altered by changes in heart rate or increases in extracellular potassium (9). Sodium-calcium exchange has been implicated and in a number of experiments (5,36,103) calcium gain has been modified by alterations of the intra- to extracellular sodium gradient. However, further experiments are necessary in order to show that calcium uptake via sodium-calcium exchange can occur without imposed changes in the sodium gradient. Using intracellular electrodes, Kleber (61) has shown that the sodium activity does not change for at least 15 min of ischemia. This is of interest because at this time, at temperatures between 31 and 33°C, a full recovery of function can be expected on reperfusion without there being a gain of calcium (8,9,40).

Another possible explanation for intracellular calcium gain is that calcium enters the cell as a consequence of gross disruption of the cell membrane. Certainly, when such an abnormality is present, cell death is inevitable. Calcium uptake can be shown to occur when the cell membrane is intentionally destroyed using a detergent or the calcium paradox (96).

Evidence against gross disruption as a primary mechanism comes from observations that extensive sarcolemmal disruption is a relatively late ischemic event (3,13) and that, during hypoxia, low flow ischemia, and total ischemia, the uptake of calcium can occur without extracellular markers gaining access to the intracellular space (8,9,83,114). Defects in the cell membrane can be demonstrated during ischemia by electronmicroscopy, but it is difficult to correlate them with cell death (3,55,56) because of artifacts which may occur during tissue preparation, because blebbing of the cell surface may exaggerate artifacts, and because of the problem of inhomogeneous cell populations (116). The uptake of calcium during reoxygenation or reperfusion can be inhibited by small molecules such as nickel, and by metabolic inhibitors such as cyanide and fluorocyanocarbonylphenylhydrazine (FCCP) (96). These observations provide some evidence for the idea that the uptake of calcium may be by passive diffusion into the cytosolic fluid (and then into the mitochondria) and not as a consequence of gross disruption to the membrane.

## Importance of Intracellular Calcium Concentrations

*A key factor in determining the role of calcium in hypoxic or ischemic injury is its concentration in the cytosol.* Depending on whether there is an increase or decrease in concentration, calcium may act as a major contributor to pathological processes, or alternatively it merely may be a secondary event late in the ischemic process. A number of attempts have been made to measure the cytosolic concentration of calcium. With the aequorin technique, for example, conflicting results have been obtained such that calcium concentration has been shown to remain unchanged, or to rise (63), or even fall (1). On exposure of heart muscle to the metabolic inhibitor FCCP, the consequent rise in resting tension has been shown to occur at the same time as a rise in cytosolic calcium (19). With a null point method or light-emitting agents, calcium has been reported to increase in the presence of rotenone (81,82). The differences in these results possibly may be attributable to species, to experimental design, or to inhomogeneity of cell damage. Some insight into the problem has been obtained in recent experiments in which cultured heart cells were exposed to calcium-free solutions and to FCCP and rotenone (81). Despite a five- to tenfold increase in total calcium, almost half of which went into the mitochondria, the cells did not appear to become grossly damaged since there was only a small leakage of intracellular enzymes and a decline in ATP content of only 20%. From such observations we might contend that calcium per se does not appear to be a cause of cell death. However, it should be pointed out that cytosolic calcium concentrations were not stated and that larger changes in enzyme leakage and ATP content were seen in the rotenone experiments. It is possible therefore that a "steady state" might have been reached where there was a high intracellular calcium concentration but no inward flux, so making a direct comparison with ischemic muscle inappropriate.

### Reperfusion and Calcium

Reperfusion or reoxygenation of the myocardium is associated with an increased calcium influx, the mechanism of which has already been discussed. Since early reperfusion is usually accompanied by cell recovery, *for the calcium hypothesis to be valid it is necessary to show that inhibition of the calcium uptake results in an augmented recovery and failure to recover must be accompanied by calcium accumulation.* The uptake of calcium during reperfusion can be prevented by nickel (46), acidosis (65), and metabolic inhibitors (96). In addition, the removal of calcium from the perfusate before a period of ischemia or hypoxia (65) delays the development of contracture and improves recovery. This last observation is, however, due largely to the attendant reduction in contractility and conservation of ATP, i.e., a cardioplegic effect. This can be demonstrated because the removal of calcium during hypoxia after the fall of developed tension (35,71,85) has no effect on the subsequent rise of resting tension. However, reduction of calcium at the moment of reperfusion or reoxygenation does appear to influence mechanical recovery (16,88,113), and *I would conclude that the events occurring during reperfusion, even if they are a consequence of changes which have occurred during ischemia, can influence eventual myocardial mechanical function and the likelihood of cell death.*

## "CHRONIC ISCHEMIA" AND "STUTTERING ISCHEMIA"

The clinical importance of understanding cell death is that it may provide a rational basis for the use of therapeutic manipulations to delay the onset of cell necrosis or prevent unfavorable changes arising during reperfusion. If it were possible to delay the onset of severe injury, then more time would be available to the clinician to reestablish blood flow by techniques such as angioplasty (37) and thrombolysis (32,76,104). There is also the possibility that the same protective manipulations may prevent the progression of a mild ischemic episode to myocardial infarction. In this connection there has been a longstanding debate between clinicians and biochemists over the existence of a state called "chronic" ischemia (see Chapter 2). By this is meant a new steady-state in which a biochemical event linked to the ischemic process reduces myocardial contractility. *Doubt has existed as to whether such a condition could exist as a true steady-state rather than progressing, albeit slowly, to necrosis or recovery. The concept is probably redundant because of the realization of the dynamic nature of ischemia and its prolonged consequences.* Thus, it is known that after even short periods of ischemia (less than, say, 15 min) there is a prolonged abnormality of potassium homeostasis, a persistent reduction of myocardial contractility which may last for several days or even weeks (14,47,68), and a loss of nucleotides which may take weeks to fully regenerate (101). This condition has been nicknamed a cardiac "hangover" (D. J. Hearse, *personal communication*). Repeated episodes of angina in man can lead to myocardial infarction (75); and thus stuttering ischemia, where blood flow is only transiently restored by natural thrombolysis or reduced vasoconstriction in the natural vessel or collaterals, can have an important cumulative effect. Furthermore, episodes of transient ischemia occurring every day would not permit sufficient time for complete recovery ever to occur. The process could result in cell death and patchy fibrosis, and the clinical picture would be similar to that previously called "chronic ischemia."

## CONCLUDING COMMENTS

Cell death in the myocardium is multifactorial and is dependent on the initiating cause. Disruption of the cell membrane is a late event and can be exacerbated by contracture of myocardial cells. A low ATP in the myocardium may be an additional factor contributing to cell death during continuing ischemia without reperfusion. However, the relevance of a lack of ATP when the myocardium is reperfused after a period of ischemia is less clear particularly in relation to disturbances of ionic homeostasis occurring at that time. Changes in cell membranes during hypoxia or ischemia may make them particularly sensitive to the reintroduction of oxygen with an increase in calcium permeability. The precise nature of this change in the membrane is unclear but it may involve phospholipases or oxygen free radicals, and particularly the latter during the reintroduction of oxygen. Massive calcium accumulation, once it has occurred, is incompatible with ultimate cell survival and the calcium accumulation itself will prevent cell recovery. *All of these points, together with the material discussed in earlier sections, lead me to believe that the key event in cell death is the loss of ionic homeostasis due to damage of the myocardial cell membrane.*

## REFERENCES

1. Allen, D. G., and Orchard, C. H. (1983): Intracellular calcium concentration during hypoxia and metabolic inhibition in mammalian ventricular muscle. *J. Physiol.*, 339:107–122.
2. Arnold, G., Kosche, F., Miessner, E., Neitzert, A., and Lochner, W. (1968): The importance of the perfusion pressure in the coronary arteries for the contractility and the oxygen consumption of the heart. *Pfluegers Arch.*, 299:339–356.
3. Ashraf, M., White, F., and Bloor, C. M. (1978): Ultra-structural influences of reperfusing dog myocardium with calcium-free blood after coronary artery occlusion. *Am. J. Pathol.*, 90:423–434.
4. Bechem, M., and Pott, L. (1984): K-channels activated by loss of intracellular ATP in guinea-pig atrial cardioballs. *J. Physiol.*, Proceedings of the November meeting at Queen Elizabeth College, 56P.
5. Bersohn, M. M., Philipson, K. D., Fukushima, J. Y. (1982): Sodium-calcium exchange and sarcolemmal enzymes in ischaemic rabbit hearts. *Am. J. Physiol.*, 242:C288–295.
6. Borgers, M., Thone, F., Xhonneux, R., and Flameng, W. (1982): Shifts of calcium in the ischemic myocardium. A structural analysis. In: *Protection of Tissues Against Hypoxia*, edited by A. Wallquier, M. Borgers, and W. K. Amery, pp. 365–375. Elsevier, Amsterdam.
7. Born, G. V. R., Görög, P., and Kratzer, M. A. A. (1981): Aggregation of platelets in damaged vessels. *Philos. Trans. R. Soc. Lond.*, 294:241–250.
8. Bourdillon, P. D. V., and Poole-Wilson, P. A. (1981): Effects of ischaemia and reperfusion on calcium exchange and mechanical function in isolated rabbit myocardium. *Cardiovasc. Res.*, 15:121–130.
9. Bourdillon, P. D. V., and Poole-Wilson, P. A. (1982): The effects of verapamil, quiescence and cardioplegia on calcium exchange and mechanical function in ischemic rabbit myocardium. *Circ. Res.*, 50:360–368.
10. Bricknell, O. L., Daries, P. S., and Opie, L. H. (1981): A relationship between adenosine triphosphate, glycolysis and ischaemic contracture in the isolated rat heart. *J. Mol. Cell. Cardiol.*, 13:941–945.
11. Brower, R. W., Meij, S., and Serruys, P. W. (1983): A model of asynchromous left ventricular relaxation predicting the bi-experimental pressure decay. *Cardiovasc. Res.*, 17:482–488.
12. Burt, J. M., Duenas, C. J., and Langer, G. A. (1983): Influence of polymyxin B, a probe for anionic phospholipids, on calcium binding and calcium and potassium fluxes of cultured cardiac cells. *Circ. Res.*, 53:679–687.
13. Burton, K. P., Hagler, H. K., Templeton, G. H., Willerson, J. T., and Buja, L. M. (1977): Lanthanum probe studies of cellular pathophysiology induced by hypoxia in isolated cardiac muscle. *J. Clin. Invest.*, 60:1289–1302.
14. Bush, L. R., Buja, L. M., Samowitz, W., Rude, R. E., Wathen, M., Tilton, G. D., and Willerson, J. T. (1983): Recovery of left ventricular segmental function after long-term reperfusion following temporary coronary occlusion in conscious dogs. Comparison of 2nd 4 hour occlusions. *Circ. Res.*, 53:248–263.
15. Cachelin, A. B., de Peyer, J. E., Kokubun, S., and Reuter, H. (1983): $Ca^{2+}$ channel modulations by 8-bromocyclic AMP in cultured heart cells. *Nature*, 304:462–464.
16. Chappell, S. P., Lewis, M. J., and Henderson, A. H. (1983): Myocardial reoxygenation damage can be circumvented. *J. Mol. Cell. Cardiol.*, 15(Suppl 1):329 (abstract).
17. Cobbe, S. M., and Poole-Wilson, P. A. (1980): The time of onset and severity of acidosis in myocardial ischaemia. *J. Mol. Cell. Cardiol.*, 12:745–760.
18. Corr, P. B., Lee, B. I., and Sobel, B. E. (1981): Electrophysiological and biochemical derangements in ischemic myocardium: interactions involving the cell membrane. *Acta Med. Scand.* (Suppl.), 651:59–69.
19. Dahl, G., and Isenberg, G. (1980): Decoupling of heart muscle cells: correlation with increased cytoplasmic calcium activity and with changes of nexus ultrastructure. *J. Membr. Biol.*, 53:63–75.
20. Davies, M. J., and Thomas, T. (1981): The pathological basis and microanatomy of occlusive thrombus formation in human coronary arteries. *Philos. Trans. R. Soc. Lond. (Biol.)*, 294:225–229.
21. Denton, R. M., and McCormack, J. G. (1981): Calcium ions, hormones and mitochondrial metabolism. *Clin. Sci.*, 61:135–140.

22. Dhalla, N. S., Tomlinson, C. W., Singh, J. N., Lee, S. L., McNamara, D. B., Harrow, J. A. C., and Yates, J. C. (1976): Role of sarcolemmal changes in cardiac pathophysiology. In: *The Sarcolemma: Recent Advances in Studies on Cardiac Structure and Metabolism*, Vol. 9, edited by P. E. Roy and N. S. Dhalla, pp. 377–394. University Park Press, Baltimore, Maryland.

23. Donaldson, R. M., Taggart, P., Nashat, F., Abed, J., Rickards, A. F., and Noble, D. (1983): Study of the electrophysiological effects of early or subendocardial ischaemia with intracavitory electrodes in the dog. *Clin. Sci.*, 65:579–588.

24. Drake-Holland, A. J., and Noble, M. I. M. (1983): Myocardial protection by calcium antagonist drugs. *Eur. Heart J.*, 4:823–825 (editorial).

25. Fleckenstein, A., Janke, J., Doring, H. J., and Leder, O. (1974): Myocardial fiber necrosis due to intracellular Ca overload—a new principle in cardiac pathophysiology. In: *Myocardial Biology: Recent Advances in Studies in Cardiac Structure and Metabolism*, Vol. 4, edited by N. S. Dhalla, pp. 563–580. University Park Press, Baltimore.

26. Fleckenstein, A., Janke, J., Doring, H. J., and Leder, O. (1975): Key role of Ca in the production of non-coronarogenic myocardial necrosis. In: *Pathophysiology and Morphology of Myocardial Cell Alteration: Recent Advances in Studies on Cardiac Structure and Metabolism*, Vol. 6, edited by A. Fleckenstein and G. Rona, pp. 21–32. University Park Press, Baltimore.

27. Folts, J. D., Gallagher, K., and Rowe, G. G. (1982): Blood flow reductions in stenosed canine coronary arteries: vasospasm or platelet aggregation. *Circulation*, 65:248–259.

28. Ganote, C. E. (1983): Contraction bond necrosis and irreversible myocardial injury. *J. Mol. Cell. Cardiol.*, 15:67–73.

29. Ganote, C. E., and Kaltenbach, J. P. (1979): Oxygen-induced enzyme release: early events and a proposed mechanism. *J. Mol. Cell. Cardiol.*, 11:389–406.

30. Ganote, C. E., McGarr, J., Liu, S. Y., and Kaltenbach, J. P. (1980): Oxygen-induced enzyme release. Assessment of mitochondrial function in anoxic myocardial injury and effects of the mitochondrial uncoupling agent 2, 4-dinitrophenol (DNP). *J. Mol. Cell. Cardiol.*, 12:387–408.

31. Ganote, C. E., and Sims, M. A. (1983): Physical stress-mediated enzyme release from calcium deficient hearts. *J. Mol. Cell. Cardiol.*, 15:421–429.

32. Ganz, W., Buchbinder, N., Marcus, H., Mondkar, A., Maddahi, J., Charuzi, Y., O'Connor, L., Shell, W., Fishbein, M. C., Kass, R., Miyamoto, A., and Swan, H. J. C. (1981): Intracoronary thrombolysis in evolving myocardial infarction. *Am. Heart J.*, 101:4–13.

33. Gordon, L. M., Sauerheber, R. D., and Esgate, J. A. (1978): Spin label studies on rat liver and heart plasma membranes: effects of temperature, calcium and lanthanum on membrane fluidity. *J. Supramol. Struct.*, 9:299–326.

34. Gorman, M. W., and Sparks, H. V. (1982): Progressive coronary vasoconstriction during relative ischaemia in canine myocardium. *Circ. Res.*, 51:411–420.

35. Green, H. L., and Weisfeldt, M. L. (1977): Determinants of hypoxic and post-hypoxic myocardial contracture. *Am. J. Physiol.*, 232:526–533.

36. Grinwald, P. M. (1982): Calcium uptake during post-ischemic reperfusion in the isolated rat heart: influence of extracellular sodium. *J. Mol. Cell. Cardiol.*, 14:359–365.

37. Grüntzig, A. R., Senning, A., and Siegenthaler, W. E. (1979): Non-operative dilatation of coronary-artery stenosis: percutaneous transluminal coronary angioplasty. *N. Engl. J. Med.*, 301:61–68.

38. Guarnieri, C., Flamigni, F., and Calderera, C. M. (1980): Role of oxygen in the cellular damage induced by re-oxygenation of hypoxic heart. *J. Mol. Cell. Cardiol.*, 12:797–808.

39. Gudbjarnason, S., Mathes, P., and Ravens, K. G. (1970): Functional compartmentalisation of ATP and creatine phosphate in most muscle. *J. Mol. Cell. Cardiol.*, 1:325–329.

40. Harding, D. P., and Poole-Wilson, P. A. (1980): Calcium exchange in rabbit myocardium during and after hypoxia: effect of temperature and substrate. *Cardiovasc. Res.*, 14:435–445.

41. Harris, P. (1975): A theory concerning the course of events in angina and myocardial infarction. *Eur. J. Cardiol.*, 3:157–163.

42. Hearse, D. J. (1977): Reperfusion of the ischemic myocardium. *J. Mol. Cell. Cardiol.*, 9:605–616.

43. Hearse, D. J. (1979): Oxygen deprivation and early myocardial contractile failure: a reassessment of the possible role of adenosine triphosphate. *Am. J. Cardiol.*, 44:1115–1121.

44. Hearse, D. J., Humphrey, S. M., and Bullock, G. R. (1978): The oxygen paradox and the calcium paradox: two facets of the same problem? *Cardiology*, 10:641–663.

45. Henry, P. D., Schuchlieb, R., Davis, J., Weiss, E. S., and Sobel, B. E. (1977): Myocardial

contracture and accumulation of mitochondrial calcium in ischemic rabbit heart. *Am. J. Physiol.*, 233:H677–H684.

46. Hess, M. L., Okabe, E., and Kontos, H. A. (1981): Proton and free oxygen radical interaction with the calcium transport system of cardiac sarcoplasmic reticulum. *J. Mol. Cell. Cardiol.*, 13:767–772.
47. Heyndrickx, G. R., Millard, R. W., McRitchie, R. J., Maroko, P. R., and Vatner, S. F. (1975): Regional myocardial functional and electrophysiological alterations after brief coronary artery occlusion in conscious dogs. *J. Clin. Invest.*, 56:978–985.
48. Higgins, T. J. C., Bailey, P. J., and Allsopp, D. (1981): The influence of ATP depletion on the action of phospholipase C on cardiac myocyte membrane phospholipids. *J. Mol. Cell. Cardiol.*, 13:1027–1030.
49. Hirche, H. J., Franz, C., Bös, L., Bissig, R., Lang, R., and Schramm, M. (1980): Myocardial extracellular $K^+$ and $H^+$ increase and noradrenaline release as possible causes of early arrhythmias following acute coronary artery occlusion in pigs. *J. Mol. Cell. Cardiol.*, 12:579–593.
50. Holubarsch, C., Alpert, N. R., Goulette, R., and Mulieri, L. A. (1982): Heart production during hypoxic contracture of rat myocardium. *Circ. Res.*, 51:777–786.
51. Humphrey, S. M., Gavin, J. B., and Herdson, P. B. (1980): The relationship of ischemic contracture to vascular reperfusion in the isolated rat heart. *J. Mol. Cell. Cardiol.*, 12:1397–1406.
52. Ito, Y., and Chidsey, C. A. J. (1972): Intracellular calcium and myocardial contractility. IV. Distribution of calcium in the failing heart. *J. Mol. Cell. Cardiol.*, 4:507–517.
53. Jacobus, W. E., Pores, I. H., Lucas, S. K., Clayton, H. K., Weisfeldt, M. L., and Flaherty, J. T. (1982): The role of intracellular pH in the control of normal and ischaemic myocardial contractility: a [31]P nuclear magnetic resonance and mass spectrometry study. In: *Intracellular pH: Its Function, Regulation and Utilization in Cellular Functions*, edited by R. Neccitelli and D. W. Deamer, pp. 537–565. Alan Liss, New York.
54. Jasmin, G., and Solymoss, B. (1975): Preventions of hereditary cardiomyopathy in the hamster by verapamil and other agents. *Proc. Soc. Exp. Biol. Med.*, 149:193–198.
55. Jennings, R. B., Ganote, C. E., and Reimer, K. A. (1975): Ischemic tissue injury. *Am. J. Pathol.*, 81:179–198.
56. Jennings, R. B., Hawkins, H. K., Lowe, J. E., Hill, M. C., Klottman, S., and Reimer, K. A. (1978): Relation between high energy phosphate and lethal injury in myocardial ischemia in the dog. *Am. J. Pathol.*, 92:187–214.
57. Jennings, R. B., and Reimer, K. A. (1981): Lethal myocardial ischemic injury. *Am. J. Pathol.*, 102:241–255.
58. Jennings, R. B., Steenbergen, C., Kinney, R. B., Hill, M. L., and Reimer, K. A. (1983): Comparison of the effects of ischaemia and anoxia on the sarcolemma of the dog heart. *Eur. Heart J.*, (Suppl.) 4:123–137.
59. Katz, A. M., and Messineo, F. C. (1981): Lipid-membrane interactions and the pathogenesis of ischemic damage in the myocardium. *Circ. Res.*, 48:1–16.
60. Katz, A. M., and Reuter, H. (1979): Cellular calcium and cardiac cell death. *Am. J. Cardiol.*, 44:188–190.
61. Kleber, A. G. (1983): Resting membrane potential, extracellular potassium activity and intracellular sodium activity during acute global ischaemia in isolated perfused guinea pig hearts. *Circ. Res.*, 52:442–456.
62. Klein, H. H., Schaper, J., Puschmann, S., Nienaber, C., Kreuzer, H., and Schaper, W. (1981): Loss of canine myocardial nicotinamide adenine dinucleotides determines the transition from reversible to irreversible ischemic damage of myocardial cells. *Basic Res. Cardiol.*, 76:612–621.
63. Klein, I., Snowdowne, K., and Borle, A. (1982): Studies of intracellular free calcium in isolated heart cells. *J. Cell. Biol.*, 85:376a (abstract).
64. Kloner, R. A., Ganote, C. E., and Jennings, R. B. (1974): The "no reflow" phenomenon after temporary coronary occlusion in the dog. *J. Clin. Invest.*, 54:1496–1508.
65. Lakatta, E. G., Nayler, W. G., and Poole-Wilson, P. A. (1979): Calcium overload and mechanical function in posthypoxic myocardium: biphasic effect of pH during hypoxia. *Eur. J. Cardiol.*, 10:77–87.
66. Langer, G. A., and Nudd, L. M. (1982): Effects of cations, phospholipases and neuroaminidase on calcium binding to "gas-dissected" membranes from cultured cardiac cells. *Circ. Res.*, 53:482–490.
67. Laustiola, K., Metsa-Katela, T., and Vapaatalo, H. (1979): Mechanism of early changes in

contractility during hypoxia in spontaneously beating rat atria. *J. Mol. Cell. Cardiol.*, 11(Suppl. 2):33.

68. Lavallée, M., Cox, D., Patrick, T. A., and Vatner, S. F. (1983): Salvage of myocardial function by coronary artery reperfusion 1, 2 and 3 hours after occlusion in conscious dogs. *Circ. Res.*, 53:235–247.

69. Lebedev, A. V., Levitsky, D. O., and Loginov, V. A. (1982): Oxygen as an inducer of divalent cation permeability through biological and model lipid membranes. In: *Advances in Myocardiology 3*, edited by E. Chazov, V. Siminov, and N. S. Dhalla, pp. 425–438. Plenum, New York.

70. Lehninger, A. L., Reynafarje, B., Vercesi, A., and Tew, W. P. (1978): Transport and accumulation of calcium in mitochondria. *Ann. NY Acad. Sci.*, 307:160–176.

71. Lewis, M. J., Grey, A. C., and Henderson, A. H. (1979): Determinants of hypoxic contracture in isolated heart muscle preparations. *Cardiovasc. Res.*, 13:86–94.

72. Lewis, M. J., Housmans, P. R., Claes, V. A., Brutsaert, D. L., and Henderson, A. H. (1980): Myocardial stiffness during hypoxic and reoxygenation contracture. *Cardiovasc. Res.*, 14:339–344.

73. Ljunggren, B., Schutz, H., and Siesjö, B. K. (1974): Change in energy state and acid-base parameters of the rat brain during complete compression ischaemia. *Brain Res.*, 73:277–289.

74. Lossnitzer, K., Janke, J., Hein, B., Stauch, M., and Fleckenstein, A. (1975): Disturbed calcium metabolism: a possible pathogenetic factor in the hereditary cardiomyopathy of the Syrian hamster. In: *Pathophysiology and Morphology of Myocardial Cell Alteration: Recent Advances in Studies on Cardiac Structure and Metabolism*, edited by A. Fleckenstein and B. Roma, pp. 563–580. University Park Press, Baltimore.

75. Maseri, A., L'Abbate, A., Baroldi, G., Chierchia, S., Marzilli, M., Ballestra, A. M., Severi, S., Parodi, O., Biagini, A., Distante, A., and Pesola, A. (1978): Coronary vasospasm as a possible cause of myocardial infarction. *N. Engl. J. Med.*, 299:1271–1277.

76. Mathey, D. G., Kuck, K. H., Tilsner, V., Krebber, H. J., and Bleifeld, W. (1981): Non-surgical coronary artery recanalisation after acute transluminal infarction. *Circulation*, 67:489–497.

77. McCord, J. M., and Roy, R. S. (1982): The pathophysiology of superoxide: roles in inflammation and ischaemia. *Can. J. Physiol. Pharmacol.*, 60:1346–1352.

78. McDonald, T. F., Hunter, E. G., and MacLeod, D. P. (1971): Adenosine triphosphate partition in cardiac muscle with respect to transmembrane electrical activity. *Pfluegers Arch.*, 322:95–108.

79. McDonald, T. F., Hunter, E. G., and MacLeod, D. P. (1971): Adenosine triphosphate partition in cardiac muscle with respect to transmembrane electrical activity. *Pfluegers Arch.*, 322:95–108.

80. Morgenstern, M., Noack, E., and Köhler, E. (1972): The effects of isoprenaline and tyramine on the $^{45}$calcium uptake, the total calcium content and the contraction force of isolated guinea-pig atria in dependence on different extracellular hydrogen ion concentrations. *Naunyn-Schmiedebergs Arch. Pharmacol.*, 274:125–137.

81. Murphy, E., Aiton, J. F., Horres, C. R., and Lieberman, M. (1983): Calcium elevation in cultured heart cells: its role in cell injury. *Am. J. Physiol.*, 245:C136–C321.

82. Murphy, E., and Lieberman, M. (1983): Cystolic free Ca in chick heart cells: its role in cell injury. *J. Mol. Cell. Cardiol.*, 15(Suppl. 1):83 (abstract).

83. Nakanishi, T., Nishioka, K., and Jarmakani, J. M. (1982): Mechanism of tissue $Ca^{2+}$ gain during reoxygenation after hypoxia in rabbit myocardium. *Am. J. Physiol.*, 242(3):H437–H449.

84. Nayler, W. G., Grau, A., and Slade, A. (1976): A protective effect of verapamil on hypoxic heart muscle. *Cardiovasc. Res.*, 10:650–662.

85. Nayler, W. G., Yepez, C. E., and Poole-Wilson, P. A. (1978): The effect of β-adrenoceptor and $Ca^{2+}$ antagonist drugs on the hypoxia-induced increase in resting tension. *Cardiovasc. Res.*, 12:666–674.

86. Nayler, W. G., and Williams, A. (1978): Relaxation in heart muscle: some morphological and biochemical considerations. *Eur. J. Cardiol.*, 7(Suppl):35–50.

87. Noma, A. (1983): ATP-regulated $K^+$ channels in cardiac muscle. *Nature*, 305:147–148.

88. Ogilby, J. D., and Apstein, C. S. (1983): Reversal of reperfusion injury with post-ischemia EDTA pulse therapy. *J. Mol. Cell. Cardiol.*, 15(Suppl. 1):330.

89. Ogunro, E. A., Ferguson, A. G., and Lesch, M. (1980): A kinetic study of the pH optimum of canine cardiac cathepsin D. *Cardiovasc. Res.*, 14:254–260.

90. Opie, L. H. (1983): High energy phosphate compounds. In: *Cardiac Metabolism*, edited by A. J. Drake-Holland, and M. I. M. Noble, pp. 279–307. John Wiley, New York.

91. Papahadjopoulos, D. (1978): Calcium-induced phase changes and fusion in natural and model

membranes. In: *Membrane Fusion. Cell Surface Reviews*, edited by G. Porst and G. L. Nicolson, pp. 765–790. Elsevier/North-Holland, Amsterdam.

92. Parr, D. R., Wimhurst, J. M., and Harris, E. F. (1975): Calcium-induced damage of rat heart mitochondria. *Cardiovasc. Res.*, 9:366–372.
93. Pine, M. B., Caulfield, J. B., Bing, O. H. L., Brooks, W. W., and Abelman, W. H. (1979): Resistance of contracting myocardium to swelling with hypoxia and glycolytic blockade. *Cardiovasc. Res.*, 13:215–224.
94. Poole-Wilson, P. A., Bourdillon, P. D., and Harding, D. P. (1979): Influence of contractile state on the size of the extracellular space in isolated ventricular myocardium. *Basic Res. Cardiol.*, 74:604–610.
95. Poole-Wilson, P. A. (1983): Angina—pathological mechanisms, clinical expression and treatment. *Postgraduate Med. J.*, 59(Suppl 3):11–21.
96. Poole-Wilson, P. A., Harding, D. P., Bourdillon, P. D. V., Tones, M. A. (1984): Calcium out of control. *J. Mol. Cell. Cardiol.*, 16:175–187.
97. Powell, W. J., Dibona, D. R., Flores, J., and Leaf, A. (1976): The protective effect of hyperosmotic material in myocardial ischemia and necrosis. *Circulation*, 54:603–615.
98. Rao, P. S., Cohen, M. V., and Mueller, H. S. (1983): Production of free radicals and lipid peroxides in early experimental myocardial ischaemia. *J. Mol. Cell. Cardiol.*, 15:713–716.
99. Rau, E. E., Shine, K. I., and Langer, G. A. (1977): Potassium exchange and mechanical performance in anoxic mammalian myocardium. *Am. J. Physiol.*, 232:H85–H94.
100. Reichel, H. (1976): The effect of isolation on myocardial properties. *Basic Res. Cardiol.*, 71:1–16.
101. Reimer, K. A., Hill, M. L., and Jennings, R. B. (1981): Prolonged depletion of ATP and of the adenine nucleotide pool due to delayed resynthesis of adenine nucleotides following reversible myocardial ischemic injury in dogs. *J. Mol. Cell. Cardiol.*, 13:229–239.
102. Reimer, K. A., Lowe, J. E., Rasmussen, M. M., and Jennings, R. B. (1977): The wavefront phenomenon of ischemic cell death. I. Myocardial size vs. duration of coronary occlusion in the dog. *Circulation*, 56:786–794.
103. Renlund, D. G., Gerstenblith, G., Lakatta, E. G., Jacobusd, W. E., Kallman, C. H., and Weisfeldt, M. L. (1982): Dependence of mechanical and biochemical myocardial recovery on extracellular sodium during ischaemia. *Circulation*, 66II:158 (abstract).
104. Rentrop, K. P., Blanke, H., Karsch, K. R., Kaiser, H., Kostering, H., and Leitz, K. (1981): Selective intracoronary thrombolysis in acute myocardial infarction and unstable angina pectoris. *Circulation*, 63:307–317.
105. Ringer, S. (1883): A further contribution regarding the influence of the different constituents of the blood on the contraction of the heart. *J. Physiol.*, 4:29–42.
106. Romson, J. L., Hook, B. G., Kunkel, S. L., Abrams, G. D., Shork, M. A., and Lucchesi, B. R. (1983): Reduction of the extent of ischemic myocardial injury by neutrophil depletion in the dog. *Circulation*, 67:1016–1023.
107. Rona, G., Chappel, C. I., Balazs, T., and Gaudry, R. (1959): An infarct-like myocardial lesion and other toxic manifestations produced by isoprotenerol in the rat. *Arch. Pathol.*, 67:443–455.
108. Rowe, G. T., Manson, N. H., Carlan, M., and Hess, M. L. (1983): Hydrogen peroxide and hydroxyl radical mediation of activated leukocyte depression of cardiac sarcoplasmic reticulum. Participation of the cycloxygenase pathway. *Circ. Res.*, 53:584–591.
109. Sayen, J. J., Sheldon, W. F., Pierce, G., Kuo, P. T. (1958): Polarographic oxygen, the epicardial electrocardiogram and muscle contraction in experimental acute regional ischaemia of the left ventricle. *Circ. Res.*, 6:779–798.
110. Sharma, A. D., Saffitz, J. E., Lee, B. I., Sobel, B. E., and Corr, P. B. (1983): Alpha adrenergic-mediated accumulation of calcium in reperfused myocardium. *J. Clin. Invest.*, 72:802–818.
111. Shen, A. C., and Jennings, R. B. (1972): Kinetics of calcium accumulation in acute myocardial ischemic injury. *Am. J. Pathol.*, 67:441–452.
112. Shen, A. C., and Jennings, R. B. (1972): Myocardial calcium and magnesium in acute ischaemic injury. *Am. J. Pathol.*, 67:417–434.
113. Shine, K. I., and Douglas, A. M. (1983): Low calcium reperfusion of ischemic myocardium. *J. Mol. Cell. Cardiol.*, 15:251–260.
114. Shine, K. I., Douglas, A. M., and Ricchiuti, N. V. (1978): Calcium, strontium and barium movements during ischemia and reperfusion in rabbit ventricle: implications for myocardial preservation. *Circ. Res.*, 43:712–720.

115. Shine, K. I., Serena, S. D., and Langer, G. A. (1971): Kinetic localisation of contractile calcium in rabbit myocardium. *Am. J. Physiol.*, 221:1408–1417.
116. Steenbergen, C., Deleeuw, G., Barlow, C., and Chance, B. (1977): Heterogeneity of the hypoxic state in perfused rat heart. *Circ. Res.*, 41:606–615.
117. Tobian, L., and Duke, M. (1969): Increased calcium and water concentration in the left ventricle of hypertensive rats. *Am. J. Physiol.*, 217:522–524.
118. Tones, M. A., Letts, G., Fleetwood, G., and Poole-Wilson, P. A. (1983): Failure to demonstrate a pathological role for leukotriene D$_4$ in hypoxic rabbit myocardium. *J. Mol. Cell. Cardiol.*, 15(Suppl 1):409.
119. Tones, M. A., and Poole-Wilson, P. A. (1983): Effect of lysophosphatidylcholine on cellular integrity and calcium uptake in rabbit myocardium. *Eur. Heart J.*, 4(Suppl E):73.
120. Tranum-Jensen, J., Janse, M. J., Fiolet, J. W. T., Krieger, W. J. G., D'Alnoncourt, C. N., and Durrer, D. (1981): Tissue osmolality, cell swelling, and reperfusion in acute regional myocardial ischemia in the isolated porcine heart. *Circ. Res.*, 49:364–381.
121. Ventura-Clapier, R., and Vassort, G. (1981): Rigor tension during metabolic and ionic rises in resting tension in rat heart. *J. Mol. Cell. Cardiol.*, 13:551–561.
122. Vogel, W. M., Apstein, C. S., Briggs, L. L., Gaasch, W. H., and Ahn, J. (1982): Acute alterations in left ventricular diastolic chamber stiffness. Role of the "erectile" effect of coronary arterial pressure and flow in normal and damaged hearts. *Circ. Res.*, 51:465–478.
123. Webb, S., Canepa-Anson, R., Fox, K., Rickards, A. F., and Poole-Wilson, P. A. (1983): Evidence that myocardial potassium loss during ischaemia in man precedes electrocardiographic changes and chest pain. *Clin. Sci.*, 65:24P.
124. Webb, S. C., Rickards, A. F., Poole-Wilson, P. A. (1983): Coronary sinus potassium concentration recorded during coronary angioplasty. *Br. Heart J.*, 50:146–148
125. Weglicki, W. B., Waite, B. M., and Stam, A. C. (1972): Association of phospholipase A with a myocardial membrane preparation containing the (Na$^+$ + K$^+$)-Mg$^{2+}$-ATPase. *J. Mol. Cell. Cardiol.*, 4:195–201.
126. Weiss, J., and Shine, K. I. (1981): Extracellular K$^+$ accumulation during early myocardial ischaemia. Implications for arrhythmogenesis. *J. Mol. Cell. Cardiol.*, 13:699–704.
127. Whalen, D. A., Hamilton, D. G., Ganote, C. E., and Jennings, R. B. (1974): Effect of a transient period of ischaemia on myocardial cells. *Am. J. Pathol.*, 74:381–397.
128. Wildenthal, K. (1978): Lysosomal alterations in ischaemic myocardium: result or cause of myocellular damage? *J. Mol. Cell. Cardiol.*, 10:595–604.
129. Winegrad, S., and Shanes, A. M. (1962): Calcium flux and contractility in guinea pig atria. *J. Gen. Physiol.*, 45:371–394.
130. Wrogeman, K., and Dena, S. D. J. (1976): Mitochondrial calcium overload: a general mechanism for cell necrosis in muscle diseases. *Lancet*, 1:672–674.
131. Zimmerman, A. N. E., and Hulsman, W. C. (1966): Paradoxical influence of calcium ions on the permeability of the cell membranes of the isolated rat heart. *Nature*, 211:646–647.

*Therapeutic Approaches to Myocardial Infarct Size Limitation*, edited by D. J. Hearse and D. M. Yellon. Raven Press, New York © 1984.

# 4

# Where Is the Salvable Zone?

## Michiel J. Janse

*Department of Cardiology and Experimental Cardiology, Academisch Medisch Centrum, 1105 AZ Amsterdam, Netherlands*

In the past decade, many clinical and experimental studies have been conducted to determine whether the eventual size of an evolving myocardial infarct could be limited. Certain expressions have almost become household words in cardiac departments, such as "jeopardized myocardium," "tissue salvage," "myocardial protection," "infarct size reduction," and one sometimes wonders if an advertising agency has been consulted in selecting these words. *Many concepts are now accepted as truths*, and, for example, in our hospital, many young clinicians believe that sodium nitroprusside reduces infarct size because creatine kinase levels were found to be lower, and short-term mortality was less in patients with acute myocardial infarction who had been treated with that substance than in patients who received a placebo (6). Since it cannot be denied that short- and long-term mortality are higher in patients with large infarcts, and that complications are more frequent, it seems logical that measures that reduce mortality and decrease the number of complications do so by reducing infarct size. One can understand why some clinicians think one is indulging in silly word-play when one expresses one's feeling that the only way in which the size of an infarct can be reduced is by shrinkage of the connective tissue within the area of dead cells.

It is not my intention to discuss here whether the administration of sodium nitroprusside, or any other drug, to patients in the acute phase of an evolving myocardial infarction is useful (2,6,21) or, if so, by which mechanisms such drugs act. Rather, I discuss some of the experimental evidence related to "tissue salvage," and concentrate on the three border zones: the lateral, the epicardial, and the endocardial. What is the nature of these border zones? Can tissue in any of these border zones be salvaged, and, if so, is this always beneficial?

## LATERAL BORDER ZONE

One of the concepts that played an important role in the attempts to reduce infarct size was the notion that in the acute phase of regional myocardial ischemia, the central ischemic area is surrounded by a shell of tissue in which the ischemic injury is less severe than in the center. This assumed mass of tissue has become universally known as "the border zone." Cells in this lateral border zone could be prevented from becoming irreversibly injured by measures that would increase collateral blood flow and/or reduce oxygen consumption.

Before describing some of the experiments in which it was sought to find out if such a border zone really exists, it is useful to consider methodological problems and problems concerning definitions (see also Chapter 2).

### Definitions and Complications

The first difficulty arises with the use of the word ischemia. An area may be ischemic in the sense that it receives less blood flow than normal, but, depending both on the degree of flow reduction and the energy requirements of the tissue involved, the flow may be sufficient to maintain normal function. Only at a certain threshold flow, which may differ in various circumstances, will the ischemic region begin to show functional abnormalities. The demarcation between ischemic and normal tissue is thus dependent on the functional index that one chooses to measure. Indicators for ischemia that have been used include: changes in myocardial $Po_2$, $Pco_2$, and pH; in fluorescence caused by changes in tissue levels of NAD and NADH; in tissue levels of high energy phosphates and lactate; in extracellular potassium concentration; in ratios for various ions; in local extracellular electrograms; in transmembrane potential; in local contractility; in local blood flow; and in morphology: *The detection of ischemia can, therefore, be a question of technique.* An additional difficulty is that no correlative studies have been done to compare all possible indicators for ischemia (see Chapter 2).

Another aspect to consider is reversibility. In the dog, for example, the threshold flow value below which cells cannot survive has been estimated to be between 30 and 40% of normal flow (12). *It is, however, conceivable that apart from a threshold flow value which determines whether or not cells will become necrotic, several other threshold flow values exist in relation to various cellular activities.* For example, electrical activity might persist at a level of flow reduction where contractile function has already ceased. *Thus, at a certain site and at a certain time, functional abnormalities may be detected; however, one cannot necessarily predict whether the tissue in question will die or survive. On the other hand, one cannot be absolutely certain that surviving cells will necessarily have normal function.*

As discussed in Chapter 2, Hearse and Yellon (15) have made the important distinction between "jeopardized" and "condemned" tissue. In jeopardized tissue, cells receive a flow that is less than optimal and several functions can be impaired, but flow is sufficient for the cells to remain viable for a long time. Cellular injury is reversible because the ischemia is not very severe. In condemned tissue, the cells are also reversibly injured, but, here, flow is so reduced that cell death is inevitable unless reperfusion occurs very rapidly, perhaps within 30 min. A border zone which could be salvaged should thus be defined as a spatially identifiable zone of reversibly injured cells in which the cells are jeopardized.

## Problems of Measurement

At first sight many studies, using different techniques, support the existence of a lateral border zone surrounding a central core of condemned or already infarcted tissue, in which the cells are injured to a lesser degree than those in the center. Zones of intermediate $Po_2$, of moderate morphological changes, of intermediate ratios of various ions, of intermediate changes in extracellular potentials, and of moderately reduced blood flow have been found and usually interpreted as evidence for the existence of a lateral border zone.

As pointed out by Hearse and Yellon (15), one must take into account the limitations of the techniques. Thus, the width of a border zone in which transitions in flow, metabolism, or electrophysiology are detected depends on the resolving power of the technique (for example, the distance between recording sites or the location of biopsy samples). Furthermore, when a biopsy specimen is homogenized and analyzed for activity of radioactive microspheres (to obtain an estimate of local blood flow), or for tissue content of high energy phosphates and lactate (to obtain an index for local metabolism), intermediate values between those of normal and central ischemic tissue can be explained in two ways (Fig. 1). Either a homogeneous population of cells is present which has an intermediate degree of ischemic injury, or a mixed population of normal and ischemic cells exists in which the ischemic cells are as severely damaged as those in the center of the infarct.

*Many studies, including our own, in which the resolution of the experimental techniques was such that differences could be detected over very small distances support the latter explanation,* and I describe briefly some of our experiments to illustrate this point.

## Interface Characterization

Both in porcine hearts *in situ*, and in isolated porcine hearts perfused according to the Langendorff technique with a 1:1 mixture of blood and modified Tyrode solution, we attempted to correlate the electrophysiological, metabolic, and histochemical changes induced by coronary artery occlusion (18). Intramural and epicardial direct current extracellular electrograms were recorded from the left ventricle

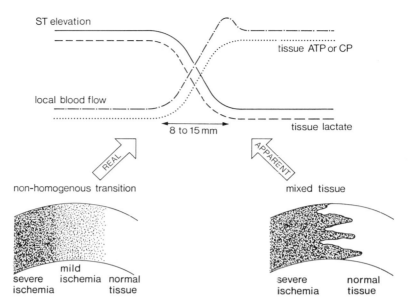

**FIG. 1.** Nature of the Lateral Interfaces of Injury. How a real or apparent lateral border zone may arise.

at sites 4 mm apart. In Fig. 2, it can be seen how 8 min after occlusion of the left anterior descending coronary artery, the extracellular complexes at A and B show marked ischemic changes. The depression of the TQ segment is fully developed and reaches values in the order of − 10 to − 15 mV. This TQ-segment depression is caused by the partial depolarization of the resting membrane potential of ischemic cells. In diastole, there is a potential difference between the intracellular compartments of ischemic and normal cells, and, consequently, an intracellular current flows from ischemic towards normal cells. This current crosses the cell membranes and causes current sinks in the ischemic area (negative extracellular potential) and current sources in the normal myocardium (positive extracellular potential). Intrinsic deflections have either disappeared or become very small, indicating that local action potentials are absent or have very small amplitudes and are incapable of propagating.

The electrograms at site C are typical of the electrophysiologic boundary zone: TQ-segment depression and ST-segment elevation are present, but their magnitude is less than in recordings located 4 mm nearer the ischemic center; large intrinsic deflections indicate the presence of large amplitude action potentials while adjacent recordings moving towards the center show absence of, or very small, intrinsic deflections.

Electrodes at sites D, E, and F are in normal myocardium and show slight reciprocal TQ-segment elevation and ST-segment depression caused by the local current circuits between ischemic and normal tissue.

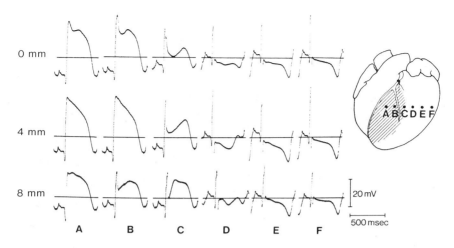

**FIG. 2.** The Electrophysiological Boundary Zone. Epicardial and intramural direct current electrograms (at 0, 4, and 8 mm from the epicardial surface) 8 min after occlusion of the left anterior descending coronary artery in a pig heart. Electrodes **A** to **F** were in a row, separated by 4 mm *(see inset)*. The *straight line* represents the direct current potential of the aortic root. **A** and **B** are ischemic tissue; **C** is electrophysiological boundary; and **D, E,** and **F** are normal. (From ref. 18, with permission.)

In the porcine heart, the position of the electrophysiological boundary zone remains constant throughout a 2-hr period following coronary artery occlusion.

A correlation between electrical and metabolic changes was made by taking transmural, cylindrical biopsies of 3 mm diameter from the recording sites, and determining tissue content of ATP, creatine phosphate, and lactate. At any time after coronary artery occlusion, biopsies from the electrophysiological border zone showed values which were intermediate between those from the central ischemic zone and normal myocardium. The only conclusion that could be made from these findings was that, within the limits of the technique, there was a good correlation between electrophysiological and biochemical measurements.

When a coronary artery has been occluded for about 1 hr, the glycogen has gradually disappeared from ischemic cells, and in biopsies taken from the electrophysiological border zone, a sharp and irregular demarcation between glycogen-depleted and glycogen-containing cells could be seen (Fig. 3). Fully stained cells were adjacent to unstained cells, but small areas could be found where a few cells with intermediate glycogen lay between dark- and light-stained cells. The distances parallel to the epicardial surface where both glycogen-depleted and glycogen-containing zones interdigitated, were in the order of 4 to 9 mm.

*We had the occasion to study an isolated, revived human heart in the same way as the porcine hearts and obtained similar results:* The electrophysiological border zone correlated with the metabolic border, and within the border zone the same sharp and irregular demarcation between glycogen-depleted and glycogen-containing cells was found.

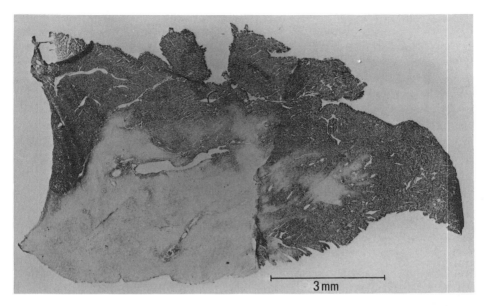

3 mm

**FIG. 3.** The Anatomy of the Lateral Boundary. Glycogen distribution in a large transmural biopsy taken to incorporate the lateral electrophysiological boundary zone after 1 hr of coronary artery occlusion. *Light areas* indicate glycogen-depleted cells; *dark areas* indicate glycogen-filled cells. (From ref. 18, with permission.)

*These results indicate that the lateral border zone consists of a mixed population of normal and ischemic cells.* Additional support for this interpretation was obtained by recording with microelectrodes from a circular area with a diameter of about 5 mm, which by extracellular recording was identified as the electrophysiological boundary. As shown in Fig. 4, resting membrane potentials and action potential amplitudes from cells in the transition zone could show all gradations between completely normal to severely ischemic.

Studies by many other investigators, using different techniques in different animal species, also showed that in the border zone the demarcation between ischemic and normal cells is sharp, following an irregular profile such that peninsulas of normal and ischemic cells interdigitate (8,14,16,28). For example, studies utilizing the NADH fluorescence technique to visualize the demarcation between anoxic and normoxic cells have shown that the transition zone between anoxic and normoxic cells is in the order of 0.1 mm, a depth to which oxygen could be delivered by diffusion. These studies indicate that in metabolic terms a cell either operates aerobically or anaerobically, and that there is no in-between state (1,13,25).

From our studies thus far, it could not be excluded that the ischemic cells in the boundary zone were less injured than those in the ischemic center, and the possibility therefore existed that reperfusion could reverse injury in the boundary zone

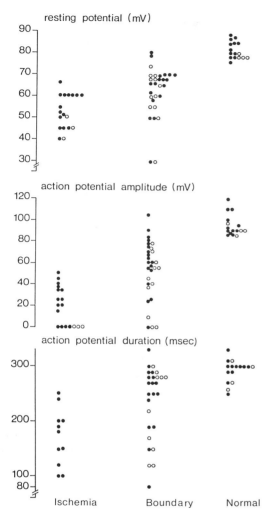

**FIG. 4.** Transmembrane Potentials in the Electrophysiological Boundary Zone. Values of resting membrane potential, action potential amplitude, and action potential duration at ischemic, boundary, and normal sites. The results from 18 experiments are pooled. *Solid circles* indicate measurements made between 15 min and 2 hr of occlusion, *open circles* are values found after a 1-hr period of reperfusion following a 2-hr occlusion. In ischemic and boundary areas, some cells showed no response at low resting membrane potentials. Note that in the transition zone, both during occlusion and after reperfusion, all gradations between normal and unresponsiveness occur. (From ref. 18, with permission.)

while being ineffective in the ischemic center. After a 2-hr period of coronary artery occlusion, reperfusion did not result in recovery of electrophysiological, metabolic, or histochemical changes in either the boundary zone or the center, and therefore it was concluded that with the experimental conditions employed, the ischemic cells in the boundary zone were just as severely injured after a 2-hr period of occlusion as those in the central ischemic area. It may be that for reperfusion after shorter periods of ischemia, a difference may exist in the reversibility of injury in the boundary and in the center, *but I would consider this unlikely. Once the threshold is reached, and cells cannot maintain aerobic metabolism, the fate for ischemic cells is the same regardless of their location.*

## CAN THE LATERAL BORDER BE SHIFTED?

The possibility may arise where the severity of ischemia within an area of injury is sufficiently mild that, under favorable circumstances, normal function is maintained despite the deprivation of flow. If conditions deteriorate, for example, a further diminution of flow or increase in oxygen requirement, the affected cells may develop functional abnormalities such that the initial sharp line of demarcation between cells with normal flow and those with ischemic flow shifts its position to that between severely ischemic dying cells and mildly ischemic, but living, cells. Cells in such a "border zone" could therefore be designated "jeopardized" while conditions remain optimal, but become "condemned" and die when conditions deteriorate. It is obvious that such a "border zone" could only arise in hearts with preexisting collateral connections between the major coronary arteries, and it is in this respect that species differences become particularly important.

### Species Differences

The pig has no preexisting collaterals to speak of, whereas in canine hearts they can be abundant. *The normal human heart resembles more the porcine than the canine heart, but in chronic coronary artery disease, substantial collateral collections can develop (10,23).*

One may ask whether collateral circulation may increase during the first hours of coronary artery occlusion, and thus perhaps shift the lateral border towards the ischemic center? *The answer, in respect to the lateral boundary in the absence of any intervention would appear to be no.* Thus, in the dog, due to its preexisting collateral supply, there is a residual blood flow in the central ischemic area of about 20% of normal. This flow, however, does not change between 5 min and 2 hr following coronary occlusion (29). The same conclusion applies to the position of the electrophysiological interface (18) indicating, in both instances, that any preexisting collaterals are fully recruited during the first minutes of ischemia. Although spontaneous shifts of flow and electrophysiological interface location do not appear to occur under standardized conditions, interventions such as changes in perfusion pressure may, as discussed later, in some instances offer some possibility.

### Electrophysiological Studies

We performed experiments in which it was attempted to alter collateral flow and document changes in the position of the lateral boundary zone. Isolated hearts of both pigs and dogs were perfused according to the Langendorff technique. During occlusion of either the left anterior descending branch or the circumflex branch, the position of the electrophysiological border zone was determined by simultaneous recording of 60 direct current extracellular electrograms. By changing the perfusion pressure to the rest of the heart during an occlusion, and thus changing eventual collateral flow to the area at risk, we attempted to shift the position of the electrophysiological boundary, i.e., to increase or decrease the area from which extracellular potentials showed ischemic changes. In several experiments, biopsies were also taken in order to confirm that the electrophysiological interface at any instant coincided with the metabolic interface (19).

Examples of such experiments are shown in Figs. 5 and 6. Figure 5 shows isopotential maps of a rectangular epicardial area (44 by 16 mm) from which 60 direct current electrograms were simultaneously recorded. On the left, two maps from an isolated pig heart are seen 10 min after occlusion of the left anterior descending coronary artery when perfusion pressure to the nonoccluded vessels was high, and after 15 min of occlusion when perfusion pressure had been reduced for 5 min. In both instances, the position of the electrophysiological interface was the same, as was the distribution of negative and positive TQ-segment potentials on both sides of the border. In contrast, in the dog heart, shown on the right side, reduction of perfusion pressure between 10 and 15 min after occlusion of the left anterior descending branch resulted in a considerable shift of the electrical interface and also increased positive T-Q potential levels on the nonischemic side of the boundary.

Figure 6 shows activation patterns from the same hearts. For time zero, an arbitrary point during the TQ segment was chosen, and isochronic lines were drawn at 10-msec intervals. Areas of conduction block are shaded. In the pig heart, the

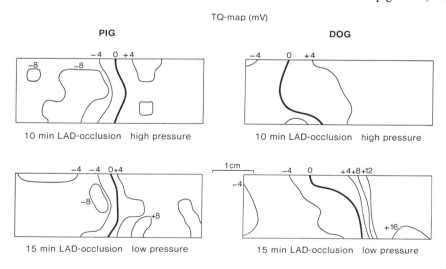

**FIG. 5.** The Lateral Electrophysiological Boundary Can Be Shifted in Dogs but Not in Pigs. Rectangular area from which 60 direct current extracellular electrograms were simultaneously recorded on the anterolateral aspect of the left ventricular wall of a dog heart *(right panels)* and of a pig heart *(left panels)*. Isopotential maps are shown from the T-Q segment of beats propagated from the atrium at various times during occlusion of the left anterior descending coronary artery (LAD). The 0 mV line indicates the position of the electrophysiologic interface. This interface remains constant in the pig heart when the perfusion pressure is changed from a high to a low value, but is shifted in the dog heart. (From ref. 19, with permission.)

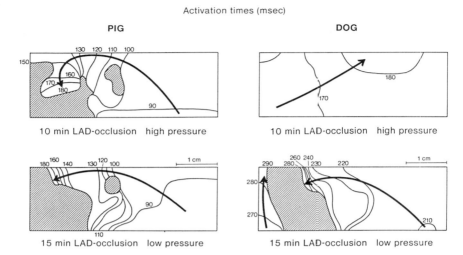

**FIG. 6.**    The Lateral Electrophysiological Boundary Can Be Shifted in Dogs but Not in Pigs. The same experiments as illustrated in Fig. 5 showing the sequence of activation of the area covered by the multiple electrode. Isochrones separate areas activated within the same 10-msec interval (time 0 was an arbitrary point in the TQ interval; values are in msec; *shaded areas* are zones of conduction block). Note that the lowering of the perfusion pressure does not influence the activation pattern in the pig heart, whereas it has a great effect in the dog heart. (From ref. 19, with permission.)

pattern of activation is hardly altered by changing the perfusion pressure during the occlusion, but in the dog heart the pattern is profoundly changed: conduction within the ischemic zone is markedly delayed, a large part has become inexcitable, and the direction of the wavefront changed when perfusion pressure was lowered 10 min after occlusion.

In hearts where the zone showing ischemic changes became larger after lowering the perfusion pressure, the boundary could be shifted back to its original position by raising the perfusion pressure. The ischemic area could never be made smaller by increasing perfusion pressure above normal. In other words, we could not reduce the ischemic area, only increase it.

The position of the electrophysiological boundary during occlusion of the left anterior descending artery and the circumflex branch is illustrated in Fig. 7 so as to summarize our findings in eight porcine and eight canine hearts. In six pig hearts and in one dog heart, the electrophysiological interface had the same position when, at equal perfusion pressures, either the left anterior descending branch or the circumflex branch was occluded. In these hearts, the interface could not be shifted. In seven dog hearts and two pig hearts, the two interfaces were separated by an area in which normal electrograms were recorded during the occlusion of either artery. In hearts with such a "gap" between boundaries, a shift in the position of the interface could be accomplished by manipulation of the perfusion pressure.

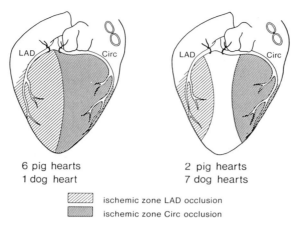

6 pig hearts
1 dog heart

2 pig hearts
7 dog hearts

▨ ischemic zone LAD occlusion

▨ ischemic zone Circ occlusion

**FIG. 7.** Differences Between and Within Species. Schematic representation of the position of the electrophysiologic interface during left anterior descending (LAD) and circumflex (Circ) arterial occlusion. This interface could have the same position when either the LAD or circumflex branch was occluded (this was the case in 6 pig hearts and 1 dog heart); or an intermediate area was present where normal potentials were recorded during occlusion of each artery (7 dog hearts, 2 pig hearts). In this last group the electrophysiologic interface could be shifted by changing collateral flow; in the first group it could not. (From ref. 19, with permission.)

The distance over which this shift occurred varied considerably: In one pig heart, only the configuration of extracellular potential changed, and within the limits of the technique, no change in the position of the zero mV isopotential line during the TQ segment could be observed. In some dog hearts, the zero mV isopotential line shifted over several centimeters. In some hearts, the coronary arteries were injected with barium sulphate gelatin, and the presence of collaterals could be confirmed in dog hearts showing large shifts in interface position. Similarly, the absence of collaterals could be shown in pig hearts in which the interface remained in one position.

Although this experimental model was rather "unphysiological," because it was a Langendorff-perfused, isolated heart performing no external work, and because the reduction in perfusion pressure was rather drastic, several conclusions can be made. First, our findings show that *despite clear species differences, there are also marked variations among hearts of the same species:* Some pigs behaved like dogs, some dogs like pigs. As indicated by Schaper and co-workers (24) this emphasizes the need to use individual hearts as their own control. Second, the possibility arises that the sharp interface between ischemic and normal cells may be shifted by measures that decrease collateral flow. This could be particularly important in regional ischemia caused by subtotal coronary artery occlusion. Reduction of preload and reduction of afterload (but not to the extent that coronary perfusion will be diminished) might salvage myocardium, not so much by "reducing infarct size" but by preventing a developing infarction from reaching its maximal size.

## TRANSMURAL BORDER ZONES

Combined electrophysiological and morphological studies have shown that an infarction caused by permanent coronary artery occlusion is sandwiched between two zones of surviving cells with abnormal electrophysiological properties: an *endocardial border zone* consisting of Purkinje cells and muscle cells lying between the infarct and the cavity, and an *epicardial border zone* between infarct and epicardium (9,27). These border zones are the sites where arrhythmias in the later stages of coronary artery occlusion arise.

Not all condemned cells die at the same moment after coronary occlusion, and with time a "wavefront of cell death" spreads towards both the endocardium and epicardium (9,22). When finally the infarction is "transmural," there often are still rims of surviving tissue, which, although salvaged, may do more harm than good.

### Endocardial Border Zone

After 1 hr of coronary occlusion, there is a rim of tissue, about 5 mm thick, separating the dead intramural cells from the ventricular cavity. These cells show structural ischemic changes but produce normal action potentials. Later, many of these cells die, and by 6 hr there is a layer of 2 to 4 ventricular cells and 2 to 4 layers of subendocardial Purkinje cells surviving between infarct and cavity. These fibers not only have ultrastructural ischemic abnormalities (lipid deposits, reduced glycogen content, etc.) but also have abnormal action potentials.

Initially, the subendocardial cells survive because they are provided with oxygen and nutrients via diffusion from the cavity, or possibly from retrograde perfusion through sinusoidal channels. Purkinje fibers stand a better chance to survive because they are better able to withstand hypoxic conditions than muscle cells. Dangman et al. (3) elegantly demonstrated that in the first 24 hr after coronary occlusion, the surviving Purkinje fibers overlying infarcted muscle receive no blood from the capillary system. These authors isolated canine hearts 24 hr after coronary artery occlusion and perfused them through the coronary arteries via a donor dog. Extracellular subendocardial electrograms from the infarcted zone showed distinct deflections caused by the activity of Purkinje fibers. When potassium chloride was injected into the coronary arteries, electrical activity in the normal myocardium ceased because the potassium chloride depolarized the coronary perfused cells and made them inexcitable. Electrical activity of the Purkinje cells remained unaltered, indicating absence of coronary flow. When these experiments were performed in hearts with older infarcts (3 days to 4 weeks), the surviving Purkinje fibers were depolarized after intracoronary potassium chloride administration, indicating that, with time, capillary flow is restored to surviving subendocardial cells.

Endocardial recordings in patients with chronic myocardial infarction and recurrent, life-threatening ventricular tachycardia, have shown that the endocardial border zone is the source of arrhythmias (4,17). Our own preliminary results *(unpublished)* with isolated preparations resected at the site of earliest activity during ventricular tachycardia in such patients have shown that both normal and abnormal action potentials can be recorded from ventricular myocardial cells lying underneath the thick fibrous endocardial scar. In histological preparations, strands of surviving muscle cells are separated from each other by bundles of connective tissue, and vessels are present. This suggests that, whatever the cause for initial survival, the myocardial cells in the subendocardium of the infarct are still alive many months after the onset of infarction because of the development of a subendocardial circulation. The cells may be alive, but it is questionable whether all is well.

Impulse conduction in these isolated preparations is slow, even in areas displaying perfectly normal action potentials. It is tempting to suggest that the abnormal architecture, with strands of connective tissue interspersed between small bundles of surviving muscle, is one of the causes for abnormal impulse conduction. In addition, abnormalities in cellular coupling may also exist. The slow conduction within the surviving subendocardial network may be an important factor in setting the stage for reentry, which could be the cause for the tachycardias. It must be emphasized that, at this stage, we do not know the mechanism for the recurrent tachycardia in patients with chronic myocardial infarction. Nor do we know what the anatomical characteristics are of the subendocardial border zone in the small subset of patients with myocardial infarction that do develop recurrent ventricular tachycardia, compared to patients remaining free from malignant arrhythmias. Still, it seems justified to say that the surviving subendocardial cells are too few in number, and too dispersed, to have any contractile function. They may have just the electrophysiological properties for reentry (or other arrhythmogenic mechanisms) to occur and seriously jeopardize the life of the patient.

## Epicardial Border Zone

After coronary artery occlusion in the dog heart, a layer of muscle cells frequently survives in the epicardium, and this layer may be several millimeters thick. These cells are kept alive as a consequence of the existence of epicardial collateral anastomoses (27). Ventricular tachycardias can be induced in such hearts by applying premature stimuli to the ventricles, or by driving the heart at rapid rates. The underlying mechanism for these arrhythmias is reentry within the epicardial border zone (7,27). As is the case for the endocardial border zone, action potentials from the surviving subepicardial cells may be completely normal, but conduction is very slow and fragmented. This impairment of conduction can be attributed to the development of fibrosis and separation of muscle bundles along their longitudinal axes which acts to diminish side-to-side cell connections. Many aspects of the electrical instability of the surviving epicardial border zone still remain to be resolved. For example, it is not known whether dogs in which ventricular tachyarrhythmias can be induced by premature stimulation of the ventricles also develop such arrhythmias spontaneously. Several years ago, we studied dogs with small infarcts which had tissue in both the subendocardium and subepicardium which had survived for many months, sometimes for even more than a year after the initial coronary artery occlusion. These dogs were apparently healthy, and although no ambulatory electrocardiographic recording was performed, no spontaneous life-threatening arrhythmias occurred. It was, however, possible in all animals, to induce reproducible ventricular fibrillation by applying two premature stimuli to the surviving tissue within the infarct. Under these circumstances multiple extracellular recordings provided evidence for slow and fragmented conduction through the surviving strands, and for reentry being responsible for the triggering of arrhythmias (5). In contrast, I have never been able to induce ventricular arrhythmias in normal dogs, even when applying five successive premature stimuli (provided the stimuli did not have an excessively high intensity). Thus, although the dogs with small infarcts, and surviving muscle at endocardial and epicardial border zones, were electrically unstable, this did not necessarily mean that they were at a high risk for sudden death due to the spontaneous development of ventricular fibrillation.

*In order to be able to promote tachycardias there appears to be a certain critical thickness for the epicardial border zone since if the layer is too thin, or if the layer is thicker than 100 cells, reentry does not occur (11). It would appear that measures which would salvage a greater number of subepicardial cells might be beneficial in so far as there may be a reduction in the vulnerability to arrhythmias.*

One way of salvaging subepicardial cells is reperfusion. It is generally agreed that complete reversal of ischemia-induced functional abnormalities throughout the ischemic zone is only possible when reperfusion occurs within approximately 30 min. However, myocardial cells have been salvaged by reperfusion of tissue which had been ischemic for as long as 2 hr. Although immediately after reperfusion contractile function barely improved, at later stages contractile function returned to the previously ischemic area, presumably because of resorption of initial edema and because viable cells hypertrophied (26). The structure of such a reperfused infarct is, however, different from an infarct resulting from a permanent occlusion of a coronary artery. No accurate delineation of the infarct is possible, the lateral borders being extremely irregular, and throughout the infarct regions of viable myocardium are interspersed with patches of necrotic cells (20). Although, in some dogs, reperfusion after a 2-hr period of ischemia resulted in very small infarcts in which no tachyarrhythmias could be induced, it appeared that in reperfused infarcts, arrhythmias are induced more frequently and more easily than in infarcts caused by permanent coronary occlusion.

*It, therefore, appears that, as far as electrical stability is concerned, tissue salvage may be both beneficial and dangerous. If thin layers of myocardial cells survive, they will contribute little to the contractile function of the heart but may place the individual at high risk to fatal arrhythmias. In such situations, it might have been better if all the ischemic cells had died.*

On the other hand, if a thick layer of subepicardial muscle can be salvaged, overall contractile function may be improved and arrhythmias should be unlikely to occur. The most important factor, apart from the site of coronary occlusion, which determines whether the surviving epicardial border zone is thick or thin, is most likely the amount and the capacity of preexisting collateral anastomoses (see

Chapter 5). Given the great variability in collateral vessels in individual hearts, studies designed to salvage myocardium should preferably use the same hearts as controls, by sequentially occluding two coronary arteries of the same size in different circumstances (24).

## CONCLUDING COMMENTS

It is now well established that there is no quantitatively significant lateral border zone of intermediate ischemia separating the core of severe ischemia from the surrounding normal tissue. Instead, the lateral interface is characterized by a sharp transition between ischemic and normal cells. This interface runs along an irregular profile from the endocardium to the epicardium with peninsulas of ischemic and normal cells intermingling. An intermediate zone of a few cells may exist, and here oxygen may reach ischemic cells by diffusion. In animals with preexisting collaterals, the lateral electrophysiological boundary may be shifted when substantial decreases in collateral flow occur, and restoration of collateral flow may result in shifting back the lateral electrophysiological interface to its original position. However, major collateral-dependent differences may occur between and within species.

During evolving infarction, and also when the infarct has reached its final size, an intramural mass of necrotic cells is sandwiched between a thin endocardial border zone, consisting mostly of surviving Purkinje cells and an epicardial border zone of surviving muscle cells. Both of these tissue zones may act as a source of arrhythmias. However, when the epicardial border zone is either thinner than several cell layers, or thicker than about 100 cells, it ceases to be an arrhythmogenic zone. During maintained ischemia, the thickness of the epicardial zone depends on the extent of preexisting collaterals. The size of this zone can increase if early reperfusion can be achieved. Reperfusion can, however, also convert a nonarrhythmogenic infarct into a tissue mass which is prone to develop arrhythmias. Thus, if the surviving rim of epicardial cells is not thicker than about 100 cells, or if intramurally viable cells are interspersed with necrotic cells, reentrant arrhythmias will occur far more easily than in a transmural infarct which has no, or very few, surviving epicardial cells. I would contend that as far as arrhythmias are concerned, cells in the infarcted zone may be better dead than alive, unless a sizeable homogeneous subepicardial layer survives, in which case tissue salvage can be truly beneficial.

## REFERENCES

1. Barlow, C. H., and Chance, B. (1976): Ischemic areas in perfused rat hearts: measurements by NADH fluorescence photography. *Science*, 193:909–910.
2. Cohn, J. N., Franciosa, J. A., Francis, G. S., Archibald, D., Tristani, F., Fletcher, R., Montero, A., Cintron, G., Clarke, J., Hager, D., Saunders, R., Cobb, F., Smith, R., Loeb, H., and Settle, H. (1982): Effect of short-term infusion of sodium nitroprusside on mortality rate in acute myocardial infarction, complicated by left ventricular failure: results of a Veterans Administration cooperative study. *N. Engl. J. Med.*, 306:1129–1135.
3. Dangman, K. H., Wang, H. H., and Wit, A. L. (1979): Effects of intracoronary potassium chloride

on electrograms of canine Purkinje fibers in six-hour to four-week old myocardial infarcts: an indication of time dependent changes in collateral blood flow. *Circ. Res.*, 44:392–405.

4. De Bakker, J. M. T., Janse, M. J., Van Capelle, F. J. L., and Durrer, D. (1983): Endocardial mapping by simultaneous recording of endocardial electrograms during cardiac surgery for ventricular aneurysm. *J. Am. Coll. Cardiol.*, 2:947–953.

5. Durrer, D., Van Dam, R. T., Freud, G. E., and Janse, M. J. (1971): Reentry and ventricular arrhythmias in local ischemia and infarction in the infarct dog heart. *Proc. Kon. Ned. Akad. Wetensch. (Amsterdam Series)*, C74:321–334.

6. Durrer, J. D., Lie, K. I., Van Capelle, F. J. L., and Durrer, D. (1982): Effect of sodium nitroprusside on mortality in acute myocardial infarction. *N. Engl. J. Med.*, 306:1121–1128.

7. El-Sherif, N., Mehra, R., Gough, W. B., and Zeiler, R. H. (1982): Ventricular activation pattern of spontaneous and induced ventricular rhythms in canine one-day-old myocardial infarction. Evidence for focal and reentrant mechanism. *Circ. Res.*, 51:152–166.

8. Factor, S. M., Sonneblick, E. H., and Kirk, E. S. (1978): The histologic border zone of acute myocardial infarction—islands or peninsulae. *Am. J. Pathol.*, 92:111–120.

9. Fenoglio, J. J., Jr., Karaqueuzian, H. S., Friedman, P. L., Albala, A., and Wit, A. L. (1979): Time course of infarct growth towards the endocardium after coronary occlusion. *Am. J. Physiol.*, 236:H356–370.

10. Fulton, W. F. M. (1965): *The Coronary Arteries.* Charles C Thomas, Springfield, Illinois.

11. Gardner, P., Ursell, P. C., Fenoglio, J. J., Jr., Allessie, M. A., Bonke, F. I. M., and Wit, A. L. (1981): Structure of the epicardial border zone in canine infarct is a cause of reentrant excitation. *Circulation*, 64(Suppl. IV):IV-320.

12. Gottwik, M., Zimmer, P., Wusten, B., Hoffmann, M., Winkler, B., and Schaper, W. (1979): Experimental myocardial infarction in a closed-chest canine model. Observations on temporal and spatial evolution over 24 hours. *Basic Res. Cardiol.*, 74:233–239.

13. Harken, A. H., Barlow, C. H., Harden, W. R., and Chance, B. (1978): Two and three dimensional display of myocardial ischemic "border zone" in dogs. *Am. J. Cardiol.*, 42:954–959.

14. Harken, A. H., Simpson, M. B., Haselgrove, J., Wetstein, L., Harden, W. R., and Barlow, C. H. (1981): Early ischemia after complete coronary ligation in the rabbit, dog, pig and monkey. *Am. J. Physiol.*, 241:H202–210.

15. Hearse, D. J., and Yellon, D. M. (1981): The "border zone" in evolving myocardial infarction. Controversy or confusion? *Am. J. Cardiol.*, 47:1321–1334.

16. Hirzel, H. O., Sonneblick, E. H., and Kirk, E. S. (1977): Absence of a lateral border zone of intermediate creatine phosphokinase depletion surrounding a central infarct 24 hours after acute coronary occlusion in the dog. *Circ. Res.*, 41:673–683.

17. Horowitz, L. N., Josephson, M. E., and Harken, A. H. (1980): Epicardial and endocardial activation during sustained ventricular tachycardia in man. *Circulation*, 61:1227–1238.

18. Janse, M. J., Cinca, J., Morena, H., Fiolet, J. W. T., Kleber, A. G., De Vries, G. P., Becker, A. E., and Durrer, D. (1979): The "border zone" in myocardial ischemia. An electrophysiological, metabolic and histochemical correlation in the pig heart. *Circ. Res.*, 44:576–588.

19. Janse, M. J., and Wilms-Schopman, F. (1982): Effects of changes in perfusion pressure on the position of the electrophysiologic border zone in acute regional ischemia in isolated perfused dog and pig heart. *Am. J. Cardiol.*, 50:74–82.

20. Karagueuzian, H. S., Fenoglio, J. J., Jr., Weiss, M. B., and Wit, A. L. (1979): Protracted ventricular tachycardia induced by premature stimulation of the canine heart after coronary artery occlusion and reperfusion. *Circ. Res.*, 44:833–846.

21. Passamani, E. R. (1982): Nitroprusside in myocardial infarction. *N. Engl. J. Med.*, 306:1168–1170 (editorial).

22. Reimer, K. A., Lowe, J. E., Rasmussen, M. N., and Jennings, R. B. (1977): The wavefront phenomenon in ischemic cell death. I. Myocardial infarcts size vs duration of coronary occlusion in dogs. *Circulation*, 56:786–794.

23. Schaper, W. (1971): *The Collateral Circulation of the Heart.* North-Holland, Amsterdam.

24. Schaper, W., Hoffmann, M., Muller, K. D., Genth, K., and Carl, M. (1979): Experimental occlusion of two small coronary arteries in the same heart. A new validation method for infarct size manipulation. *Basic Res. Cardiol.*, 74:224–229.

25. Simpson, M. B., Harden, W. R., Barlow, C. H., and Harken, A. H. (1979): Visualization of the distance between perfusion and anoxia along an ischemic border. *Circulation*, 60:1151–1155.

26. Theroux, P., Ross, J., Jr., Franklin, D., Kemper, W. S., and Sasayama, S. (1978): Coronary

arterial reperfusion. Early and late effects on regional myocardial function and dimensions in conscious dogs. *Am. J. Cardiol.*, 38:599–606.

27. Wit, A. L., Allessie, M. A., Fenoglio, J. J., Jr., Bonke, F. I. M., Lammers, W. J. E. P., and Smeets, J. (1981): Significance of the endocardial and epicardial border zones in the genesis of myocardial infarction arrhythmias. In: *Cardiac Arrhythmias, A Decade of Progress*, edited by D. C. Harrison and G. K. Hall, pp. 39–68. Medical Publishers, Boston.

28. Yellon, D. M., Hearse, D. J., Crome, R., Grannel, J., and Wyse, R. K. H. (1981): Characterization of the lateral interface between normal and ischemic tissue during acute myocardial infarction. *Am. J. Cardiol.*, 47:1233–1239.

29. Yellon, D. M., Hearse, D. J., Crome, R., and Wyse, R. K. H. (1983): Temporal and spatial characteristics of evolving cell injury during regional myocardial ischemia in the dog: the "border zone" controversy. *J. Am. Coll. Cardiol.*, 2:661–670.

*Therapeutic Approaches to Myocardial Infarct Size Limitation*, edited by D. J. Hearse and D. M. Yellon. Raven Press, New York © 1984.

# 5

# Experimental Infarcts and the Microcirculation

## Wolfgang Schaper

*Department of Cardiology, Max-Planck-Institut, D-6350 Bad Nauheim, West Germany*

In 1965, the Soviet scientist Lavin traveled through West Africa and stopped at Dr. Grayson's laboratory in Lagos, Nigeria. He persuaded Dr. Grayson to occlude coronary arteries in the African green monkey, to measure tissue blood flow with heat clearance, and to assess the degree of myocardial damage. A report of this study appeared in *The Lancet* in 1966 (5) and it contained the startling conclusion that the region of underperfusion was larger than the anatomic area of perfusion of the occluded coronary artery. This was attributed to spasm of the adjoining microcirculation and it was shown that the injection of lidocaine and other drugs relieved this spasm.

    This article triggered a lot of activity. Rees and Redding (14,15) used radioactive Xenon-133 clearance techniques to show that there was no indication of spasm in acute and subacute coronary artery ligation. We reported (18) that *the size of the ensuing infarct 24 hr after coronary ligation was indeed smaller than the perfusion area of the occluded coronary artery, thereby reestablishing in an animal model an old observation made by many pathologists in the infarcted human heart at autopsy.* Two years after our study, an often-cited paper by Braunwald's group (11) claimed that the myocardium made ischemic by coronary occlusion could be salvaged from infarction by a variety of drugs.

It was probably a wise decision of the Braunwald group not to include risk region measurements or blood flow studies in their experiments as the earlier papers did, because these methods experienced remarkable refinements in the years to come. Braunwald's empirical "screening" approach with simple methods certainly provided a strong stimulus for the progress in methodology.

## TOOLS OF THE TRADE: METHODS AND MODELS

A bewildering variety of techniques for the direct and indirect assessment of myocardial damage existed in the early days of infarct sizing. This made it difficult, if not impossible, to compare results, let alone extrapolate the findings to the human situation. Over the years, the variety of methods has decreased and today only a relatively short discussion is needed to describe: how to measure the area at risk of infarction; how to measure infarct size with morphologic techniques; and how to measure residual perfusion. It is, of course, sometimes desirable to add other measurements or to analyze metabolic intermediates, *but risk region and infarct size measurements of the highest possible precision are a must and cannot be replaced.*

### A Beastly Choice

Experimental models have been developed in dogs, pigs, rats, rabbits, and guinea pigs, but *only rarely is it stated what kind of clinical situation investigators are mimicking in the design of their models.* To some investigators it is self-evident that, when using the rat coronary artery ligation model, they intend to study acute coronary occlusion in young human males with no previous history of coronary artery disease; but not all investigators who use the rat model are aware of this. Others study acute coronary occlusion in the guinea pig unaware of the growing evidence that myocardial infarction is not a necessary consequence of occlusion in that species. Some investigators believe that anesthesia interferes with the process of infarction and with the drugs they are going to administer, and they prefer chronically instrumented animals. I agree that some types of anesthesia, such as pentobarbitone, are evil, but other types, for example, morphine-chloralose, may be perfectly acceptable.

### A Chronic Problem

Chronic instrumentation looks good in print, but we do not really know in what way the trauma, healing processes, adhesions, foreign bodies, and possible partial denervation change the process we are going to study. Bloor (1) demonstrated years ago that chronic instrumentation increases the number and caliber of anatomically demonstrable collaterals which may seriously interfere with the speed and extent of infarction. In this context it is of note that Becker's group (2) reports relatively small infarcts in chronically instrumented animals. The small print in the method section often states that the chronically instrumented animals were given morphine during the actual coronary occlusion. This is difficult to understand because acute coronary occlusion does not produce pain reactions in the dog (21); in other words, there should be no need for an analgesic. *This practice actually combines the disadvantages of anesthesia and chronic instrumentation.* It is possible to exploit some of the effects of chronic instrumentation. Cobb's group (12), for example, has shown that chronic instrumentation could increase collateral flow but that this was highly variable among dogs. This large scatter in baseline values was then used to reveal a close linear correlation between infarction and residual flow.

## MEASUREMENT OF INFARCTS AFTER SHORT OCCLUSIONS, OR: THE "FORMAZAN FOLLIES"

### Importance of Timing Your Steps

*Very often it is not appreciated how difficult it is to measure the size of an infarct using morphologic methods after short coronary artery occlusions.* With light microscopy, coronary occlusion must have lasted for about 12 hr before an infarct can even be detected, but at this time it would still be too early for exact size measurements, which really require 24 or 48 hr. It is for this reason that in many cases of sudden death, myocardial infarcts cannot be detected; the patient probably died from ventricular fibrillation, a typical early symptom of ischemia. Under such conditions, there may not even be time for the cells to die from ischemia proper, let alone undergo the critical reactions of cell death.

*In experimental coronary occlusions, infarct diagnosis with morphologic methods is much easier because one can use reflow to speed up the processes of vital reactions. Reflow is believed to hasten the decay of dead myocytes and to salvage those not dead at the moment of reflow (22). Although this is a tenable conclusion, I show later that it may require some minor qualification.* With light microscopic techniques, reperfusion must be maintained for about 12 hr before infarct size measurements can be made. This has the double disadvantage that the animal must withstand not only the insult of the operation, the occlusion and the reperfusion, but must also survive the following night.

### Methods and Mechanisms

The observation by us and other authors (8,9,17), that incubation of freshly sliced, reperfused myocardium in tetrazolium solutions produces reliable estimates of infarct size represented a definite improvement over other methods. The tetrazolium procedure is dependent on the ability of tetrazolium salts to act as electron acceptors and the fact that, in infarcted tissue, dehydrogenase-mediated electron transport is dramatically reduced. As a consequence of electron acceptance tetrazolium changes its structure to a bright red or deep purple dye which precipitates over normal tissue (with intact enzymes). It does not precipitate over infarcted tissue. Discriminative staining (no dye over the infarct but precipitate over ischemic-living and nonischemic tissue) could arise under three different conditions: (a) the absence of substrate for the dehydrogenase enyzmes; (b) the absence of coenzymes for NAD-dependent dehydrogenases; and (c) the absence of the dehydrogenase enzymes themselves. *We have shown recently (9) that in experimental infarcts after short occlusions it is the NAD cofactor that becomes the limiting factor and not lack of dehydrogenase activity or substrate*, adequate supplies of the latter almost invariably being present. There are four pieces of evidence which support this view: (a) the addition of NAD or NADH causes the immediate precipitation of dye over previously unstained infarcts; (b) incubation with succinate also causes the dye to precipitate over previously unstained infarcted tissue; this occurs because succinate dehydrogenase activity does not need NAD as a coenzyme; (c) direct measurement of the tissue activity of various dehydrogenases and other enzymes (e.g., lactate dehydrogenase, malate dehydrogenase, and creatine phosphokinase) reveals that considerable enzyme activity persists in the tissue up to 32 hr after coronary artery occlusion; (d) direct measurement of nicotinamide adenine dinucleotide content of infarcted tissue shows a drastic reduction due to the splitting of the coenzyme by glycohydrolase (13).

Two of the many available tetrazolium salts have gained wide acceptance for infarct size studies, these are triphenyltetrazolium chloride (TTC) and para-nitrobluetetrazolium (pNBT), each of which offers distinct advantages and disadvantages. TTC, for example, is able to permeate through the cell membrane; it can be injected intravenously or it can be infused into the coronary arteries. It can thus gain very good access to the tissue and its enzymes. Unfortunately, after intravenous infusion it will cause the death of the animal because it is an electron acceptor and causes the bypassing of oxidative phosphorylation. With pNBT staining, infusion is not possible because the compound cannot cross the cell membrane. It therefore has the disadvantage that it can only act on cut surfaces of cells. However, with the pNBT stain infarct edges look particularly distinct and are sharper than those seen with TTC staining.

*The tetrazolium method, when used without reperfusion, becomes discriminative between 3 and 4 hr after coronary occlusion and it can be trusted at about 6 hr after occlusion. With reperfusion, infarcts can be demonstrated after only 20 min of occlusion depending on animal species and hemodynamic circumstances.* These infarcts are, however, usually small and spotty and are generally located only in the subendocardium. After 90 min of occlusion, well defined infarcts can often be demonstrated if reperfusion is employed. Without reperfusion there is no way of knowing exactly how large an infarct will be. This, of course, generates some uncertainty over the problems and complications of reperfusion damage.

## PROBLEMS OF REPERFUSION DAMAGE

Reperfusion of ischemic tissue produces several effects which, on first sight, may be interpreted as reperfusion-induced damage. These include: (a) ventricular tachycardia and fibrillation; (b) hemorrhagic infarction; and (c) considerable ultrastructural destruction of the tissue which appears to be much less damaged prior to reflow.

A careful consideration of these effects reveals that reperfusion-induced arrhythmias are maximal after relatively short occlusion times, say 20 min, at which time there is very little, if any, permanent tissue damage. This effect can therefore be dismissed as an indicator of reperfusion injury. Hemorrhagic infarction can also be dismissed on the basis that it is a very late phenomenon which usually does not occur earlier than 4 to 6 hr after occlusion and reperfusion. Hemorrhagic infarction is a consequence of irreversible ischemic injury in the microvasculature which is generally believed to die later than the myocytes (25); however, this view has been disputed by some investigators (see Chapter 7). The third indicator, reperfusion-induced increases in ultrastructural damage, is less readily dispelled. If one examines canine myocardium after a period of coronary occlusion thought to be sufficient to induce permanent damage (this time may vary greatly depending on species, anesthesia, hemodynamic status, etc.), then the tissue injury appears to be very heterogeneous. Cells with severe but reversible injury can, for example, be seen to be situated next to irreversibly damaged cells. Upon reperfusion, these differences become amplified such that irreversibly injured cells now exhibit an advanced state of destruction, usually with severe contracture bands, whereas reversibly injured now look essentially normal. Thus, although reperfusion may rapidly and extensively alter the degree of tissue injury, it may not alter the ratio of dead to living cells. To investigate this possibility, we have counted the number of cells classified as irreversibly injured (by ultrastructural criteria) in biopsies obtained from dog hearts just before and 10 min after reperfusion (26); we found no difference. In another related experiment (6), we have tried to determine if reperfusion after 3 or 6 hr of coronary occlusion inflicts damage on cells which were not classified as dead immediately prior to reflow. If reperfusion damage really exists, then one would expect to find that infarcts in the reperfused group are larger than those in the nonreperfused group. We, therefore, occluded two coronary arteries in the same heart, but released the occlusion in only one. There was no difference in the ultimate infarct size of the reperfused and nonreperfused beds. *Even hemorrhagic infarction, which always occurs with reflow after 6 or more hours of occlusion did not increase infarct size. All the above evidence leads me to conclude that reperfusion is a very powerful salvaging agent in reversibly injured cells, but it can also accelerate destruction in cells which are already dead at the time of reflow.*

## RISQUÉ REMARKS ON RISK REGIONS

Infarct size depends in the first place on the size of the occluded coronary artery and the bed which it serves. Since coronary anatomy varies within a given species, and from species to species, a standardization must be found which is better than "the LAD was occluded about halfway down between the base and apex." *The amount of muscle normally supplied by the occluded artery is the only acceptable base of reference with which the size of the infarct must be compared.*

## Postmortem Injection

There are several ways to measure risk regions. The oldest, and still one of the best, is postmortem injection of the coronary tree. It probably originated from Spalteholz' work, was revived by Kalbfleisch (7) for the human heart, reintroduced by us in 1969 (18) for infarct and risk region measurements in the dog (24), and widely used by Becker's group (2) and by Marcus and colleagues (10). The difficulty with the postmortem injection method is that two different techniques, angiography and surface photography (for the formazan stain), are used for the measurement of the size of the infarct and the risk region.

## Autoradiography

Two other methods for risk region measurement are in current use, these are autoradiography of heart slices obtained after the injection of suitably labeled radiomicrospheres and the injection of dyes plus tetrazolium. With the microsphere method, technetium-labeled albumin microspheres of high specific activity are injected so as to microembolize predominantly in the normally perfused muscle. The high specific activity guarantees short exposure, but a short half-life for the isotope may often necessitate that the microspheres can only be given at the end of the experiment, often at a time when collateral blood flow has increased. This, of course, may cause problems of interpretation particularly in experiments with long ischemic intervals because the label may enter the anatomical risk region. This could result in infarcts larger than the apparent "functional" risk region being observed. Agents which have been reported to decrease infarct size expressed as a fraction of functional risk region must then have exerted their actions without changing perfusion of the risk region. *It is difficult to comprehend how a drug can allow heart muscle to survive when a major blood flow deficit is maintained.*

An improved version of microsphere autoradiography has been described by Downey and colleagues (4). In this procedure, cerium-141-labeled microspheres are injected immediately after coronary occlusion. This isotope emits $\beta$ as well as $\gamma$ rays, and the $\beta$ emission is well suited for autoradiography generating on the autoradiogram a sharp point image of each microsphere rather than the blurred hazing effect seen with technetium and other isotopes. Since the cerium microspheres can be given at the beginning of ischemia and since collateral flow is lowest immediately after occlusion, a risk region as defined by this method corresponds more closely to the anatomic region. Another advantage with this method is that it can easily be applied to small rodents where it is difficult, if not impossible, to use postmortem angiography.

## *In Vivo* Dye Injection

The injection of dyes (Evans blue or Monastral blue) into arteries supplying normal myocardium and the injection of TTC into the peripheral occluded coronary artery at the same pressure and time produces a pleasing picture with the Anglo-American colors: blue (nonischemic), red (ischemic-surviving), and white (infarct). It has the advantage that infarct size, as well as perfusion area, are obtained from the same color transparency. The disadvantages are: (a) if both dyes are not perfused from the same pressure source, the risk region may vary; in addition it is critical that the infusion catheters are of the same length and bore; (b) cannulation of the peripheral end of the occluded coronary artery is sometimes difficult and this may mean that some side branches may not be perfused; (c) the method only works with TTC, which is the tetrazolium dye of second choice; unfortunately, it does not work with pNBT. We overcame this problem in my laboratory by perfusing the distal arterial end with a modified Krebs-Ringer solution. This is infused at the same pressure and the time as the Monastral blue. The heart is then cut into slices and incubated in pNBT.

## EXPERIMENTAL INFARCTION ACROSS THE ANIMAL KINGDOM, OR: HOW GUINEA PIGS WIN THE RAT RACE

The choice of animal model for the study of myocardial infarction is difficult because it demands a fairly good knowledge about the human disease that one wants to investigate in the laboratory. *More often than not the correct choice of the animal model comes with hindsight and is not the result of good design.* Thus, after carrying out extensive studies in dog and man, I, too, had nothing more specific in mind than the general biological interest of a bird watcher when I set out to investigate the consequences of coronary occlusion in the rat, guinea pig, rabbit, cat, and pig.

### Spectrum of Collateral Flow

In choosing an animal species, the first difficulty that one encounters is anesthesia. It is not possible to use the same anesthetic procedure in all species, each one responds differently to different anesthetic agents. Another difficulty lies in the measurement of the risk region. Thus, in larger species such as the pig, cat, and rabbit, we found it best to use an angiographic method; whereas, in smaller species, we found it necessary to use cerium-141 autoradiography (4). Despite these imposed differences, we have undertaken a study in which infarct size (measured by pNBT), risk zone size, and collateral flow were measured in a number of species after 22.5, 45, 90, and 180 min of coronary occlusion. In these studies, occlusion was always followed by reperfusion. *The results (Fig. 1) indicated that there was a wide species-dependent spectrum in the speed and the extent of infarction.* Rapid and complete infarction occurred in the rabbit, pig, and rat (the rat is not shown in Fig. 1 as it was identical to the rabbit). Infarction proceeded at a slower rate in the dog and the cat and infarction was not complete. The guinea pig does not exhibit any infarction at all. *An interesting finding is that these major*

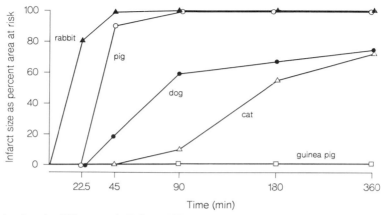

**FIG. 1.** Species Differences in Collateral Flow and the Rate of Development of Infarction. Infarct size, expressed as a percent of the area at risk in relation to the duration of elapsed ischemia (followed by reperfusion) in the rabbit, pig, dog, rat, and guinea pig. The rat (not shown) follows the identical profile to the rabbit.

*differences in the speed and extent of infarction correlated rather well with the volume of collateral blood flow* as measured with radioactive tracer microspheres. In the rat, rabbit, and pig, collateral flow was not significantly different from zero flow. In the dog and the cat it was measurable but was significantly lower than normal flow. In the guinea pig collateral flow was not significantly different from normal control flow. This latter finding agrees well with observations of Rosen (16) who reported a lack of surface NADH-fluorescence following coronary artery occlusion in the guinea pig. We have studied hearts from two other species that produced large transmural infarcts with very low collateral blood flows. These were the sheep and the pony. Very similar results have been obtained with the baboon (3) and the wild boar (19).

## Putting Man in His Place

*The critical question arising from the abovementioned studies is where in this spectrum of collateral flow does the human heart lie? In answer to this, I would contend that human coronary disease encompasses the entire spectrum shown in Fig. 1.*

Human coronary heart disease covers an enormous time span, with acute onset ventricular fibrillation it may be over in as little as 30 sec, but with stable effort-dependent angina pectoris it may last for 30 years. It is known that acute *myocardial infarction in young human males often occurs without premonitory symptoms, it results in large transmural infarctions which may produce aneurysms. It is extremely likely that such infarctions are caused by acute coronary occlusions in previously undamaged vessels. In this diseased condition there is no time for the collateral circulation to develop.* By contrast, in other disease states, coronary atherosclerosis may proceed slowly enough for the development of collaterals; under these conditions complete coronary occlusion may not be of any consequence to the subtended myocardium for a long period of time. It is only when the arteries, from which collaterals originate, become occluded one after another, that the heart may finally succumb. Complete chronic occlusions of the left main coronary artery have been reported without infarctions.

*It would, therefore, seem logical to me that if we want to study acute occlusion without the advantages of collateral protection, we should do it in the rat, rabbit, pig, sheep, baboon, or pony. However, if we want to study subendocardial infarction in the presence of collateral blood flow, we should use dogs and cats. Should we want to study angina of effort in a laboratory model, then coronary occlusion in the working, stimulated guinea pig heart may be the model of choice.*

## SUPPLY-SIDE ECONOMICS

Earlier studies of myocardial protection emphasized the reduction of oxygen demand as a means to narrowing the gap between energy supply and energy demand (11). *Many of the investigations based on this philosophy had no clear idea about the magnitude of the supply side, and most of them failed to show in quantitative terms the extent to which any intervention had actually narrowed the gap.* Furthermore, many studies were carried out in animal species such as the pig or the rat in which the supply-demand hypothesis did not apply because of the clear lack of any supply. It is very difficult for me to understand why the reduction of oxygen demand in normally perfused myocardium should be beneficial to nonperfused ischemic muscle. It would seem to me that it is important to know as much as possible about the supply-side and then concentrate on improving it. This necessitates accurately measuring collateral blood flow in ischemic myocardium. This can, however, be achieved with radioactive tracer microspheres, provided the number and size of spheres injected has an acceptable relationship to the extent of collateral blood flow. In my experience, a blood flow of approximately 5 ml/min/ 100 g tissue is a threshold value below which it becomes difficult to discern flow from random analytical noise (26). If blood flow is approximately this level, then an inordinate number of microspheres must be injected and a large volume of tissue must be analyzed. *These conditions are usually difficult, if not impossible, to match in the rat, rabbit, and even the pig heart* (23). *The only species where collateral blood flow can be measured with acceptable precision (because of the amount of flow and tissue available) is the dog heart.* Table 1 shows typical values for collateral flow in anesthetized open-chest dogs. It can be seen that collateral flow increases considerably with time over a period of between about 6 and 24 hr. This correlates well with our early observations (19) that there is a corresponding increase in the diameter of these vessels. *If conditions exist where there is measurable blood flow extending from the subepicardium into midmyocardium, then the supply-demand concept is, I believe, tenable, and strategies designed to enhance supply or reduce demand can be meaningfully tested. The ultimate goal should, however, be to enhance the growth rate of collateral vessels in order that myocardial protection can be achieved on a permanent basis.*

TABLE 1. *Collateral blood flow*[a]

| Time after occlusion | 1 hr postoperation | 6 hr postoperation | 24 hr postoperation |
|---|---|---|---|
| Subepicardium | 27.8 ± 3.4 | 29.5 ± 2.6 | 47.7 ± 6.5 |
| Midmyocardium | 12.2 ± 1.6 | 11.0 ± 2.0 | 18.4 ± 1.9 |
| Subendocardium | 7.9 ± 1.3 | 5.8 ± 2.6 | 7.9 ± 6.5 |

[a]ml/min/100 g in closed chest dog.

## COLLATERAL BLOOD FLOW: TOO MUCH TO DIE, TOO LITTLE TO LIVE?

Hearse and Yellon, in Chapter 2 of this book, have raised the question of chronic cell injury and the possibility that flow reductions and tissue injury may be such that cells remain acontractile but do not deteriorate to necrosis. Using a similar type of argument it may be possible to envisage a situation where collateral flow, at least during the early stages of ischemia, may be just sufficient to support a low level of contractile performance, but that this makes no major contribution to pump function and only acts to deplete energy reserves and hasten cell death. Under such circumstances one might conceive of a situation where the deliberate suppression of contractile function in the ischemic zone during early ischemia could preserve cells such that, following the growth of new collateral vessels, they might make a real contribution to myocardial function. Consideration of such a possibility requires a knowledge of the relationship between the amount of oxygen available in the collateral supply and the contractile activity that this will support.

A close look at the oxygen supply available via the collateral vessels reveals that it is, indeed, quite substantial and should suffice to maintain the integrity of cellular structure. A blood flow of 25 ml/min/100 g delivers about 5 ml of $O_2$/min/100 g of which about 4 ml can be extracted. Nonbeating heart muscle however needs only about 1.5 ml. If it is stimulated (but not contracting) it needs, depending on rate, approximately a further 1 ml. Levels of collateral supply of this magnitude are in keeping with reality and can probably explain why in the dog heart, for example, the subepicardial third of the tissue is often spared from infarction. Flow to the subendocardial segment is probably too low and in any event requirements are, as discussed in Chapter 8, considerably higher and probably make cell death inevitable. In the midmyocardial third, the situation is such that the tissue usually dies. I would argue, however, that with the collateral flow available to it, and various anaerobic energy-producing processes [such as glycolysis and substrate level phosphorylation from glutamate and aspartate after transamination (23)] that this midmyocardial tissue should not die. Why blood flow and anaerobic energy transduction does not keep more muscle alive probably relates to the fact that ischemic muscle wastes most of the oxygen in futile attempts at contraction. I can envisage (although it is yet to be conclusively proven) that ischemic muscle is under even heavier stimulation (possibly by catecholamines and calcium ions) than is normally perfused muscle. It appears to me that if it were possible to selectively depolarize and prevent contraction in an ischemic zone, without causing depression in the normal muscle, that we may be able to exploit the theoretical ability of low levels of collateral to prevent cell death while new collateral vessels develop.

## CONCLUDING COMMENTS

*It appears to me that research aimed at preventing the deterioration of ischemia into infarction has lost some of its appeal and that this has occurred at a time when the tools of our trade are present, honed, and refined.* One possible reason for this strange situation (which already influences the funding policies of some government agencies) may be that too much was tried too early by too many whose enthusiasm was more developed than their methods. A more prudent, down-to-earth approach, using the right methods, inevitably looks unexciting on paper and may be called "re-search" in the literal sense, i.e., doing things over again but doing it better than the first time and in a more sober mood. Another reason may be the feeling that the rewards of our endeavors will be much less than anticipated and that the hypothesis is extremely difficult to prove in a clinical situation.

*My own experiments have shown that measurable, residual perfusion of ischemic myocardium is a condition* sine qua non: *Without this residual perfusion myocardial protection is not possible.* The supply-demand concept is meaningless without measurable supply. However, if this condition is met and significant residual flow exists then *the progression from ischemia to infarction can be greatly retarded* by reducing the myocardial as well as the total body oxygen demand. Reduction of oxygen demand for the entire organism is important because it will reduce cardiac stimulation. *However, despite this, in my laboratory, we have not been successful in reducing infarct size after an abrupt and a permanent coronary artery occlusion.* With gradual and progressive coronary stenosis leading to complete occlusion within 3 days infarctions can, however, be avoided (20).

*Permanent myocardial salvage in the presence of permanent occlusion would appear to me to be feasible if we can maintain a state of low myocardial oxygen demand for a sufficiently long period to allow adequate collateral enlargement to occur (20).* While such an approach would appear to hold promise we cannot dismiss the possibility that these delaying tactics might also act to reduce the stimulus for vascular growth. Clearly, new and exciting areas of investigation await our attention.

## REFERENCES

1. Bloor, C. M. (1974): Functional significance of the coronary collateral circulation. *Am. J. Pathol.*, 76:561.
2. Blumenthal, D. S., Hutchins, G. M., Jugdutt, B. I., and Becker, L. C. (1981): Salvage of ischemic myocardium by dipyridamole in the conscious dog. *Circulation*, 64:915–923.
3. Bruyneel, K. J. J., and Opie, L. H. (1973): The value of warning arrhythmias in the prediction of ventricular fibrillation within one hour of coronary occlusion. Experimental studies in the baboon. *Am. Heart J.*, 86:373–384.
4. Downey, J. M., Chambers, D., and Wilkerson, R. D. (1982): The inability of isoproterenol or

propranolol to alter the lateral dimensions of experimentally induced myocardial infarcts. *Basic Res. Cardiol.*, 77:486–498.

5. Grayson, J., and Lapin, B. A. (1966): Observations on the mechanisms of infarction in the dog after experimental occlusion of the coronary artery. *Lancet*, I:1284–1288.
6. Hofmann, M., Hofmann, M., Genth, K., and Schaper, W. (1980): The influence of reperfusion on infarct size after experimental coronary artery occlusion. *Basic Res. Cardiol.*, 75:572–582.
7. Kalbfleisch, H. (1975): Eine Methode zur postmortalen Grossenbestimmung der Versorgungsgebiete einzelner Herzkranzarterein. *Z. Kardiol.*, 64:987.
8. Klein, H. H., Puschmann, S., Schaper, J., and Schaper, W. (1981): The mechanism of the tetrazolium reaction in identifying experimental myocardial infarction. *Virchows Arch. [Pathol. Anat.]*, 393:287–297.
9. Klein, H. H., Schaper, J., Puschman, S., Nienaber, C., Kreuzer, H., and Schaper, W. (1981): Loss of canine myocardial nicotinamide adenine dinucleotides determines the transition from reversible to irreversible ischemic damage of myocardial cells. *Basic Res. Cardiol.*, 76:612–621.
10. Marcus, M. L. (editor) (1983): *The Coronary Circulation in Health and Disease.* McGraw-Hill, New York.
11. Maroko, P. R., Kjekshus, J. K., Sobel, B. E., Watanabe, T., Covell, J. W., Ross, J., and Braunwald, E. (1971): Factors influencing infarct size following experimental coronary artery occlusions. *Circulation*, 41:67–82.
12. Murdock, R. H., Jr., Harlan, D. M., Moris, J. J., III, Pryor, W. W., Jr., and Cobb, F. R. (1983): Transitional blood flow zones between ischemic and nonischemic myocardium in the awake dog. Analysis based on distribution of the intramural vasculature. *Circ. Res.*, 52:451–459.
13. Nunez, R., Calva, E., Briones, E., and Lopez-Soriano, F. (1974): Nicotinamide coenzymes in heart and coronary blood during myocardial infarction. *Am. J. Physiol.*, 226:73–76.
14. Rees, R. J., and Redding, V. J. (1967): Anastomotic blood flow in experimental myocardial infarction. *Cardiovasc. Res.*, 1:169–178.
15. Rees, R. J., and Redding, V. J. (1968): Experimental myocardial infarction by Wedge method: early changes in collateral flow. *Cardiovasc. Res.*, 2:43–53.
16. Rösen, R., Marsen, A., and Klats, W. (1984): Local myocardial perfusion and epicardial NADH-fluorescence after coronary artery ligation in the isolated guinea pig heart. *Basic Res. Cardiol.*, 79:59–67.
17. Sandritter, W., and Jestädt, R. (1958): Triphenyltetrazoliumchlorid (TTC) als Reduktionsindikator zur makroskopischen Diagnose des frischen Herzinfarkts. *Verh. Dtsch. Ges. Pathol.*, 41:165–170.
18. Schaper, W., Remijsen, P., and Xhonneux, R. (1969): The size of myocardial infarction after experimental coronary artery occlusion. *Z. Kreislaufforschg.*, 58:904–909.
19. Schaper, W. (editor) (1971): *The Collateral Circulation of the Heart.* Elsevier/North-Holland, Amsterdam.
20. Schaper, W., DeBrabander, M., and Lewi, P. (1971): DNA-synthesis and mitoses in coronary collateral vessels of the dog. *Circ. Res.*, 28:671–679.
21. Schaper, W., and Pasyk, S. (1976): Influence of collateral flow on the ischemic tolerance of the heart following acute and subacute coronary occlusion. *Circulation*, 53(3):I-57–I-62.
22. Schaper, W., and Schaper, J. (1977): The coronary microcirculation. *Am. J. Cardiol.*, 40:1008–1012.
23. Schaper, W. (editor) (1979): *The Pathophysiology of Myocardial Perfusion.* Elsevier/North-Holland, Amsterdam.
24. Schaper, W., Frenzel, H., and Hort, W. (1979): Experimental coronary artery occlusion. I. Measurement of infarct size. *Basic Res. Cardiol.*, 74:46:53.
25. Schaper, J., Schwarz, F., Kittstein, H., Kreisel, E., Winkler, B., and Hehrlein, F. W. (1980): Ultrastructural evaluation of the effect of global ischemia and reperfusion on human myocardium. *Thorac. Cardiovasc. Surg.*, 28:337–342.
26. Schaper, W., Schaper, J., and Hoffmeister, H. M. (1984): Pathophysiology of the coronary system. In: *Handbook of Experimental Pharmacology*, vol. 76, Antianginal Drugs, edited by U. Abshagen. Springer, Heidelberg *(in press)*.
27. Taegtmeyer, H. (1978): Metabolic response to cardiac hypoxia. Increased production of succinate by rabbit papillary muscle. *Circ. Res.*, 43:808–815.

*Therapeutic Approaches to Myocardial Infarct Size Limitation*, edited by D. J. Hearse and D. M. Yellon. Raven Press, New York © 1984.

# 6

# What Factors Influence Coronary Flow?

## Melvin L. Marcus

*Department of Internal Medicine, Cardiovascular Division, University of Iowa, Iowa City, Iowa 52242*

The coronary circulation is regulated by five basic mechanisms: metabolic control, autoregulation, neural modulation, myogenic regulation, and humoral control. The relative importance of these factors under normal conditions has been well defined. Metabolic regulation is dominant, myogenic modulation may not exist, and the other three factors (autoregulation, neural control, and humoral regulation) are of intermediate importance. Under pathophysiological conditions the relative roles of these control mechanisms may be altered considerably. For example, in the presence of a severe coronary stenosis (greater than 95% luminal obstruction), small decreases in perfusion pressure, coronary vasodilation, or increases in sympathetic tone can profoundly influence myocardial perfusion (19,24,49,53).

Recent reviews of coronary physiology (2,15,38) provide a detailed account of the current state of knowledge in this field. The purpose of this chapter is to summarize succinctly what is known and to call attention to new and emerging concepts concerning fundamental mechanisms that regulate coronary blood flow.

## METABOLIC FACTORS THAT REGULATE
## CORONARY BLOOD FLOW

Under physiological conditions the dominant factor that modulates coronary vascular resistance is myocardial metabolism. Over a broad range, in all cardiac chambers, there is a strikingly parallel relationship between changes in myocardial metabolism as assessed by measurements of myocardial oxygen consumption and changes in myocardial perfusion (11,31,58) (Fig. 1). Furthermore, any perturbation that affects oxygen delivery to the myocardium, such as changes in hemoglobin concentration (27,55), or hemoglobin oxygen affinity (10) will lead to compensatory changes in coronary vascular resistance that tend to prevent the development of ischemia.

Although the parallel relationship between myocardial metabolism and coronary blood flow has been recognized for decades, the tightness of this coupling has recently been emphasized. Step changes in myocardial metabolism can alter coronary vascular resistance in a fraction of a second (52). Also, maximal coronary dilation can be marshalled in 15 to 20 sec in several animal species (6,13) and in man (35). *Thus, full gain of the system can be realized in a short time interval.*

On a macroscopic scale, the broad outlines of the relationship between myocardial metabolism and coronary blood flow have been well established. Mechanisms that fine-tune oxygen delivery to the myocardium at the level of the microvasculature remain to be defined. Several studies have emphasized that under normal conditions in small subsegments of the myocardium, oxygen consumption and myocardial perfusion are markedly heterogenous (12,57). Little is known about

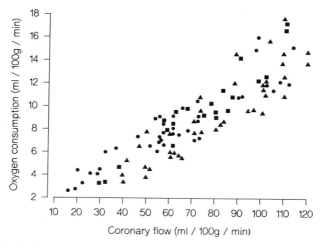

**FIG. 1.** The Relationship Between Left Ventricular Myocardial Oxygen Consumption and Left Ventricular Coronary Blood Flow. Over a broad range there is a close correlation between left ventricular myocardial oxygen consumption and left ventricular coronary blood flow. *Square:* experimental procedure (hemorrhage or intravenous epinephrine); *triangle:* intracoronary infusion of 2,4-dinitrophenol; *circle:* control. (From ref. 2, with permission.)

the regulation of capillary density, permeability, or microcirculatory hemodynamics in the beating left ventricle. I expect that a recent technological development by Nellis et al. (44) will allow investigators to measure directly diameter, intraluminal pressure, and flow in the coronary microcirculation of the untethered beating left ventricle. *Application of this technology should, I believe, lead to rapid expansion of knowledge in this area.*

A relatively new concept involving metabolic regulation of coronary blood flow relates to ascending coronary dilation. Several investigators have noted that selective downstream coronary dilation promptly produces dilation of the large proximal coronary arteries (18,25). Although the magnitude of the ascending dilation is modest and may not have a significant influence on total coronary vascular resistance, the mechanism responsible for this phenomenon is intriguing. *Furthermore, it is possible that in the presence of a severe coronary obstruction, ascending coronary dilation could significantly affect coronary hemodynamics by contributing to the dynamic behavior of certain types of coronary obstructive lesions (19).*

## Coronary Reactive Hyperemia

When a coronary vessel is transiently occluded, the myocardium in the perfusion field of the occluded artery becomes profoundly ischemic and the downstream coronary vessels dilate. When the occlusion is released, normal perfusion pressure is restored to a dilated coronary bed. As a consequence, coronary blood flow increases enormously and then gradually returns to control. This response sequence is referred to as coronary reactive hyperemia. In the normal coronary circulation, the magnitude of the coronary reactive hyperemic response is dependent on the duration of the coronary occlusion and coronary driving pressure (8). In small mammals such as the rat, maximal coronary reactive hyperemia occurs following a 5- to 10-sec coronary occlusion (56). In larger mammals such as the dog (6) and pig (13) a 15- to 20-sec coronary occlusion is needed to elicit a maximal coronary reactive hyperemic response.

Recent studies have defined the quantitative characteristic of coronary reactive hyperemia in humans (35). In man, maximal coronary reactive hyperemic responses are produced by a 20-sec coronary occlusion (35) (Figs. 2 and 3). Peak coronary blood flow velocity increases to five- to sixfold following release of a 20-sec coronary occlusion. Coronary reactive hyperemia in humans is found to be similar in the right and left ventricles both in males and females. Furthermore, the magnitude of the response is age-independent in the absence of superimposed disease (37). *Even though the coronary reactive hyperemic response is somewhat artificial, it is my opinion that understanding the basic mechanisms responsible for this response will greatly enhance our appreciation of fundamental factors that regulate coronary blood flow. Unfortunately, the mechanisms responsible for the coronary reactive hyperemic response remain elusive.*

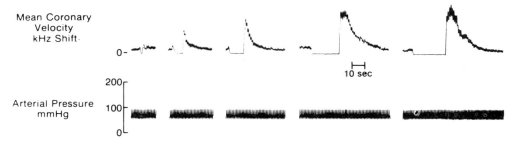

**FIG. 2.** Coronary Reactive Hyperemic Responses in a Patient. The responses were obtained from a right ventricular branch of the right coronary artery. The coronary artery was angiographically normal and the right ventricle was also normal. Transient coronary occlusion did not alter arterial pressure or heart rate. In this patient, the maximal reactive hyperemic response occurred following a 20-sec coronary occlusion. (From ref. 35, with permission.)

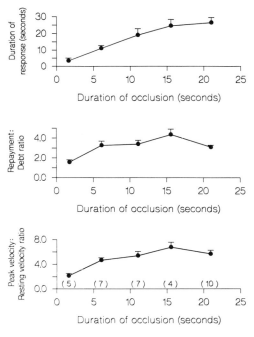

**FIG. 3.** Quantitative Characteristics of Coronary Reactive Hyperemic Responses in Humans. Duration of response, repayment ratio, and peak-to-resting velocity ratio all increase as a function of the duration of the coronary occlusion. Maximal responses occur with an occlusion of 15 to 20 sec. The integers above the zero line in the *bottom panel* refer to the number of patients studied at each occlusion time. In all patients the coronary vessel studied was angiographically normal and perfused a normal ventricle. Responses of the right and left coronary vessels were similar. (From ref. 35, with permission.)

## Mediators of Metabolic Coronary Vasodilation

The coupling between myocardial oxygen consumption and coronary vascular resistance must be mediated by one or more substances. Although many such mediators have been proposed (for example, potassium, prostaglandins, adenosine) the quest for the major mediator continues with no end in sight.

## Potassium

*Although the potassium ion can modulate coronary resistance, the magnitude and temporal course of changes in the interstitial level of potassium that accompany alterations in myocardial metabolism are inadequate to explain the accompanying alterations in coronary vascular resistance (9,32,33).*

## Prostaglandins

A substantial volume of evidence supports the concept that various prostaglandins have powerful effects on coronary flow (40). At the same time, the notion that prostaglandins or prostacyclins are the primary mediators that couple changes in myocardial metabolism to changes in coronary vascular resistance is steeped in controversy (1,17,26,45). *There is no convincing evidence, at present, that prostaglandins or prostacyclins play a major role in modulating coronary vascular responses to changes in myocardial metabolism.*

## Adenosine

For nearly two decades, Berne and his numerous disciples have championed the notion that adenosine plays a key role in coupling changes in myocardial metabolism to alterations in coronary vascular resistance (2). Although this hypothesis is attractive, recent studies with adenosine deaminase (48) cast serious doubt on the relative importance of adenosine as a key mediator. This issue will probably not be resolved until a technological breakthrough allows investigators to directly measure adenosine concentrations in the interstitial fluid surrounding coronary resistance vessels. *Despite 20 years of intensive investigation, in my view, the adenosine hypothesis remains unproven.*

## AUTOREGULATION IN THE CORONARY CIRCULATION

In many organs including the heart, changes in perfusion pressure are not associated with parallel changes in flow. This occurs because when a step change in coronary driving pressure is introduced, within a few seconds compensatory changes in downstream coronary resistance effectively buffer the change in arterial pressure, and consequently alterations in flow are attenuated. In the left ventricle, autoregulation is effective over a relatively broad range (50–60 mm Hg to 130–150 mm Hg) (3,22,41). As discussed in Chapter 8, at pressures below 50 mm Hg or above 150 mm Hg, further step changes in coronary driving pressure are accompanied by nearly parallel changes in flow (3,22,41).

Although autoregulation exists in the coronary circulation, for two reasons this phenomenon is more complex than in other organs. First, if the coronary vessels are not perfused separately from a reservoir system, changes in coronary perfusion pressure will almost always be associated with changes in left ventricular pressure. Since left ventricular pressure has a major influence on myocardial metabolism, a step change in coronary driving pressure in the intact circulation will almost always activate two mechanisms (metabolic and autoregulation), both of which can significantly modulate coronary vascular resistance. Second, in the left ventricle, autoregulation is much more effective in the subepicardial layers than in the subendocardial layers (Fig. 4) (22). The differences in autoregulation across the left ventricular wall have major implications concerning the effects of a coronary stenosis or occlusion on transmural myocardial perfusion. A severe coronary stenosis or occlusion invariably decreases downstream coronary perfusion pressure. *Because autoregulation is less effective in the subendocardial layers of the left ventricle, a coronary stenosis or occlusion will have more severe effects on subendocardial perfusion than subepicardial perfusion.*

The effectiveness of autoregulation has recently been quantified by using an index in which following a step change in pressure, the resulting change in flow in milliliters per minute is divided by the change in pressure in mm Hg. An index of unity would indicate the absence of autoregulation and a value of zero would imply perfect autoregulation. Within the autoregulatory range (60–130 mm Hg) in the anesthetized dog, autoregulation in the left ventricle is far from perfect and typically an index of 0.4 to 0.6 is observed (8).

A study by Murray and Vatner (43) suggests that autoregulation is nonexistent in the coronary circulation perfusing the right ventricle. This observation would suggest that there exists a fundamental difference between autoregulation in the right and left ventricles. A recent study by Willhoite et al. challenges this notion (59). Willhoite found that autoregulation in the right and left ventricles was about equally effective.

### Extravascular Compressive Forces

During cardiac contraction the heart compresses and twists the coronary vasculature. These external forces contribute to coronary vascular resistance. *Under normal conditions, 15% of coronary vascular resistance can be attributed to extravascular compressive forces.* In addition to augmenting total coronary vascular

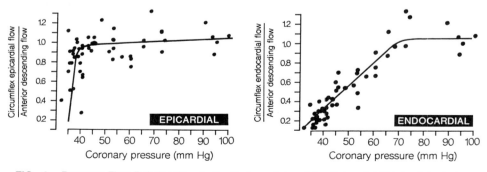

**FIG. 4.** Pressure-Flow Relationships in the Endocardial and the Epicardial Thirds of the Left Ventricular Myocardium. The ability of the epicardial vessels to autoregulate is substantially greater than that of the endocardial vessels. (From ref. 22, with permission.)

resistance, cardiac contraction significantly alters the phasic character of coronary blood flow. During systole, coronary blood flow in the epicardial coronary vessels is diminished and represents both capacitive and true forward flow. In the intramural coronary arteries, flow is negative in midsystole (5). Thus, in midsystole, coronary blood flow is "forward" in epicardial arteries and "backward" in intramural arteries. The presence of simultaneous forward and backward flow in two vascular segments that are in series implies that there must be a capacitor interposed between them. The characteristics of the coronary capacitor are currently under intensive investigation.

## NEURAL CONTROL OF THE CORONARY CIRCULATION

Neural control mechanisms in the coronary circulation have always been difficult to elucidate because the nerves have direct and indirect effects on coronary blood flow. Furthermore, the indirect effects of neural activation (change in cardiac metabolism secondary to alterations in heart rate, myocardial contractility, and arterial pressure) often dominate. Nonetheless, in the past decade much has been learned about neural control of the coronary circulation.

### Effects of Sympathetic Nerves on Coronary Flow

#### Direct and Indirect Effects

Stimulation of sympathetic nerves produces a marked increase in left ventricular myocardial oxygen consumption because heart rate, aortic pressure, and myocardial contractility are substantially augmented by sympathetic activation. This increase in cardiac metabolism engenders a substantial decrease in coronary vascular resistance. Thus, the *indirect effects* of sympathetic nerve stimulation are associated with coronary dilation. In contrast, the *direct effects* of sympathetic nerve stimulation produce modest coronary constriction. The net result of sympathetic nerve stimulation is transient coronary constriction followed by profound coronary dilation (see Fig. 5) (20). This biphasic response occurs because direct constrictor effects of sympathetic nerve stimulation become manifest a few seconds before the indirect dilator effects.

#### Receptor Sites

Coronary vessels contain $\beta_1$, $\beta_2$, $\alpha_1$, and $\alpha_2$ receptors. Physiological studies indicate that $\beta_1$ receptors have a negligible direct effect on coronary vasomotor tone. $\beta_2$-Receptor coronary dilation is modest and probably of little physiologic importance (39). In contrast, activation of $\alpha_1$ receptors can produce physiologically significant decreases in coronary blood flow (39). In addition, the release of norepinephrine by sympathetic nerves supplying the coronary vasculature is influenced by $\alpha_2$ receptors (29). *Although sympathetic nerve stimulation has discernable effects on coronary blood flow* in vivo, *the magnitude of the responses is meager*

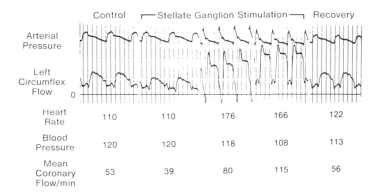

| | Control | ⌐Stellate Ganglion Stimulation⌐ | | Recovery |
|---|---|---|---|---|
| Heart Rate | 110 | 110 | 176 | 166 | 122 |
| Blood Pressure | 120 | 120 | 118 | 108 | 113 |
| Mean Coronary Flow/min | 53 | 39 | 80 | 115 | 56 |

**FIG. 5.** Effects of Stellate Ganglion Stimulation on Left Circumflex Coronary Artery Flow in a Chronically Instrumented Awake Dog. During the first few seconds following nerve stimulation there was no change in heart rate or arterial pressure, but a decrease in coronary blood flow. Thereafter, heart rate, arterial pressure, and coronary blood flow increased substantially. Thus, sympathetic nerve stimulation produces a biphasic effect on coronary blood flow; initial coronary vasoconstriction followed by coronary dilation. Heart rate is reported in beats/min; mean arterial pressure in mm Hg; mean coronary flow in ml/min. (From ref. 20, with permission.)

*compared to the extent of coronary modulation that occurs in response to metabolic factors.*

### Coexisting Influences

During the past few years, several situations have been described in which the effects of sympathetic nerve stimulation on coronary vessels are magnified or compete effectively with metabolically mediated changes in coronary blood flow. Hypercholesterolemia (47) and severe coronary obstruction (24) magnify the effects of sympathetic nerve stimulation on coronary blood flow. Furthermore, during exercise, α-adrenergic activation limits coronary dilation (42), and during maximal coronary dilation secondary to adenosine infusion, coronary vessels can constrict in response to α-receptor activation (28). Lastly, coronary atherosclerosis may amplify coronary constrictor effects of sympathetic nerve stimulation. This occurs for two reasons. First, a severe stenosis will limit metabolic dilation, and thereby the vasoconstrictor component of sympathetic activation will be unopposed. In a sense, the obstruction serves as a resistance amplifier. Second, data from my institution *(unpublished)* suggests that dietary-induced atherosclerosis in the cynamolgus monkey may sensitize coronary vessels to the vasoconstrictor effects of the α-agonist phenylephrine. The conditions noted above point to the importance of discovering situations in which the effects of sympathetic nerve stimulation may be intensified.

### Effects of Vagal Stimulation on Coronary Flow

Vagal stimulation produces indirect coronary constriction because the associated marked decrease in heart rate and slight decline in myocardial contractility decrease myocardial oxygen consumption (15). If the heart is paced, the direct coronary dilator effects of vagal stimulation are demonstrable (14). Recent studies indicate that infused acetylcholine (21) produces more dilation of coronary vessels in the subendocardium of the left ventricle than in the subepicardium. Also, it has been demonstrated that acetylcholine infusion dilates both large conduit and small resistance vessels (7).

### Reflex Control of Coronary Flow

Four reflexes have been shown to influence coronary vasomotor tone: the baroreceptor reflex, the chemoreceptor reflex, the pulmonary inflation reflex, and the Bezold-Jarisch reflex. *These reflex influences on the coronary circulation are generally modest with one exception—the pulmonary inflation reflex (54).* In the awake dog, a spontaneous deep breath is associated with a substantial increase in coronary flow which is mediated by alterations in the autonomic nervous system. Recent studies by Wilson et al. (60), utilizing a unique intraluminal coronary Doppler catheter, have shown that in conscious humans pulmonary inflation has no appreciable effect on coronary flow. This implies that major species differences exist with regard to certain reflex control mechanisms in the coronary circulation. *In my opinion, further investigations concerning reflex control of the coronary circulation in humans in the presence and absence of coronary atherosclerosis are likely to yield important new insight.* The availability of methods of measuring phasic coronary blood flow velocity in individual coronary vessels will greatly facilitate such investigations.

### Central Control of Coronary Flow

*The most exciting new aspect of neural control mechanisms that regulate coronary blood flow concerns central control of the coronary circulation.* Recent experiments suggest that the electrical stimulation of the lateral hypothalamus in the cat can produce a substantial increase in coronary vascular resistance which competes effectively with metabolic dilator responses (4). Other studies also suggest that central control of the coronary circulation may be important. For example, Pasyk et al. (46) have demonstrated that the injection of fentanyl, an opioid blocker, into the lateral ventricle of an awake dog produces profound coronary vasoconstriction that may be mediated by the release of vasopressin. These initial studies with regard to central control of the coronary circulation are of interest and should stimulate additional research in this area.

## MYOGENIC REGULATION OF CORONARY BLOOD FLOW

Myogenic regulation implies control of vasomotor tone by intrinsic mechanisms within the blood vessel wall. Although myogenic mechanisms are important in the regulation of flow to organs other than the heart (30), *it is my contention that to date no convincing data have been published that demonstrate myogenic responses contribute significantly to the regulation of coronary blood flow.*

## HUMORAL CONTROL OF CORONARY BLOOD FLOW

Numerous substances circulating in the blood or released from tissues have the capacity to influence coronary vasomotor tone. This area has recently been reviewed in detail (36). *Thus far, only three classes of humoral agents (catecholamines, angiotensin, and thyroid hormone) have been shown unequivocally to influence coronary vasomotor tone under physiologic or pathophysiological conditions (36).* It is also likely that vasopressin may modulate coronary vascular resistance under certain circumstances (36).

*A new concept concerning humoral control of the coronary circulation has recently come to light. Studies of isolated coronary vascular rings* in vitro *have shown that the coronary endothelium may modulate coronary vascular muscle responses to several humoral substances including acetylcholine, serotonin, and thrombin (16).* When the coronary endothelium is intact, administration of acetylcholine into the tissue bath causes the coronary vascular rings to relax; when the endothelium is mechanically removed, acetylcholine produces coronary constriction in the isolated coronary ring preparation. Although these *in vitro* studies are interesting, many questions in this area remain to be answered. Most importantly, these studies need to be extended to an intact preparation so that the importance of the endothelium:smooth muscle interaction can be examined under conditions when other mechanisms that modulate coronary vascular resistance are operative. In addition, the *in vitro* studies with vascular rings obtained from large conduit coronary vessels need to be extended to much smaller coronary vessels since it is the smaller vessels that primarily regulate coronary vascular resistance.

*It is possible that the endothelium:smooth muscle interaction plays a role in the pathogenesis of coronary spasm.* Clinicians are well aware that the intensity and incidence of coronary spasm is greatest under conditions when coronary endothelial damage is likely to exist, i.e., immediately postcoronary angioplasty and in the early days and weeks following acute myocardial infarction. In the setting of a damaged coronary endothelium, humoral or possibly neural control mechanisms may be sufficiently augmented to significantly contribute to the pathogenesis of coronary spasm. Thus, the interaction between endothelium and coronary vascular muscle may have significant pathophysiological implications.

## MECHANISMS THAT REGULATE CORONARY COLLATERAL FLOW

*Whenever regulation of coronary collateral flow is discussed, it is critical to define the type of collateral being considered.* In a broad sense, *coronary collaterals are categorized as native collaterals or developed or mature collaterals.* Native collaterals are present from birth. These thin-walled, tiny vessels (usually less than 100 μm) link the large conduit coronary vessels to each other. The resistance via these native coronary collaterals is 30 to 40 times greater than the minimal resistance of the normal coronary vasculature (Fig. 6) (50,51).

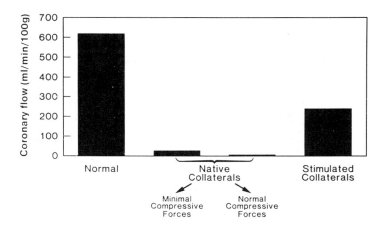

**FIG. 6.** Coronary Flow During Maximal Coronary Dilation in Normal Coronary Vessels (Normal), Native Collaterals, and Mature Stimulated Collaterals. All flows were measured at a coronary perfusion pressure of 100 mm Hg. The data emphasize the minimal capacity of native collaterals. The maximal flow that can be delivered by mature stimulated collaterals is less than half of that which can be delivered by normal collateral channels. (From refs. 50 and 51, with permission.)

Mature or developed coronary collaterals can be quite large (1–3 mm in diameter) relatively thick-walled vascular channels. These vessels develop in response to ischemia (50,51).

### Regulation of Resistance in Native Coronary Collateral Vessels

Resistance in native coronary collateral vessels is markedly influenced by extravascular compressive forces such as alteration in heart rate and arterial pressure (50,51). *The resistance in native coronary collateral vessels is exquisitely sensitive to changes in extravascular compressive forces. If these extravascular compressive forces are kept constant, most studies indicate that coronary resistance in native collaterals is unalterable (50,51). In particular, no drug has been shown to effectively diminish resistance in native coronary collateral vessels by altering the tone of these collateral channels.* If, however, a pharmacological agent influences extravascular compressive forces, this will indirectly change native coronary collateral resistance. Such changes are usually very small.

Recent observations by Harrison et al. (23) suggest that ischemia may decrease coronary resistance in the native coronary collateral vessels modestly. This effect of ischemia on the resistance of flow through native coronary collaterals appears not to be related to alterations in extravascular compressive forces which occur as a consequence of ischemia.

### Regulation of Resistances in Mature Coronary Collateral Vessels

Under ideal conditions, maximal flow via mature coronary collaterals is 60 to 75% of that which can be achieved in the normal coronary vasculature. Furthermore, perfusion of myocardial tissue that is collateral-dependent is responsive to metabolic stimulation. For example, in the dog, flow to a zone served by a mature collateral circulation can increase fourfold in response to strenuous exercise (Fig. 7) (34). Although studies of this type suggest that the mature coronary collaterals may be responsive to various types of stimuli, it is always difficult to determine whether or not changes in coronary vascular resistance that occur in zones served by mature coronary collateral vessels occur as a consequence of dilation of the collateral channels or dilation of the resistance vessels distal to the collateral channel. The coronary collateral channels are in series with the normal downstream coronary vessels. Hence, it is difficult to separate effects on the coronary collateral per se versus the distal vasculature when measurements of tissue perfusion are employed. Such measurements reflect the aggregate function of the entire vascular bed. It is known that perfusion to myocardial segments served by mature collaterals can be varied substantially by pharmacological manipulation and by activating control mechanisms that regulate the normal coronary circulation (50,51). *It is uncertain how much of the observed response is related to changes in resistance in the collateral channels themselves versus alterations in the tone of the distal coronary vasculature.*

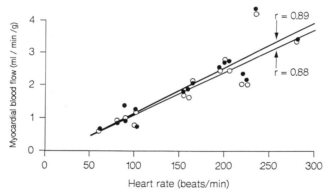

**FIG. 7.** Effects of Exercise on Myocardial Blood Flow: A normally perfused area of the left ventricle (*open circle:* anterior papillary muscle region) and a collateral-dependent area of the left ventricle (*solid circle:* posterior papillary muscle region). The collateral circulation to the posterior papillary muscle was stimulated to develop by gradual occlusion of the circumflex coronary artery with an implanted Ameroid constrictor months prior to the exercise study. The data indicate that the blood flow to the two regions was equal during exercise to heart rates of almost 300 beats/min. In almost all the animals studied, the maximal flow rates achieved were less than 3 ml/min/g. During exercise, mean arterial pressure increases. Hence, at a flow of 3 ml/g/min and an increase in mean arterial pressure, calculated coronary vascular resistance would probably be twofold greater than minimal coronary vascular resistance that could be achieved in the dog. The decrease in coronary vascular resistance achieved in this exercise study is about equal to the maximal capacity of coronary collateral vessels to dilate (see Fig. 6). Thus, the data in Fig. 6 and this figure are consistent. (From ref. 34, with permission.)

## FUTURE DEVELOPMENTS

During the past two decades knowledge concerning the regulation of the coronary circulation in experimental animals has vastly expanded. In the coming years many technological advances [for example, fast computerized tomography, nuclear magnetic resonance, intraluminal coronary Doppler catheters (see Chapter 9)] will permit clinical investigators to perform detailed studies of the coronary circulation in humans. Such studies will undoubtedly contribute substantial new knowledge concerning the regulation of the coronary circulation under normal and pathological conditions.

## CONCLUDING COMMENTS

A broad outline of the factors that regulate coronary flow on a macroscopic level in normal animals is now available. Metabolic mechanisms are dominant and autoregulation is of considerable importance. Neural and humoral effects are detectable and myogenic control is yet to be demonstrated. Regulation of myocardial perfusion at the microvascular level remains uncharted and the biochemical mediator primarily responsible for modulating coronary vascular resistance is elusive. Knowledge concerning the regulation of coronary flow in humans is modest, and an understanding of the effects of disease states on coronary regulation in patients is in its infancy. As the new technological breakthroughs currently available are applied to fundamental questions concerning control of the coronary circulation, further understanding of mechanisms which regulate coronary blood flow in humans will rapidly emerge.

## REFERENCES

1. Alexander, R. W., Kent, K. M., Pisano, J. J., Keiser, H. R., and Cooper, T. (1975): Regulation of postocclusive hyperemia by endogenously synthesized prostaglandins in the dog heart. *J. Clin. Invest.*, 55:1174–1181.
2. Berne, R. M., and Rubio, R. (1979): Coronary circulation. In: *Handbook of Physiology*, Vol. 1, Section 2, edited by R. M. Berne, p. 873–952. American Physiological Society, Bethesda.
3. Boatwright, R. B., Downey H. F., Bashour, F. A., and Crystal, G. J. (1980): Transmural variation in autoregulation of coronary blood flow in hyperperfused canine myocardium. *Circ. Res.*, 47:599–609.
4. Bonham, A. C., Gutterman, D. D., Marcus, M. L., Gebhart, G. F., and Brody, M. J. (1984): Electrical stimulation in the hypothalamus evokes coronary vasoconstriction (abstract). *Fed. Proc.*, 43:425.
5. Chilian, W. M., and Marcus, M. L. (1982): Phasic blood flow velocity in intramural and epicardial coronary arteries. *Circ. Res.*, 50:775–761.
6. Coffman, J. D., and Gregg, D. E. (1960): Reactive hyperemia characteristics of the myocardium. *Am. J. Physiol.*, 199:1143–1149.
7. Cox, D., Hintze, T., and Vatner, S. F. (1981): Effects of acetylcholine on large coronary vessels in conscious dogs. *Fed. Proc.*, 40:707.
8. Dole, W. P., Montville, W. J., and Bishop, V. S. (1981): Dependency of myocardial reactive hyperemia on coronary artery pressure in the dog. *Am. J. Physiol.*, 240:H709–H715.
9. Driscol, T. E., and Berne, R. M. (1957): Role of potassium in regulation of coronary blood flow. *Proc. Soc. Exp. Biol. Med.*, 96:505–508.

10. Duvelleroy, M. A., Martin, J. L., Teisseire, B., Gauduel, Y., and Duruble, M. (1980): Abnormal hemoglobin oxygen affinity and the coronary circulation. *Bibl. Haematol.*, 46:70–80.
11. Eckenhoff, J. E., Hafkenschiel, J. H., Landmesser, C. M., and Harmel, M. (1947): Cardiac oxygen metabolism and control of the coronary circulation. *Am. J. Physiol.*, 149:634–649.
12. Falsetti, H. L., Carroll, R. J., and Marcus, M. L. (1975): Temporal heterogeneity of myocardial blood flow. *Circulation*, 52:848–853.
13. Fedor, J. M., McIntosh, D. M., Rembert, J. C., and Greenfield, J. C. (1978): Coronary and regional myocardial blood flow response to transient ischemia in awake domestic pigs. *Am. J. Physiol.*, 4:H435–H444.
14. Feigl, E. O. (1969): Parasympathetic control of coronary blood flow in dogs. *Circ. Res.*, 25:509–519.
15. Feigl, E. O. (1983): Coronary physiology. *Physiol. Rev.*, 63(1):1–205.
16. Furchgott, R. F. (1983): Role of endothelium in responses of vascular smooth muscle. *Circ. Res.*, 53:557–573.
17. Giles, R. W., and Wilcken, D. E. L. (1977): Reactive hyperemia in the dog heart: Inter-relations between adenosine, ATP, and aminophylline and the effect of indomethacin. *Cardiovasc. Res.*, 11:113–121.
18. Gould, K. L., and Kelly, K. O. (1982): Physiological significance of coronary flow velocity and changing stenosis geometry during coronary vasodilation in awake dogs. *Circ. Res.*, 50:695–704.
19. Gould, K. L. (1980): Dynamic coronary stenosis. *Am. J. Cardiol.*, 45:286–292.
20. Granata, L., Olsson, R. A., Huvos, A., and Gregg, D. E. (1965): Coronary inflow and oxygen usage following cardiac sympathetic nerve stimulation in unanesthetized dogs. *Circ. Res.*, 16:114–120.
21. Gross, G. J., Buck, J. D., and Warltier, D. C. (1981): Transmural distribution of blood flow during activation of coronary muscarinic receptors. *Am. J. Physiol.*, 240:H941–H946.
22. Guyton, R. A., McClenathan, J. H., Newman, G. E., and Michaelis, L. L. (1977): Significance of subendocardial S-T segment elevation caused by coronary stenosis in the dog. *Am. J. Cardiol.*, 40:373–380.
23. Harrison, D. G., Barnes, D. H., and Marcus, M. L. (1983): Modulation of coronary collateral resistance by ischemia. *Clin. Res.*, 31:705A (abstract).
24. Heusch, G., and Deussen, A. (1983): The effects of cardiac sympathetic nerve stimulation on perfusion of stenotic coronary arteries in the dog. *Circ. Res.*, 53:8–15.
25. Hintz, T. H., and Vatner, S. F. (1984): Reactive dilation of large coronary arteries in conscious dogs. *Circ. Res.*, 54:50–57.
26. Hintz, T. H., and Kaley, G. (1977): Prostaglandins in the control of blood flow in the canine myocardium. *Circ. Res.*, 40:313–320.
27. Holtz, J, Bassenge, E., von Restorff, W., and Mayer, E. (1976): Transmural differences in myocardial blood flow and in coronary dilatory capacity in hemodiluted conscious dogs. *Basic Res. Cardiol.*, 71:36–46.
28. Johannsen, U. J., Mark, A. L., and Marcus, M. L. (1982): Responses to cardiac sympathetic nerve stimulation during maximal coronary dilation produced by adenosine. *Circ. Res.*, 50:510–517.
29. Johanssen, U. J., Mark, A. L., and Marcus, M. L. (1982): Alpha-2 receptors modulate coronary responses to sympathetic nerve stimulation. *Circulation*, (Suppl. II)66:153.
30. Johnson, P. C. (1980): The myogenic response. In: *Handbook of Physiology*, edited by D. F. Bohr, A. P. Somlyo, and H. V. Sparks, Jr. American Physiological Society, Bethesda.
31. Khouri, E. M., Gregg, D. E., and Rayford, C. R. (1965): Effect of exercise on cardiac output, left coronary flow and myocardial metabolism in the unanesthetized dog. *Circ. Res.*, 17:427–437.
32. Kline, R. P., and Morad, M. (1978): Potassium efflux in heart muscle during activity: Extracellular accumulation and its implications. *J. Physiol. (Lond.)*, 280:537–558.
33. Kunze, D. L. (1977): Rate-dependent changes in extracellular potassium in the rabbit atrium. *Circ. Res.*, 41:122–127.
34. Lambert, P. R., Hess, D. S., and Bache, R. J. (1977): Effect of exercise on perfusion of collateral-dependent myocardium in dogs with chronic coronary artery occlusion. *J. Clin. Invest.*, 59:1–7.
35. Marcus, M., Wright, C., Doty, D., Eastham, C., Laughlin, D., Krumm, P., Fastenow, C., and Brody, M. (1981): Measurements of coronary velocity and reactive hyperemia in the coronary circulation of humans. *Circ. Res.*, 49:877–891.
36. Marcus, M. L. (1982): Humoral control of the coronary circulation. In: *The Coronary Circulation in Health and Disease*, pp. 15–190. McGraw-Hill, New York.

37. Marcus, M. L. (1982): Metabolic regulation of coronary blood flow. In: *The Coronary Circulation in Health and Disease*, Part 3, pp. 65–92. McGraw-Hill, New York.
38. Marcus, M. L. (1982): *The Coronary Circulation in Health and Disease*. McGraw-Hill, New York.
39. McRaven, D. R., Mark, A. L., Abboud, F. M., and Mayer, H. E. (1971): Responses of coronary vessels to adrenergic stimuli. *J. Clin. Invest.*, 50:773–778.
40. Moncada, S., Flower, R. J., and Vane, J. E. (1980): Prostaglandins, prostacycline, and thromboxane A$_2$. In: *The Pharmacological Basis of Therapeutics*, edited by L. Goodman and A. Gilman, pp. 668–681. MacMillan, New York.
41. Mosher, P., Ross, J., Jr., McFate, P. A., and Shaw, R. F. (1964): Control of coronary blood flow by an autoregulatory mechanism. *Circ. Res.*, 14:250–259.
42. Murray, P. A., and Vatner, S. F. (1979): Alpha-adrenoceptor attenuation of the coronary vascular response to severe exercise in the conscious dog. *Circ. Res.*, 45:654–660.
43. Murray, P. A., and Vatner, S. F. (1981): Carotid sinus baroreceptor control of right coronary circulation in normal, hypertrophied, and failing right ventricles of conscious dogs. *Circ. Res.*, 49:1339–1349.
44. Nellis, S. H., Liedtke, A. J., and Whitesell, L. (1981): Small coronary vessel pressure and diameter in an intact beating rabbit heart using fixed-position and free-motion techniques. *Circ. Res.*, 49:342–354.
45. Owen, T. L., Ehrhart, I. C., Weidner, W. J., et al. (1975): Effects of indomethacin on local blood flow regulation in canine heart and kidney. *Proc. Soc. Exp. Biol. Med.*, 149:871–876.
46. Pasyk, S., Walton, J., and Pitt, B. (1981): Central opioid mediated coronary and systemic vasoconstriction in the conscious dog. *Circulation*, 64(Suppl. 4):41.
47. Rosendorff, C., Hoffman, J. L. E., Verrier, E. D., Rouleau, J., and Boerboom, L. E. (1981): Cholesterol potentiates the coronary artery response to norepinephrine in anesthetized and conscious dogs. *Circ. Res.*, 48:320–329.
48. Saito, D., Steinhart, C. R., Nison, D. G., and Ollsson, R. A. (1981): Intracoronary adenosine deaminase reduces canine myocardial reactive hyperemia. *Circ. Res.*, 49:1262–1267.
49. Santamore, W. P., and Walinsky, P. (1980): Altered coronary flow responses to vasoactive drugs due to coronary arterial stenosis in the dog. *Am. J. Cardiol.*, 45:276.
50. Schaper, W. (1971): *The Collateral Circulation of the Heart*. Elsevier, New York.
51. Schaper, W., and Wusten, B. (1979): Collateral circulation. In: *The Pathophysiology of Myocardial Perfusion*, edited by W. Schaper. Elsevier/North Holland, Amsterdam.
52. Schwartz, G. G., McHale, P. A., and Greenfield, J. C. (1982): Coronary vasodilation after a single ventricular extra-activation in the conscious dog. *Circ. Res.*, 50:38–46.
53. Schwartz, J. S., Caryle, P. F., and Cohn, J. N. (1979): Effect of dilation of the distal coronary bed on flow and resistance in severely stenotic coronary arteries in the dog. *Am. J. Cardiol.*, 43:219–224.
54. Vatner, S. F., and McRitchie, R. J. (1975): Interaction of the chemoreflex and the pulmonary inflation reflex in the regulation of coronary circulation in conscious dogs. *Circ. Res.*, 37:644–673.
55. von Restorff, W., Hofling, B., Holtz, J., and Bassenge, E. (1975): Effect of increased blood fluidity through hemodilution on coronary circulation at rest and during exercise in dogs. *Pfluegers Arch.*, 357:15–24.
56. Wangler, R. D., Peters, K. G., Marcus, M. L., and Tomanek, R. J. (1982): Effects of duration and severity of arterial hypertension on cardiac hypertrophy and coronary vasodilator reserve. *Circ. Res.*, 51:10–18.
57. Weiss, H. R., and Sinha, A. K. (1978): Regional oxygen saturation of small arteries and veins in the canine myocardium. *Circ. Res.*, 42:119–126.
58. White, C. W., Kerber, R. E., Weiss, H. R., and Marcus, M. L. (1981): Effect of atrial fibrillation on wall stress, oxygen consumption and perfusion of the left atrium. *Circulation*, (Suppl. 2)64:IV–65 (225).
59. Willhoite, D. J., Harrison, D. G., Barnes, D., and Marcus, M. L. (1984): Comparison of myocardial blood flow autoregulation in the right and left ventricles (abstract). *Fed. Proc.*, 43:1084.
60. Wilson, R. F., Marcus, M. L., Laughlin, D. E., Hartley, C. G., and White, C. W. (1984): The pulmonary inflation reflex: its physiologic significance in conscious humans (abstract). *Fed. Proc.*, 43:1003.

*Therapeutic Approaches to Myocardial Infarct Size Limitation*, edited by D. J. Hearse and D. M. Yellon. Raven Press, New York © 1984.

# 7

# What Happens in the Microcirculation?

## Harald Tillmanns and Wolfgang Kübler

*Medizinische Universitatsklinik Heidelberg, Department of Kardiology, 6900 Heidelberg 1, West Germany*

As is clear from many of the contributions to this book, the microcirculation and its response to ischemia is a critical determinant of the nature and extent of ischemic injury. *Despite the central role played by the microcirculation, we remain relatively ignorant about many aspects of its functional and morphological responsiveness to ischemia.* Thus, although it is well known that, at a macroscopic level, coronary artery disease in patients or coronary occlusion in animals causes major disturbances of myocardial perfusion, the nature of these hemodynamic changes at the level of the microcirculation is far from clear. We are also short of morphological information and, whereas structural alterations have been described for extended ischemia, very little is known about the critical changes in microvascular structure and function during early, reversible ischemic injury.

In considering the nature and the manipulation of ischemic injury, a number of key points relating to the microcirculation must be resolved. For example, is the reduction in coronary vascular reserve or coronary flow at rest, in the presence of a critical coronary artery stenosis, a consequence of reduced blood flow velocity in individual capillaries or is it due to a decrease in the number of capillaries perfused? *In this chapter we endeavor to answer such questions by describing the current state of knowledge concerning key microvascular changes occurring at various stages of the ischemic process.*

## ANATOMICAL CHARACTERISTICS OF THE MICROCIRCULATION

In recent years there has been a growing interest in defining the manner in which myocardial capillary patterns have developed and adapted to the functions and requirements of the heart. Data (5,30) on the structure of the terminal vascular bed are still somewhat limited. In reviewing this anatomical information, it is necessary to consider both afferent and efferent vessels, i.e., the arterioles and the venules.

### Arterioles

Arterioles that have diameters of less than 100 μm usually originate as branches at right angles from the smallest intramyocardial arteries. The arterioles then approach the nearest heart muscle fiber (obliquely or perpendicularly to fiber direction) or they proceed to more distant fiber bundles (30). The various branches given off by the main arteriole then run parallel to the muscle fibers, different branches running in other, the same, or opposite directions. The more arterioles that divide and extend their branches in the three spatial dimensions, then the shorter become the vascular segments, which run perpendicular to the cardiac muscle fibers (30). *This arteriolar branching pattern would appear to provide the best method for very dense capillarization of tissue.* It is important that each muscle fasciculus is supplied by more than one arteriole and this often occurs from different arterial sources.

Originating from deeper myocardial layers, the arterioles extend to the cardiac surface. The smaller $A_3$ arterioles and the terminal $A_4$ arterioles (diameter less than 15 μm) (Table 1) branch dichotomously such that one branch proceeds in the original direction, while the other bends back on itself and travels in the opposite direction parallel to the muscle fiber.

TABLE 1. *Coronary arteriolar branching order and dimensions*

| Vessel category | Maximum diameter (μm) | Minimum diameter (μm) |
|---|---|---|
| $A_1$ (small artery) | 300 | 101 |
| $A_2$ | 100 | 31 |
| $A_3$ | 30 | 16 |
| $A_4$ (terminal arteriole) | 15 | 8 |

## Capillaries

### Topography

The arrangement of capillaries in the left and right ventricle of the mammalian and the human heart appears to be primarily parallel, with the vessels lying on either side of the cardiac muscle fibers (3,14,30,44,46). *However, despite this alignment with the fibers, various interconnections between capillaries do occur; these so-called intercapillary anastomoses form loops of different lengths* (see Fig. 1) (44,46). In addition to connecting neighboring parallel vessels, these transverse capillary anastomoses also connect more distant vessels (5,30,46).

### Perfusion Interfaces

Capillary distribution patterns have an important bearing on the existence, or nonexistence, of border zones of intermediate injury, as discussed in Chapter 2 and by several authors (18,21,25). There are two microvascular arrangements, which, theoretically, could account for such a region of intermediate damage. First, pronounced interdigitation of unconnected capillaries originating from different arterial sources, and, second, extensive anastomoses between capillaries derived from separate arterial supply vessels.

Using different colors of silicone rubber (Microfil), injected into two coronary arteries of the dog heart at the same time and at the same pressure, Factor and colleagues (11) were unable to demonstrate either interdigitation or intercapillary anastomoses. *These authors therefore concluded that, at least for the dog heart, the perfusion field of a single coronary artery terminates as an endcapillary network.* In contrast to this, injection studies by Ludwig (30) and Brown (5) and *our own* in vivo *microscopic investigations in the rat and cat heart have demonstrated many capillaries continuously proceeding to more distant capillary beds which may be part of another circulatory unit.* This spatial arrangement of capillaries implies that heart muscle fibers may be flanked by segments of different capillaries which do not necessarily originate from the same coronary arterial source (30). *Further investigations are needed to clarify this controversial and critically important issue.*

### Densities, Diameters, and Distances

Capillary density and diffusion distance are the two important determinants for the transport action of oxygen nutrients and metabolites to the myocardial cell. An increase in diffusion distances may result in a decrease in myocardial $Po_2$, especially under conditions where an increase in diffusion distance is associated with a rise of myocardial oxygen consumption and/or a diminution of myocardial blood flow (37).

Using fluorescence microscopic techniques combined with the intravenous injection of, for example, fluoresceine isothiocyanate-tagged high-molecular dextran,

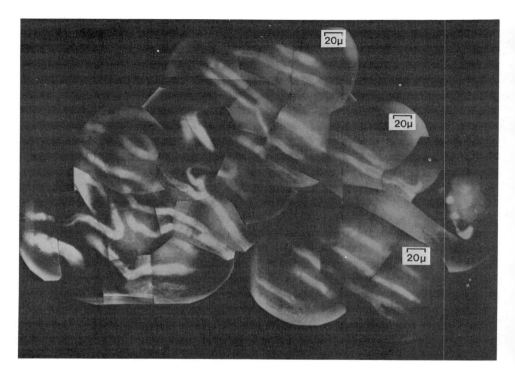

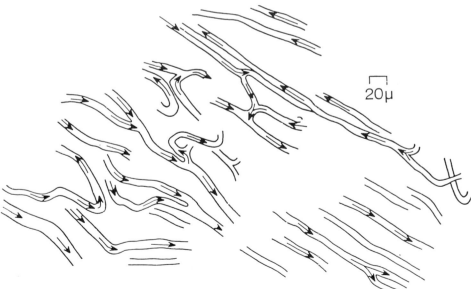

**FIG. 1.** Capillary Distribution and Flow. **Top:** *In vivo* fluorescence photomicrograph of capillaries from the left ventricular epicardium of the rat. The capillaries are filled with fluorosceine-tagged high-molecular dextran. This montage of photographs was obtained from a sequence of television tape recordings. **Bottom:** Flow directions in the capillaries derived from the above photograph.

the proximity and diameters of myocardial capillaries, as well as the direction of blood flow, can be readily visualized *in vivo* (44,46,48). *In this way, capillary diameter in the epicardium of the beating rat heart can be shown to average 5.7 ± 1.0 μm.* Similarly, it can be shown that, during systole, capillary diameter in the superficial layers of the rat and dog heart declines by about 25% (46). *In vivo* microscopic data of this type are in good agreement with diameter measurements obtained by postmortem injection techniques (3,41).

*The distances between perfused capillaries in the rat and dog ventricle when visualized by fluorescent dextran has been found to average 18 μm* (44,49) and the calculated capillary density in the cat, dog, and rat heart is in the order of 2,480 to 3,420/mm$^2$. Again, these results are generally consistent with data obtained by other investigators using postmortem injection procedures (3,19,37) or stop-motion photomicrographs of the beating rat heart (33). The capillary density values obtained by postmortem analyses do tend to be somewhat higher than those obtained by *in vivo* microscopic procedures, this is probably due to tissue shrinkage at postmortem. *It is generally agreed, however, that myocardial capillary densities vary relatively little, ranging, for example, from 2,000 capillaries/mm$^2$ in man and guinea pig to 3,700 capillaries/mm$^2$ in bats.*

### Directionality of Blood Flow

Blood flow in adjacent capillaries in the dog, rat, and turtle heart is often observed to occur in the same direction. However, countercurrent flow is also frequently noted in neighboring capillaries, particularly if they are joined together by large connecting loops (see Fig. 1) (44,46). Assessment of the extent of cocurrent and countercurrent flow in adjacent capillaries in the rat heart has yielded a ratio of 1.3:1; similar ratios have been reported for the dog and turtle heart (46). *These data support the concept that mixed countercurrent flow systems provide optimal myocardial oxygen supply (31).*

### Venules

*The venous end of the myocardial microcirculation has its own distinctive pattern, thus enabling the venules to be easily distinguished from arterioles.* Prior to the confluence of capillaries and postcapillaries to form a venule, the capillary network becomes denser, the meshes become closer, and more cross-bridges are observed between neighboring capillaries (30,46). Venules can also be readily differentiated from arterioles by observing flow direction at points of bifurcation. Myocardial postcapillaries and venules often show a tuft- or twig-like confluence to form a vein of relatively large caliber. Initially, venules run parallel to muscle fibers, however, they frequently lose their original directionality in order to proceed directly to larger veins (5,30).

In the following section we consider functional and morphological changes that occur in the microcirculation as a consequence of both prolonged and brief periods of ischemia and reperfusion.

## ISCHEMIA-INDUCED DISTURBANCES
## OF THE MICROCIRCULATION

### Microcirculatory Changes After Prolonged Ischemia
### and Reperfusion

*Capillary Morphology During Ischemia*

The condition of the microvascular bed in ischemic or infarcting myocardium may be a critical factor in determining the final outcome and reversibility of cellular injury. During the last two decades increasing attention has been paid to morphologic changes occurring in the microvasculature of the ischemic myocardium (2,13,22,23,26).

The first detectable alterations of capillary structure are the loss of the normally abundant endothelial pinocytotic vesicles and a marked swelling of the capillary endothelial cells. Some localized dilation of the endoplasmic reticulum can also be observed at this early stage (2,22). The swelling of the endothelial cells is consistent with the presence of intracellular edema.

After 40 to 60 min of uninterrupted ischemia, nuclear pyknosis becomes very evident; the increasing endothelial cell swelling leads to the formation of numerous endothelial blebs which project into the vessel lumen (22), and the marked swelling of endothelial cells also causes various degrees of luminal obstruction (2,22). *However, it is important to note that not all the cells are affected at the same rate or to the same extent and even after 60 min of ischemia, some endothelial cells remain apparently normal and unswollen (2).*

In the dog heart after 60 to 90 min of coronary artery occlusion, endothelial gaps, stasis of red cells, and the development of platelet and fibrin thrombi are observed (25). The accumulation of platelets in the ischemic tissue is considered to further exacerbate the impairment of microvascular flow (28,36).

Progressive intensification of various degenerative changes, particularly with respect to the continuity of endothelial lining and the integrity of endothelial cell membranes, is observed after 3 to 6 hr of coronary artery occlusion (2). As a consequence of these changes and the associated increase of capillary permeability, an increase in the protein and red cell content of cardiac lymph can be observed after these prolonged periods of myocardial ischemia (13).

*It can be concluded from the morphologic findings described above that, under conditions of severe ischemia, capillary fine structure remains intact during the reversible (5–20 min) and early irreversible phase (20–40 min) of cell injury.* During the latter period, focal myocyte death is believed to occur (22) and after 50 to 60 min of severe ischemia, most of the ischemic myocytes die. *Thus, with respect to morphology we would contend that during severe myocardial ischemia, myocyte damage occurs first; in other words, microvascular damage is not the primary contributor to myocardial cell death.*

### Capillary Changes During Reperfusion

The new therapeutic approach of systemic and intracoronary thrombolysis during acute myocardial infarction, and the introduction of coronary bypass surgery represent logical therapeutic maneuvers for the salvage of ischemic myocardium. However, clinico-pathologic studies (6) and experimental data (7) suggest that reperfusion following severe myocardial ischemia or infarction can precipitate postreperfusion hemorrhage. For example, reperfusion of myocardial tissue in pigs and dogs after 60 min or more of ischemia has been shown to result in capillary damage which gives rise to hemorrhage (7,23). Reperfusion after 3 to 6 hr of occlusion (38) has also been shown to aggravate interstitial damage.

In order to determine whether capillary injury contributes to myocyte death during severe ischemia, Jennings and colleagues (22,26) investigated the occurrence of a "no-reflow" phenomenon of the coronary microvasculature, similar to that observed in the cerebral circulation (32). After 40 min of ischemia, reperfusion of ischemic tissue could invariably be accomplished, and capillary endothelial swelling did not interfere with reflow (22,26). In contrast, after 90 min of severe ischemia, Kloner et al. (26) observed a "no-reflow" phenomenon in the dog heart. In these studies, marked swelling of endothelial cells and myocytes and even disruption of capillary integrity with concomitant extravasation of red cells and thrombosis was observed and appeared to be the main cause of reperfusion failure after prolonged myocardial ischemia (22,26). *However, it should be noted that no-reflow in myocardial capillaries has never been observed before the onset of lethal myocyte injury (22,26).*

## Microcirculatory Changes During Brief or Mild Ischemia

Although the microcirculatory consequences of severe or extended ischemia are quite well documented, relatively little is known about the consequences of mild or transient ischemia. In this section we present what information is available. This involves a consideration of changes in microvascular hemodynamics, effects on the flow characteristics of red cells and leukocytes, and an assessment of the importance of changes in capillary permeability and platelet trapping during ischemia and reperfusion.

### Microvascular Hemodynamics

In considering ischemia-induced changes in the hemodynamics of the microcirculation, we have been particularly interested in *determining whether the reduction in coronary blood flow arising from a coronary artery stenosis (16,24) is a consequence of a decrease in blood flow velocity in individual capillaries or a decrease in the number of capillaries being perfused.*

To address this question we have used (49) an *in vivo* microscopic procedure in both the cat and rat heart. Myocardial ischemia was induced by severely narrowing or temporarily occluding the left anterior descending coronary artery below the origin of the first septal branch. As expected, poststenotic myocardial areas exhibited dilatation of smaller coronary arterioles ($A_3$ and $A_4$ with diameters of less than 30 μm, Table 1). In contrast, capillary and venular diameters did not change significantly. In considering the mechanism of dilatation for the smaller $A_3$ and terminal $A_4$ arterioles, it would seem likely that this is mediated by adenosine which, in addition to other factors such as potassium, prostaglandins, bradykinin, pH, $PCO_2$ and $PO_2$, seems to be the key factor in the metabolic regulation of coronary blood flow (4,45). Within less than 1 sec after coronary artery occlusion, coronary arteriolar dilation can be observed due to the tight coupling between myocardial metabolic activity and adenosine formation on a beat-to-beat basis (4,45).

In our studies (49) we went on to show that despite arteriolar dilation, the decline in perfusion pressure resulted in a marked reduction of mean blood flow velocity in the capillaries and venules of both the cat (see Fig. 2) and rat heart (49). Consideration of pulsatile blood flow velocities in small vessels provided additional information, thus severe stenosis of the left anterior descending coronary artery provoked a flattening of the usual marked pulsatile blood flow velocity profile observed under normal conditions (46,48,49). *In poststenotic capillaries and venules of the cat and rat heart, a marked diminution of systolic red cell velocity and a less pronounced decrease in diastolic red cell velocity was observed. A similar flattening of pulsatile red cell velocity profiles was noted in poststenotic arterioles. Thus, severe stenosis of the left anterior descending coronary artery resulted in a reduction of diastolic arteriolar red cell velocity, whereas systolic arteriolar red cell velocity increased slightly.* This flattening of microvascular blood flow velocity

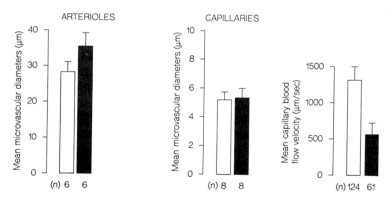

**FIG. 2.** Ischemia-Induced Functional Microcirculatory Changes in the Ventricular Myocardium of the Cat Heart. A 90% stenosis of the coronary artery was induced. The figure shows mean arteriolar diameter on the *left*, mean capillary diameter in the *middle*, mean capillary blood flow velocity on the *right*. The *open columns* represent control values, the *solid columns* are data obtained from the ischemic myocardium 1 min after coronary artery narrowing. The number of individual measurements is shown under each column; the *bars* represent the standard deviation.

profiles is probably due to the loss of contractile force induced by myocardial ischemia.

According to the diminution of systolic blood flow velocity in capillaries and venules, a marked reduction of systolic coronary venular pressure from 25 mm Hg to 12 mm Hg was noted in the ischemic myocardium. Since systolic coronary venular pressure originates from a pressure and volume wave generated by systolic compression of myocardial capillaries (48), *the fall of systolic coronary venular pressure in ischemic myocardium can easily be explained by the loss of contractile force and the reduction of blood flow in the poststenotic region.*

The drop of perfusion pressure in poststenotic arterioles induced by a severe narrowing or temporary occlusion of the supplying artery could also be shown to cause an increase in the distance between plasma-perfused capillaries, as visualized by fluorosceine-tagged high-molecular dextran (49). These data are in agreement with those of Harris et al. (17) who undertook a paired comparison of control and flow-restricted indicator dilution curves. *These authors were able to show that flow reduction decreased the absolute values of tracer capillary permeability surface area and tracer volumes. These data suggest that flow reduction has two effects which competitively affect exchange: (a) flow restriction reduces surface area by capillary decruitment; and (b) the remaining functional capillaries appear to show an increase in permeability to small molecules. The increase of functional inter-capillary distances in ischemic myocardium results in deterioration of regional myocardial oxygen supply, since, according to the Krogh model (27), a rise of diffusion distances leads to a decline of oxygen supply to the third power.*

### *Does Microvascular Spasm Exist?*

Recent years have witnessed the development of considerable interest in the existence of coronary spasm and the possibility that it might contribute to the evolution of ischemic injury. Coronary artery spasm can be provoked by the vasoconstrictor ergonovine. This compound is frequently used in both laboratory and clinical investigation (42). *We have recently used this substance to investigate whether microvascular spasm really exists.* Following the intravenous administration of ergometrine maleate we observed that the drug provoked a marked decrease (approximately 20%) in the diameter of larger $A_1$ and $A_2$ arterioles (ranging in size from 300 down to 31 $\mu$m) (Table 1) and a lesser decrease (13%) in the diameter of smaller $A_3$ arterioles (which range in size from 30 down to 16 $\mu$m). *In contrast, the diameters of terminal arterioles, capillaries, and postcapillary as well as larger collecting venules did not change significantly (47).* Ergometrine also provoked a dose-dependent reduction of capillary and venular blood flow velocity; furthermore, we also observed (47) a slight fall of capillary hematocrit (as judged by the ratio of capillaries filled with red cells to those containing solely plasma). It would seem to us that the constricting effect of ergometrine on coronary arterioles may well be of relevance in explaining the clinical phenomenon of ergometrine-induced chest pain occurring in the absence of macrovascular spasm.

## Effect of Ischemia on Capillary Flow of Blood Cells

In assessing the effects of ischemia upon the microcirculation, it is not sufficient to consider only the vessel wall since changes in blood elements may be of some importance.

### Red Cells

At any given driving pressure and vessel geometry, rate of blood flow through a single capillary is a function of viscous energy dissipation. Under normal flow conditions, the viscous energy dissipation characteristics of normal whole blood are close to those of plasma alone: this is known as Fahraeus-Lindqvist effect (12). However, this desirable blood flow characteristic may be lost if, for example, blood flow properties are impaired or the shear stresses associated with the microcirculation fall below some critical value. *Under these circumstances, red cell deformability may become a limiting factor in capillary perfusion*, and in the arterioles and venules red cell aggregation may further compromise blood flow.

In our experience with rat and cat studies (49), myocardial ischemia is characterized by a heterogeneous capillary flow pattern in respect to red cell distribution. We observed that at the early stages of ischemia a few capillaries in the ischemic region (particularly those with slow flow) exhibited an increase in capillary hematocrit which was suggestive of a leakage of plasma constituents across the capillary wall. Subsequently, 10 min after arterial ligation (in the rat) or severe artery narrowing (in the cat), the majority of poststenotic myocardial capillaries exhibited a drop of capillary hematocrit; furthermore, the red cell content of plasma-perfused capillaries also decreased (49). Thus, while under physiological conditions, approximately 78% of plasma-perfused capillaries contain red cells; in myocardial areas supplied by a stenosed vessel the ratio of capillaries filled with red cells to those containing plasma alone was markedly diminished (49). In addition, temporary myocardial ischemia was occasionally found to provoke red cell aggregation in terminal arterioles and capillaries, thereby exaggerating the severity of regional myocardial malperfusion. *We suggest that these deleterious phenomena may be explained by a reduction of red cell deformability in the presence of a diminished arteriolar perfusion pressure arising as a consequence of severe stenosis of the supplying coronary artery. Whatever the mechanism, the effect must intensify ischemia and accelerate cell death.*

### Leukocytes

Another phenomenon may also help to explain the decline in capillary hematocrit observed during myocardial ischemia. This is the observation that after several minutes of ischemia, leukocytes often appeared in slow-flow capillaries of the ischemic zone. In our experiments we found that the capillary passage time for leukocytes far exceeded that of the red cells. A possible explanation for this could be the lower deformability of white blood cells compared with red cells. Due to this lower deformability, leukocytes tend to plug capillary branches, especially under conditions of ischemia. Using an *in vivo* microscopic technique, we observed that red cell accumulation occurred upstream of a leukocyte-plugged vessel. In these circumstances we noted that capillaries downstream were still filled with fluorescent dextran, i.e., they were still experiencing plasma flow; red cells, however, were not detectable since they could not pass the leukocytes that were trapped at the capillary branch.

An augmented appearance of leukocytes has been shown by Engler et al. (10) to characterize ischemic myocardium. Those authors have suggested that leukocyte plugging might inhibit reperfusion of an ischemic area. This possibility has been supported by our *in vivo* microscopic observations which revealed that a "no-reflow" phenomenon could occur during reperfusion as a consequence of leukocyte or red cell plugging at capillary branches, especially after ischemic intervals of 15 to 20 min. *Thus, leukocyte plugging, in addition to diminished red cell deformability, may be an important contributor to regional malperfusion in the ischemic myocardium. Consequently, it would seem to us that a logical therapeutic approach to the protection of the ischemic myocardium should include an elevation of perfusion pressure so as to enhance the deformability of red cells and leukocytes. This could be combined with the use of antiinflammatory drugs to prevent leukocytes* plugging at capillary branches. Further studies are, of course, needed to demonstrate the efficacy of such a therapeutic approach.

### Changes in Capillary Permeability During Ischemia and Reperfusion

In addition to the hemodynamic and rheological changes induced by ischemia, impairment of microvascular function may arise as a consequence of changes in capillary permeability.

As discussed earlier, our *in vivo* microscopic studies of ischemic myocardium occasionally revealed an initial increase in capillary hematocrit in slow-flow capillaries which preceded the fall in capillary hematocrit observed at later injury. This initial rise may well be due to alterations of microvascular integrity, which then allow the leakage of plasma constituents across the capillary wall. In this connection we have been able to demonstrate an increase in myocardial microvascular permeability in ischemic areas of the rat heart by using a macromolecular iron-gluconate complex and Prussian blue staining. After ligation of the left anterior descending coronary artery and intravenous administration of the macromolecular complex, we were able to demonstrate depots of the complex (which has a molecular weight of approximately 10,000) in perivascular spaces after as little as 10 to 20 min of ischemia, i.e., well within the myocardial resuscitation time (29). This increase in microvascular permeability was quantified using iodine-125-labeled albumin. In these experiments we found that after 10 and 20 min of coronary artery ligation, myocardial albumin activity rose to 199% and 372%, respectively, of the value observed in control tissue. Prolongation of the ischemic period to 40 min did not result in any further increase of iodine-125 accumulation. In similar reperfusion experiments, hearts were subjected to 20 min of myocardial ischemia followed by reperfusion for 5, 10, 15, and 30 min. The results (see Fig. 3) showed that iodine-125 albumin uptake peaked at almost 400% of its control value after 10 min of reperfusion. This value then declined with increasing durations of reperfusion. *This washout of extravascular albumin indicates that the increase in microvascular permeability induced by brief periods of ischemia is reversible.*

### Myocardial Platelet Trapping

Myocardial platelet accumulation after prolonged ischemia is claimed to be an important pathogenic factor contributing to disturbances of microvascular flow (28,36). Recently, we have been interested to ascertain whether this is also an important factor during brief periods of ischemia. We have, therefore, carried out studies in which the accumulation of blood platelets labeled with tritiated diisopropylfluorophosphate was demonstrated in a qualitative manner and used as an indicator of disturbances in microvascular flow. In this study we used autoradiography to detect any increase in activity of labeled platelets in the capillaries of ischemic tissue (29). The trapping of platelets in the ischemic myocardium was quantified using chromium-51-labeled platelets. Hearts were subjected to 10 or 20 min of coronary artery ligation followed by various periods of reperfusion. We found that chromium-51 platelet activity in the previously ischemic area rose significantly during reperfusion, reaching a peak after 10 min of reperfusion. *From these studies we would conclude that, in addition to the various other factors discussed in this chapter, platelet trapping may be an important component of microvascular injury and malfunction even after very brief periods of ischemia.*

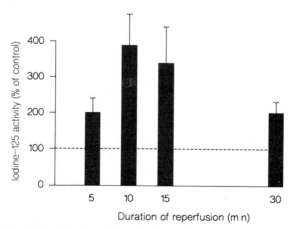

**FIG. 3.** The Effect of the Duration of Reperfusion on Changes in Vascular Permeability Induced by Brief Ischemia. Rat hearts were subjected to coronary artery ligation for 20 min followed by reperfusion for 5, 10, 15, or 30 min. The *columns* indicate the extent of extravascular uptake of iodine-125-labeled albumin expressed as a percent of its control value. Each result is the mean of 4 hearts and the *bars* represent the standard error of the mean.

### Primary Event in Irreversible Ischemic Injury:
### Myocyte or Microcirculation?

The information presented in the preceding sections indicates that after brief periods (10–20 min) of myocardial ischemia major changes occur in the flow characteristics of red cells and leukocytes, and that platelet trapping and major changes of capillary permeability can also occur. These changes, which result in marked disturbances of microcirculatory function, occur well before the onset of detectable structural changes in either the microvasculature itself or the myocytes which it supplies. *This raises the important question: Could these early microvascular changes be important determinants of ischemic injury and cell death?*

According to Kloner and Braunwald (25), the answer is no. These investigators proposed that ischemic damage arises first in the myocyte and this is followed by microvascular injury. It should be appreciated, however, that this claim is based on morphologic data and does not consider disturbances of microvascular function.

Another argument relates to the no-reflow phenomenon which is usually assumed to occur only after extended ischemia (e.g., 90 min) and is conventionally explained in terms of severe endothelial and myocyte swelling together with rupture of damaged capillaries with concomitant extravasation of red cells and thrombosis (22,25). However, we would point out that in our *in vivo* microscopic studies with brief ischemia and reperfusion we were able to generate no-reflow like effects in capillaries, and that this was due to leukocyte plugging and red cell aggregation. In these experiments the ischemia was only 10 or 20 min in duration and these microvascular no-reflow effects were observed well before the onset of capillary endothelial cell swelling. *We would argue, therefore, that microcirculatory disturbances occurring before the onset of structural changes of the microvasculature may well be the primary cause of myocardial cell death.*

## MYOCARDIAL PROTECTION VIA THE MICROCIRCULATION

As discussed in several chapters in this book, many interventions have been proposed for the reduction of infarct size. In general, these are usually pharmacological agents or metabolic manipulations aimed at the myocyte, for example, the use of β-blockers to improve myocardial energy supply:demand status and glucose infusions to promote anaerobic energy production. However, a variety of interventions can be targeted at the microcirculation and, if we are correct that the microvascular lesions contribute to cell death, then good results should be expected. In the following sections we discuss some such pharmacological interventions together with a variety of mechanical and enzymatic procedures that might be effectively used for the protection of the microcirculation.

### Coronary Vasodilators

A number of vasoactive drugs such as nifedipine, nitroglycerine, and dipyridamole have been studied extensively in the context of evolving myocardial infarction.

The results, however, can be complex and certain paradoxical situations can arise. Thus, for example, nitroglycerine and nifedipine are nowadays widely used in the treatment of patients with coronary artery disease (20). On the other hand, dipyridamole, although a potent coronary vasodilator does not relieve angina pectoris. *The basis of such apparent contradictions may be in differences in the vascular sites of action of various drugs,* and in order to identify the site of action of some of these drugs, we have used *in vivo* microscopy to study their effect on the terminal vascular bed of the cat and rat heart (50).

Intravenous nifedipine (75 $\mu$g/kg) and nitroglycerine (30 $\mu$g/kg) were found to provoke, predominantly, dilation of larger ($A_1$ and $A_2$) (Table 1) coronary arterioles, whereas intravenous dipyridamole (0.5 mg/kg) dilated the smaller ($A_3$ and $A_4$) arterioles. With all drugs, the capillary diameter remained unchanged. After administration of nifedipine and dipyridamole, a rise of capillary and venular blood flow velocity was noted; in contrast, after intravenous administration of nitroglycerine, blood flow velocity decreased. With nifedipine and dipyridamole treatment, functional intercapillary distances did not change significantly (50). However, both drugs did provoke an increase in the capillary hematocrit. From these findings we would conclude that the beneficial effect of nifedipine in patients with ischemic heart disease can be attributed to the drug's ability to dilate the larger $A_1$ and $A_2$ arterioles. *The beneficial effects of such a dilatation are reinforced by the ischemia-induced dilatation of terminal arterioles. We would, therefore, suggest that nifedipine may be the drug of choice for protection of the microvasculature during ischemia.*

### Inhibitors of Prostaglandin Synthesis

Several clinical studies have indicated that enhanced platelet aggregation and adhesion together shortened platelet survival time in patients with coronary artery disease (34). Platelet aggregates have been detected in epicardial vessels of patients who were suffering from coronary artery disease and who died suddenly (15). Furthermore, platelet accumulation has been observed in ischemic myocardium following thrombotic coronary artery occlusion (36). These clinical and experimental studies would suggest that platelet aggregation and thromboxane $A_2$ (a potent stimulator of aggregation and vasoconstriction) might cause or aggravate myocardial ischemia by provoking microcirculatory disturbances. If this is the case, then it raises the possibility that it may be possible to use appropriate agents to counteract functional microvascular impairment at the capillary level. We have investigated this possibility by studying the effect of thromboxane $A_2$ antagonist, dazoxyben, and the cyclooxygenase inhibitor, indomethacine, on microvascular permeability and platelet accumulation in the ischemic myocardium of the rat heart. Our results indicate that the increase of microvascular permeability in the ischemic and reperfused myocardium could not be influenced by inhibitors of prostaglandin synthesis. *However, the accumulation of platelets in severe ischemia (after reperfusion) could be significantly diminished by selective thromboxane $A_2$ inhibition.*

## Intermittent Coronary Sinus Occlusion

It has been shown (8,35) that coronary sinus pressure and peripheral coronary artery pressure, distal to a ligation site, increase rapidly if the coronary sinus is totally occluded. This rise of distal coronary artery pressure may arise because of increased antegrade, or retrograde flow, to the ischemic zone. Immediately after elevation of venous pressure, a capacitance change in the vasculature can be observed, i.e., the intravascular blood volume is increased (9). Using the dog hindlimb preparation, Diana and Shadur (9) were able to show that during the elevation of venous pressure, which leads to a marked increase of mean capillary hydrostatic pressure, transcapillary fluid movement is augmented.

*Applying the principle of intermittent coronary sinus occlusion, a number of studies (8,35) have reported a reduction of infarct size in the dog. It is of interest that this procedure appeared to be beneficial even when applied as late as 30 min after the onset of ischemia (8).* During intermittent coronary sinus occlusion, regional function of ischemia myocardial segments was found to improve without there being any impairment of performance in the normally contracting myocardium (35). Despite these promising experimental results, it remains to be established where intermittent coronary occlusion will find any clinical application.

## Thrombolytic Therapy

The results of recent clinical studies demonstrate that intracoronary or intravenous application of streptokinase, in patients with acute myocardial infarction, can facilitate reopening of occluded coronary arteries in the majority of cases (39,40,43). Early recanalization of vessels with total obstruction can lead to a recovery of left ventricular function (1,39,43), particularly in patients with large ischemic areas and severe depression of left ventricular function. *Such findings indicate that early successful reperfusion in patients with acute myocardial infarction can lead to a reduction of infarct size (43).*

Time of reperfusion is clearly important, and current data suggest that the success of fibrinolytic therapy requires a relatively short time interval between the onset of chest pain and the initiation of reperfusion. While estimates vary, the critical time interval for salvage of left ventricular function seems to be in the order of 4 hr in the majority of patients (39,43). The extent of collateral flow in individual patients may, however, alter this time considerably.

If clinical reperfusion is to be advocated, then it is necessary to consider the likelihood that reperfusion injury, particularly hemorrhage, may occur. Here again, the timing of the intervention would appear to be critical. On this subject clinical results are generally in good agreement with experimental findings which document the occurrence of postreperfusion myocardial hemorrhage in pigs following 1-hr occlusion of the left anterior descending coronary artery (7). In this pig study, hemorrhage was greatly reduced if the occlusion period was limited to 15 min. Early reperfusion and the presence of collaterals may protect ischemic tissue from postreperfusion hemorrhage. Clinical observations indicate that a dramatic reduction of infarct size, with concomitant improvement of prognosis, in patients with large myocardial infarctions can only be achieved by restoration of antegrade flow to the myocardial region supplied by the diseased vessel. After successful recanalization of a previously obstructed coronary artery, the rise of arteriolar perfusion pressure may result in enhanced deformability of red cells and leukocytes. The elevation of perfusion pressure may help to disperse red cell aggregates and to prevent red cells and leukocytes from plugging at capillary branches, thus improving regional myocardial oxygen supply.

## CONCLUDING COMMENTS

Early morphologic studies suggested that during severe myocardial ischemia myocardial cell damage occurred first and that microvascular disturbances were not a primary contributor to myocyte death. This viewpoint does not, however, take account of important changes of microvascular function which may occur prior to the onset of any major structural alterations. *Our experimental data on: coronary microcirculatory hemodynamics, blood flow properties of red cells and leukocytes, and platelet trapping and capillary permeability clearly demonstrate that relatively brief (10–20 min) periods of myocardial ischemia can provoke marked functional disturbances of the myocardial microvasculature.* These functional disturbances can be detected prior to morphological changes in the microvasculature or the surrounding myocytes. A "no-reflow" phenomenon at the level of the myocardial capillaries, originally observed after prolonged ischemia, can also be detected during reperfusion following brief periods (10–20 min) of ischemia; this is due to leukocyte plugging or red cell aggregation at capillary branches.

It is our opinion that of all the interventions that have been claimed to reduce myocardial infarct size, the intracoronary or intravenous application of streptokinase stands out as the most logical and promising therapeutic approach. The elevation of arteriolar perfusion pressure as a consequence of reopening of the diseased vessel may enhance deformability of red cells and leukocytes. This may help to disperse red cell aggregates and to prevent red cells and leukocytes from plugging capillaries, and so improve regional myocardial oxygen supply.

## REFERENCES

1. Anderson, J. L., Marshall, H. W., Bray, B. E., Lutz, J. R., Frederick, P. R., Yanowitz, F. G., Datz, F. L., Klausner, S. C., and Hagan, A. D. (1983): A randomized trial of intracoronary streptokinase in the treatment of acute myocardial infarction. *N. Engl. J. Med.*, 308:1312.
2. Armiger, L. C., and Gavin, J. B. (1975): Changes in the microvasculature of ischemic and infarcted myocardium. *Lab. Invest.*, 33:51–56.
3. Bassingthwaighte, J. B., Yipintsoi, T., and Harvey, R. B. (1974): Microvasculature of the dog left ventricular myocardium. *Microvasc. Res.*, 7:229.
4. Berne, R. M. (1964): Metabolic regulation of blood flow. *Circ. Res.*, 14,15 (Suppl. I):261–267.
5. Brown, R. (1965): The pattern of the microcirculatory bed in the ventricular myocardium of domestic mammals. *Am. J. Anat.*, 116:355–374.
6. Bulkley, B. H., and Hutchins, G. M. (1977): Myocardial consequences of coronary artery bypass graft surgery: a clinico-pathologic study of 53 patients. *Am. J. Cardiol.*, 39:268 (abstract).

7. Capone, R. J., and Most, A. S. (1978): Myocardial hemorrhage after coronary reperfusion in pigs. *Am. J. Cardiol.*, 41:229–266.
8. Ciuffo, A. A., Querci, A., Halperin, H., Bulkley, B. H., Shapiro, E., and Weisfeldt, M. L. (1983): Intermittent coronary sinus occlusion beginning 30 minutes after onset of ischemia: a means of profound infarct size reduction. *Circulation*, 68(Suppl. III):16.
9. Diana, J. N., and Shadur, C. A. (1973): Effect of arterial and venous pressure on capillary pressure and vascular volume. *Am. J. Physiol.*, 225:637–650.
10. Engler, R., Schmid-Schonbein, G. W., and Pavelec, R. (1981): Role of leukocyte capillary plugging in preventing myocardial reperfusion. *Circulation*, 64(Suppl. IV):138.
11. Factor, S. M., Sonnenblick, E. H., and Kirk, E. S. (1978): The histologic border zone of acute myocardial infarction: islands or peninsulas? *Am. J. Pathol.*, 92:111–120.
12. Fahraeus, R., and Lindqvist, T. (1931): The viscosity of blood in narrow capillary tubes. *Am. J. Physiol.*, 96:562–568.
13. Feola, M., and Glick, G. (1975): Cardiac lymph flow and composition in acute myocardial ischemia in dogs. *Am. J. Physiol.*, 229:44–48.
14. Fox, C. C., and Hutchins, G. M. (1972): Architecture of the human ventricular myocardium. *Johns Hopkins Med. J.*, 130:289–299.
15. Gallus, A. S. (1979): Antiplatelet drugs: clinical pharmacology and therpeutic use. *Drugs*, 18:439.
16. Gould, K. L., Lipscomb, K., and Hamilton, G. W. (1974): Physiologic basis for assessing critical coronary stenosis. Instantaneous flow response and regional distribution during coronary hyperemia as measures of coronary flow reserve. *Am. J. Cardiol.*, 33:87.
17. Harris, T. R., Gervin, C. A., Burks, D., and Custer, P. (1978): Effects of coronary flow reduction on capillary-myocardial exchange in dogs. *Am. J. Physiol.*, 234(6):H679–H689.
18. Hearse, D. J., Opie, L. H., Katzeff, I. E., Lubbe, W. F., and van der Werff, T. J., Peisach, M., and Boulle, G. (1977): Characterization of the "border zone" in acute regional myocardial ischemia in the dog. *Am. J. Cardiol.*, 40:711–726.
19. Hort, W. (1955): Quantitative Untersuchungen über die Kapillarisierung des Herzmuskels im Erwachsenen—und Greisenalter bei Hypertrophie und Hyperplasie. *Virchows Arch. Pathol. Anat.*, 327:560.
20. Hugenhotz, P. G., Michels, H. R., Serruys, P. W., and Brower, R.W. (1981): Nifedipine in the treatment of unstable angina, coronary spasm and myocardial ischemia. *Am. J. Cardiol.*, 47:163–173.
21. Janse, M. J., Cinca, J., Ganote, L. E., Morena, H., Fiolet, S. W., Kleber, A. G., de Vries, G. P., Becker, E. A., and Durrer, D. (1979): The "border zone" in myocardial ischemia. An electrophysiological, metabolic and histochemical correlation in the pig heart. *Circ. Res.*, 44:576–588.
22. Jennings, R. B., Kloner, R. A., Ganote, C. E., Hawkins, H. K., and Reimer, K. A. (1982): Changes in capillary fine structure and function in acute myocardial ischemic injury. In: *Microcirculation of the Heart. Theoretical and Clinical Problems*, edited by H. Tillmanns, W. Kübler, and H. Zebe, pp. 87–96. Springer, Berlin.
23. Jennings, R. B., Sommers, H., Smyth, G. A., Flack, H. A., and Linn, H. (1960): Myocardial necrosis induced by temporary occlusion of a coronary artery in the dog. *Arch. Pathol.*, 70:68–78.
24. Klocke, F. J. (1976): Coronary blood flow in man. *Prog. Cardiovasc. Dis.*, 19:117–166.
25. Kloner, R. A., and Braunwald, E. (1980): Observations on experimental myocardial ischemia. *Cardiovasc. Res.*, 14:371–395.
26. Kloner, R. A., Ganote, C. E., Jennings, R. B., and Riemer, K. A. (1974): The "no flow" phenomenon after temporary coronary occlusion in the dog. *J. Clin. Invest.*, 54:1496–1508.
27. Krogh, A. (1919): The number and distribution of capillaries in muscles with calculations of the oxygen pressure head necessary for supplying the tissue. *J. Physiol. (Lond.)*, 52:409.
28. Leinberger, H., Suehiro, G. T., and McNamara, J. J. (1979): Myocardial platelet trapping after coronary ligation in primates. *J. Surg. Res.*, 27:3–40.
29. Leinberger, H., Tillmanns, H., Hoppe, S., and Kübler, W. (1982): Microcirculatory impairment following transient myocardial ischemia. In: *Microcirculation of the Heart. Theoretical and Clinical Problems*, edited by H. Tillmanns, W. Kübler, and H. Zebe, pp. 98–103. Springer, Berlin.
30. Ludwig, G. (1971): Capillary pattern of the myocardium. *Meth. Achiev. Exp. Pathol.*, 5:238–271.
31. Luebbers, D. W. (1968): Die Bedeutung des Sauerstoffdruckes für die O$_2$-Versorgung des normalen

und insuffizienten Herzens. In: *Heart Failure: Pathophysiological and Clinical Aspects*, edited by H. Reindell, J. Keul, and E. Doll, p. 287. G. Thieme-Verlag, Stuttgart.

32.  Majno, G., Ames, A., II, Chaing, J., and Wright, R. L. (1967): No reflow after cerebral ischemia. *Lancet*, 2:569–570.

33.  Martini, J., and Honig, C. R. (1969): Direct measurement of intercapillary distance in beating rat heart *in situ* under various conditions of $O_2$ supply. *Microvasc. Res.*, 1:244.

34.  Mehta, J., and Mehta, P. (1979): Status of antiplatelet drugs in coronary heart disease. *JAMA*, 241:249.

35.  Mohl, W., Heimisch, W., Aigner, A., Glogar, D. H., and Wolner, E. (1983): Improvement of regional ischemic myocardial function by intermittent coronary sinus occlusion. *Circulation*, 68(Suppl. III):186.

36.  Moschos, C. B., Lahiri, K., Lyons, M., Weisse, A. B., Oldewurtel, H. A., and Regan, T. J. (1973): Relation of microcirculatory thrombosis to thrombus in the proximal coronary artery: effect of aspirin, dipyridamole and thrombolysis. *Am. Heart J.*, 86:61–68.

37.  Rakusan, K. (1971): *Oxygen in the Heart Muscle*. Charles C Thomas, Springfield, Illinois.

38.  Reimer, K. A., Lowe, J. E., Rasmussen, M. M., and Jennings, R. B. (1977): The wavefront phenomenon of ischemic cell death. I. Myocardial infarct size vs. duration of coronary occlusion in dogs. *Circulation*, 56:786–794.

39.  Rentrop, P., Blanke, H., Karsch, K. R., Rutsch, W., Schartl, M., Merz, W., Dorr, R., Mathey, D., and Kuck, K. (1982): Fruhe und spate Anderungen der linksventrikularen Funktion nach nichtchirurgischer Reperfusion im akuten Myokarinfarkt. *Z. Kardiol.*, 71:2–6.

40.  Rentrop, P., Kostering, H., Rahlf, G., Osten, H., and Keitz, K. (1979): Wiedereroffnung des Infarktgefasses durch transluminale Rekanalisation und intrakoronare Streptokinase-Applikation. *Dtsch. Med. Wochenschr.*, 104:1438.

41.  Reynolds, S. R. M., Kirsch, M., and Bing, R. J. (1958): Functional capillary beds in the beating, KCl-arrested and KCl-arrested perfused myocardium of the dog. *Circ. Res.*, 6:600.

42.  Schroeder, J. S., Bolen, J. L., Quint, R. A., Clark, D. A., Hayden, W. G., Higgins, C. B., and Wexler, L. (1977): Provocation of coronary spasm with ergonovine maleate. *Am. J. Cardiol.*, 40:487–497.

43.  Schwarz, F., Mehmel, H. C., Schuler, G., von Olshausen, K., Manthey, J., Maurer, W., Senges, J., Tillmanns, H., Lenarz, T., and Kübler, W. (1981): Die Wirkung der intrakoronaren Fibrinolysebehandlung auf die diastolische Ventrikelfunktion bei frischem Herzinfarkt. *Z. Kardiol.*, 70:583–589.

44.  Steinausen, M., Tillmanns, H., and Thederan, H. (1978): Microcirculation of the epimyocardial layer of the heart. I. A new method for *in vivo* observation of the microcirculation of superficial ventricular myocardium of the heart and capillary flow pattern under normal and hypoxic conditions. *Pfluegers Arch.*, 378:9.

45.  Thompson, C. I., Rubio, R., and Berne, R. M. (1980): Changes in adenosine and glycogen phosphorylase activity during the cardiac cycle. *Am. J. Physiol.*, 238:H389–H398.

46.  Tillmanns, H., Ikeda, S., Hanse, H., Sarma, J. S. M., Fauvel, J-M., and Bing, R. J. (1974): Microcirculation in the ventricle of the dog and turtle. *Circ. Res.*, 34:561–569.

47.  Tillmanns, H., Moller, P., Dart, A. M., Steinhausen, M., Parekh, N., and Kübler, W. (1983): Changes in myocardial microcirculatory tone during ergometrine provocation. *Circulation*, 68(Suppl. III):33.

48.  Tillmanns, H., Steinhausen, M., Leinberger, H., Thederan, H., and Kübler, W. (1981): Pressure measurements in the terminal vascular bed of the epimyocardium of rats and cats. *Circ. Res.*, 49:1202–1211.

49.  Tillmanns, H., Steinhausen, M., Leinberger, H., Thederan, H., and Kübler, W. (1981): Hemodynamics of the coronary microcirculation during myocardial ischemia. *Circulation*, 64(Suppl. IV):40 (abstract).

50.  Tillmanns, H., Steinhausen, M., Leinberger, H., Thederan, H., and Kübler, W. (1982): The effect of coronary vasodilators on the microcirculation of the ventricular myocardium. In: *Microcirculation of the Heart. Theoretical and Clinical Problems*, edited by H. Tillmanns, W. Kübler, and H. Zebe, pp. 305–311. Springer, Berlin.

*Therapeutic Approaches to Myocardial Infarct Size Limitation*, edited by D. J. Hearse and D. M. Yellon. Raven Press, New York © 1984.

# 8

# Why the Endocardium?

## James M. Downey

*Department of Physiology, University of South Alabama College of Medicine, Mobile, Alabama 36688*

*One of the most consistent and striking characteristics of the pathology of acute myocardial infarction is that the subendocardium is the most vulnerable region of the heart to necrosis* (34,60,61). In many instances, necrosis is confined to the subendocardium. Although transmural infarcts are commonly seen, focal necrosis of only the subepicardium is extremely rare. What is the basis of the increased vulnerability of the subendocardial tissue? Three obvious possibilities exist: (a) residual blood supply during ischemia is less in the subendocardium; (b) metabolic needs of the subendocardium are greater; or (c) the subendocardium is less resistant to an ischemic insult. Surprisingly, *the evidence to date would indicate that all three of these factors may well be relevant* and that the subendocardial tissue continuously faces a triple threat. In the following pages, I present current evidence and my views concerning the vulnerability of the subendocardium to myocardial infarction.

## DOES THE SUBENDOCARDIUM RECEIVE LESS BLOOD FLOW?

### Subendocardial Perfusion in the Nondiseased State

Over the years, the transmural distribution of coronary flow has been examined using many different techniques, and, during this time, the conclusions about transmural flow gradients have changed. This has been largely due to the progressive introduction of new and better measurement techniques. One of the earliest reports was the study by Love and Burch (42) in which they examined the uptake of rubidium-86 by the different layers of the heart. Rubidium-86 is a potassium analog which, when introduced into the arterial blood, passes from the capillaries to the myocytes. Once in the myocyte, it mixes with the intracellular potassium pool such that the probability of any single rubidium-86 molecule diffusing from the cell is quite low. This radioactive marker thus becomes trapped in the tissue, the amount taken up by any region being determined by blood flow to that region at the time the rubidium-86 was introduced. Love and Burch (42) found that flow was uniformly distributed between the inner and outer layers of the dog's ventricle; this conclusion was confirmed by others (10,16,43,47,49,59) who subsequently used the rubidium-86 (or radio-potassium) technique.

One limitation of the rubidium-86 technique is that the movement of tracer into the myocyte is diffusion-limited, as well as blood flow-limited (43). At physiological flow-rates, only about 80% of the rubidium-86 escapes the capillary and enters the myocyte (12), but as flow is reduced, and blood stays in the capillaries longer, there is more time to approach the equilibrium state and the percentage of extraction of rubidium-86 is increased. Since the rubidium-86 uptake is not a single-valued function of flow, its distribution across the heart wall could reflect differences in permeability as well as differences in flow. Investigators, therefore, examined other tracers that were more diffusible than rubidium-86. Paradise et al. (56) examined the uptake of tritiated water and reported an endocardial to epicardial blood flow ratio of 1·11:1 across the heart wall. Radiolabeled antipyrine (27) and xenon-133 (4) distribution have also been examined; both of these markers are highly mobile, lipid-soluble tracers and, again, inner to outer ratios of very close to unity were observed.

In 1967, Rudolph and Heymann (63) introduced the radiomicrosphere method for measurement of regional blood flow. In this method, radiolabeled microspheres of 9- or 15-μm diameter are introduced into the arterial blood. As the microspheres pass through the microcirculation they embolize the small vessels and so become trapped. Even 9-μm spheres have virtually 100% retention on a single pass through the coronary circulation. Microsphere numbers can be adjusted so that an insignificant amount of the coronary vasculature is embolized, and thus flow is not compromised as a consequence of their administration. *Microspheres have become the technique of choice for determining the transmural distribution of coronary flow,* and, in a major review, Feigl (24) recently tabulated 49 experimental studies in which the transmural distribution of the coronary flow was measured with microspheres. *The overwhelming conclusion of that review was that with normal dog heart the distribution of flow favors the subendocardium by 10 to 20% giving an endocardial to epicardial ratio of about 1·15:1.*

## Autoregulation in the Heart

The relative uniformity of coronary perfusion was surprising to early investigators who expected to find a reduced blood flow to the subendocardium. It is now known that blood flow to cardiac tissue is carefully controlled by a process termed autoregulation (Fig. 1; see Chapter 6). Autoregulation, first described in the heart by Mosher et al. (51), is the process whereby blood flow is carefully matched to the heart's metabolic requirements through adjustments of coronary tone. The balance between metabolic need and blood flow is amazingly precise (14) and occurs on a regional basis in each muscle layer (6). Because metabolism is the ultimate determinant of regional perfusion, flow tends to be independent of the physical factors (such as aortic pressure) which govern flow in most other hydraulic systems. *Only when the pressure gradient falls so low that the limits of autoregulation's ability to dilate the coronary vessels has been reached, will coronary flow be affected by such physical factors.*

*It can be concluded that regions of underperfusion cannot occur in a healthy heart having intact autoregulation and patent coronary arteries.*

### Does Coronary Artery Narrowing Cause Subendocardial Ischemia?

Myocardial infarction in the clinical setting often occurs with severely narrowed but still patent coronary arteries (22,34). With incomplete occlusion of the coronary arteries, a full spectrum of coronary blood flows, depending on the degree of narrowing, can be expected.

Griggs and Nakamura (28) demonstrated that partial occlusion of a coronary artery resulted in a selective redistribution of blood flow away from the subendocardium. They assumed that the uniform distribution of flow seen in the normally perfused dog heart was a result of coronary autoregulation, and they reasoned that partial occlusion caused coronary tone to be lost by exceeding the limits of auto-

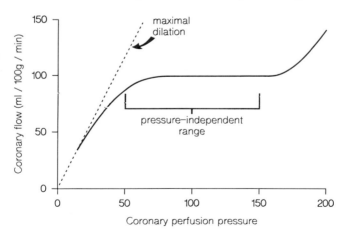

**FIG. 1.** Coronary Autoregulation. Autoregulation of blood flow in the coronary arteries causes blood flow to be independent of perfusion pressure over a wide range. Smooth muscle on the coronary vessels is coupled to the myocardial metabolic requirements by an as yet undefined mechanism. In the healthy heart this process assures an adequate blood flow to the subendocardium. (From ref. 51.)

regulation such that the mechanical influences, imposed on the coronary vessels by the contracting heart, could no longer be adequately compensated for.

Buckberg et al. (9) demonstrated that processes other than narrowing of a coronary artery, for example, aortic insufficiency, could also cause a selective depression of subendocardial perfusion. They pointed out that the one characteristic common to all maneuvers which lead to subendocardial ischemia was that they all reduced the driving pressure for flow during the diastolic period. They proposed, therefore, that due to mechanical forces on the coronary vasculature during systole, flow during that period was nonuniformly distributed away from the subendocardium, and that this nonuniform distribution had to be compensated for during diastole. Downey and Kirk (17) confirmed this theory when they demonstrated that *the systolic component of the coronary flow to the subendocardium is very low.* Forman et al. (25) further demonstrated that the *nonuniform perfusion seen with partial occlusion could indeed produce a selective ischemia of the subendocardium* such that, following coronary narrowing, the contractile function of the subendocardial fibers was found to be severely depressed while little or no functional impairment of the superficial fibers was seen.

### Mechanism for the Redistribution of Flow During Systole

Blood flow during systole experiences a nonuniform distribution that favors the subepicardium (17) and any maneuver that acts to confine coronary perfusion to the period of systole results in a selective and dramatic reduction in subendocardial flow (9,28). The nonuniformity of distribution of systolic flow is well demonstrated by the simple protocol of Russell et al. (64) who showed that when coronary perfusion is maintained from an extracorporeal source, asystole causes a sudden doubling of subendocardial flow while flow to the epicardial layers does not significantly change (see Figs. 2 and 3). Thus, *systole is associated with an impairment of subendocardial flow but has no adverse effect on the subepicardium.*

The impairment of flow during systole is the result of elevated tissue pressure in the deep layers of the heart. The precise magnitude of this compression is, at

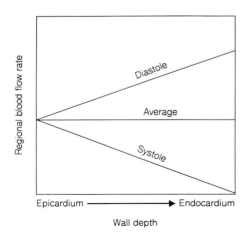

**FIG. 2.** Systolic Inhibition of Coronary Flow. The distribution of coronary blood flow during diastole is very different from that during systole. The systolic distribution is due to a gradient of mechanical compression, whereas the diastolic distribution results from a gradient of coronary tone established by autoregulation. The resulting mean flow is uniformly distributed. When autoregulation's limits are exceeded, as occurs when the coronary arteries are narrowed or occluded, then the heart can no longer compensate during diastole and selective underperfusion of the subendocardium results.

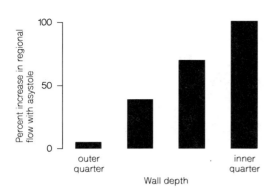

**FIG. 3.** Moment-to-Moment Distribution of Coronary Blood Flow. The inhibitory effect of systole on blood flow to the different regions of the heart can be appreciated in this figure. When coronary perfusion pressure is maintained and contraction is suddenly stopped, flow at the subendocardium doubles while that at the subepicardium is not affected. These results are interpreted to be the result of the abrupt removal of the mechanical inhibition of flow associated with systole. This response was the same for normally perfused myocardium or for ischemic collateral-dependent regions.

present, controversial, however, most agree that it is near zero at the outer surface of the heart but progressively increases with distance across the wall to reach its highest value at the subendocardium. A current point of controversy is whether the maximum value is simply equal to the pressure in the ventricular lumen (7,18,30,52) or whether it exceeds it (3,37,39,70). For the purposes of this discussion, however, it makes little difference; the effect will be the same in that *mechanical compression will severely limit blood flow to the subendocardium.*

Downey and Kirk (18) proposed that the compressive forces in the heart wall reduce local blood flow by forming vascular waterfalls similar to those described for the lung (57,58). In the waterfall model, the pressure gradient for flow in any region is simply the arterial pressure minus either the venous pressure or the tissue pressure, whichever is highest. Thus, if the arterial pressure is 100 mm Hg and the tissue pressure suddenly rises from zero to 50 mm Hg in one region, then the blood flow to that region would be halved. At the subendocardium, where systolic tissue pressure is equal to, or in excess of, arterial pressure, blood flow would stop entirely with each ejection. By contrast, in the subepicardium blood would flow continuously since in that region compression, even during systole, is quite low.

Although the waterfall hypothesis has enjoyed wide acceptance as the most likely explanation for tissue pressure-blood flow interactions, Spaan et al. (69) have offered an alternative explanation. They suggest that during systole blood vessels are pinched off, with those of the subendocardium being slower to open than those in the subepicardium. Regardless of the theory to which one subscribes, *the immediate effect of systole is clearly to divert flow away from the subendocardium. Autoregulation causes a compensatory dilation in the deep layer vessels so that the flow deficit in systole can be compensated in diastole. Thus, in the normal heart, the momentary drop in subendocardial perfusion is of no consequence.*

## Is Collateral Flow Nonuniformly Distributed Across the Heart Wall?

Our understanding of the hemodynamics of the coronary collateral circulation is fairly complete, yet *a great deal of confusion exists among cardiologists with respect to collateral blood flow and factors that control it.* When a canine coronary artery is occluded acutely, perfusion of the ischemic zone does not fall to zero but declines to some low value, usually only in the range of 10 to 20% of its preocclusion value. This residual flow arises as a consequence of naturally occurring anastomoses between the large coronary vessels. In the coronary patient, these collateral vessels often develop in response to ischemia arising from coronary artery disease, and they are often sufficiently clear to be visualized for coronary angiography. In patients with undeveloped collaterals, the collateral perfusion may be below the resolution of angiography, but, nonetheless, some collateral flow will always occur. *The existence of collaterals is important for two reasons. First, the residual perfusion will offer some metabolic support to delay, or perhaps even prevent, the death of myocytes (62) and, second, it provides a route for delivering drugs to the ischemic zone.*

*To date, the overwhelming evidence indicates that coronary collaterals act as artery-to-artery connections (38,66,75),* i.e., anastomoses interconnect major arterial branches and thus deliver blood proximal to most of the resistance vessels. *Thus, when an artery is occluded, collateral flow acts as if it were delivering blood to that artery from a single low pressure source just distal to the occlusion.* The pressure is low because the resistance of the collateral bed is many times larger than that of the ischemic bed it is supplying. The effective pressure which perfuses the ischemic segment can be measured by sampling the pressure in the segment distal to that occlusion, and, in dogs, this peripheral coronary pressure ranges from 20 to 30 mm Hg (73,75). It must be emphasized that the artery-to-artery nature of the collaterals causes all collateral blood flow to be channeled into the occluded parent artery and, thus, *there is no advantage (at least in terms of flow) for a cell to be situated at the lateral edge of an ischemic region.* Indeed, many investigators have now demonstrated that the transition from well perfused to severely ischemic tissue is very abrupt and that no gradients of flow occur at the lateral boundary of an ischemic zone (32,54,68,76) (see Chapter 2).

*There is, however, a definite gradient of collateral flow in the endocardial to epicardial plane.* Current microsphere evidence indicates that during ischemia in the dog heart, the subendocardium receives about one-third to one-half of the residual flow that is delivered to the subepicardium (13,46,62,64). In fact, collateral flow to the subepicardium in the dog is usually sufficient to ensure that the outermost layer of muscle will survive an acute occlusion of a coronary arterial branch. This spontaneous subepicardial salvage often represents between 10 and 20% of the original ischemic mass (11,45,67,77). Comparable collateral flow figures are not available for human myocardial infarction, but *recent studies (40) of human autopsy material indicate a degree of spontaneous subepicardial salvage remarkably similar to that seen in the dog.*

It has been argued that the human has less collateral function than the dog (66), however, it must be appreciated that most coronary patients have a history of either symptomatic or asymptomatic coronary artery disease such that they have already experienced significant collateral development. Therefore, it is perhaps not surprising that myocardial infarction patients have approximately the same amount of spontaneously salvaged myocardium as observed in dogs following acute occlusion of a branch of a coronary artery.

The reduced collateral blood flow received by the subendocardium can be thought of as an extension of the partial occlusion situation described previously. When effective perfusion pressure to the parent artery falls below that which can be compensated for by an autoregulation-mediated dilation, the added impairment to subendocardial perfusion will no longer be able to be compensated for and subendocardial flow will again selectively suffer. Brown et al. (8) proposed that systole occludes the collateral vessels; although this hypothesis has now been disproved (15), it should be noted, however, that systole does elevate the resistance of the ischemic bed supplied by the collateral vessels just as it does in the normally perfused segment (64). Furthermore, the systolic gradient of compression persists even when the segment is ischemic and akinetic (64).

In summary, *although the subendocardium suffers no blood flow deficit in the presence of normal coronary arteries, narrowing of the lumen or complete occlusion selectively diverts flow away from the subendocardium. This redistribution is the direct result of the added compressive forces in the subendocardial region. Because of these blood flow gradients across the heart wall, ischemia will invariably be most severe in the subendocardium.*

## ARE THE ENERGY REQUIREMENTS OF THE SUBENDOCARDIUM GREATER?

### Mechanical Models

In his classical stress analysis of the ventricle, Mirsky (48) predicted that the subendocardial fibers will undergo both exaggerated shortening and greater tension during systole. Although methodology has not been available to prove this high subendocardial stress hypothesis, Sabbah et al. (65) have presented direct evidence that during ejection, while the epicardial fibers shorten by only 10%, the subendocardial fibers shorten by 18%. Fiber tension is, of course, a major determinant of myocardial oxygen consumption; the degree of shortening is also a determinant, but to a much lesser extent. *It, therefore, seems reasonable to question whether the subendocardium may have a higher energy demand than the subepicardium. If that were to be the case, then the rate and extent of development of ischemia would effectively be enhanced.*

### Oxygen Utilization by the Subendocardium

Since autoregulation couples coronary blood flow closely to the heart's metabolic need, one would expect, in the normally perfused heart, any transmural gradient in the rate of oxygen utilization to be reflected in the transmural distribution of regional blood flow. In an earlier section, it was concluded that the blood flow to the subendocardium is probably 5% to 15% higher than that in the outer layers; this, however, is only a modest difference. The total oxygen delivery to a tissue is determined not only by the blood flow to the tissue but also by the arterial venous oxygen difference. Thus, in order to determine a true rate of oxygen consumption, it would be necessary to measure the oxygen content of the venous blood leaving each region. If one makes the assumption that the oxygen content of the venous blood is in equilibrium with the tissue that it drains, then one only needs to measure the tissue $PO_2$ in that region. This approach was first attempted by Kirk and Honig (39) who inserted platinum polarographic electrodes into the myocardium of open-chest dogs. They observed a much lower $PO_2$ in the subendocardium, a finding that has since been corroborated by Moss (50), Whalen et al. (72), and Windbury et al. (74). Tissue $PO_2$ values are in the range of 10 to 15 mm Hg in the subendocardium and 20 to 25 mm Hg in the subepicardium. Although the difference may at first seem small, it should be appreciated that *since these values lie on the steep portion of the hemoglobin dissociation curve, a 5 or 10 mm Hg difference in $PO_2$ could have a profound effect on oxygen extraction.*

The oxygen electrode work has been criticized on the ground that trauma and hemorrhage are bound to arise as a consequence of electrode insertion and that such trauma could affect blood flow and, thus, alter $PO_2$ to the region monitored by the electrode. In addition, since this trauma might be expected to be more severe when the electrode is deeply located in the tissue, the likelihood of a systematic artifact would seem to be great. To circumvent this problem, Gamble et al. (26) developed the technique of microoximetry, a method involving rapid freezing of cardiac tissue. Thin slices of the frozen tissue are viewed under a microscope and small veins are identified. A monochrometer and detector in the microscope are then used to measure the hemoglobin oxygen content in the red blood cells in that vein. *Using this technique, they confirmed a reduced $PO_2$ in the* subendocardial region of the isolated dog heart (26). More recently, Weiss (71) combined microoximetry with radiomicrospheres so that both regional flow and regional A-V oxygen differences could be measured in each animal and, in these studies, the inner to outer regional myocardial oxygen consumption ratio was found to be 1·3:1. Holtz (33), in Germany, using a similar method reported an inner to outer ratio of 1·6:1. It thus appears firmly established that *the subendocardium has a higher rate of oxygen utilization.*

## Metabolic Indicators

One of the most convincing demonstrations of the greater metabolic activity of the subendocardium can be seen in the study by Dunn and colleagues (20) who occluded the entire coronary circulation to produce total ischemia, and after a short time rapidly froze the heart and measured the regional distribution of lactate. *This waste product of ischemia was found in much higher concentration in the subendocardium, indicating more severe ischemia in that region. Since in this study coronary flow was completely eliminated, these gradients could not have been related to flow differences.* When the study was repeated in a nonworking, fibrillating heart, the transmural differences in lactate production were not found, thus adding support to the concept of an elevated work load for the subendocardial fibers (21).

## IS THE SUBENDOCARDIUM LESS TOLERANT OF ISCHEMIA?

Of the three hypotheses presented at the beginning of this chapter, the question of subendocardial tolerance to ischemia is the most difficult to address. The data concerning this subject are extremely sparse but, nevertheless, some conclusions can be drawn.

### Metabolic Gradients Across the Heart Wall

Increased subendocardial vulnerability to ischemia may reflect a reduced pool of energy-rich metabolites in that region. The content of both ATP and creatine phosphate in well-perfused hearts has been carefully examined by many groups (2,5,20,27,35,55) and none of these have reported any transmural differences in the content of either molecule. Similarly, with the exception of a report by Allison (2), neither lactate (20,35,55) nor pyruvate (29) have been reported to be nonuniformly distributed across the wall of the well-perfused heart. These, of course, are static measurements and do not give any indication of the rate at which these metabolites turn over.

*Several reports indicated that the subendocardium may have biochemically adapted to allow it to better cope with its inherent vulnerability.* For example, elevated glycogen content (1,35,36), elevated myoglobin content (31), elevated mitochondrial respiratory capability (41), and even an elevated vascularity (19) have all been reported for the subendocardium. These observations could, of course, be used to argue against any proclivity for infarction of the subendocardial tissue. However, two recent reports indicate that, in spite of these adaptations, the subendocardium may still have a lower threshold for cell death than the rest of the heart. Eng et al. (23) examined hearts in which a coronary artery was temporarily occluded, the segment distal to the occlusion was then opened to the atmosphere and blood was allowed to flow in a retrograde manner from the opened segment. Under these conditions, the collection of retrograde flow causes virtually all of the collateral flow, which was destined for the ischemic segment, to be shunted out of the severed vessel (38,75). Tissue perfusion, therefore, drops to zero, so eliminating any transmural blood flow gradients. After periods of retrograde flow between 20 min and 90 min, the artery was repaired and the dog was allowed to recover for 48 hr. The hearts were then removed. It was found that the dogs experiencing short durations of ischemia had infarcts confined to the subendocardium. With increasing durations of ischemia, the infarct progressed as a wavefront from the subendocardium to the subepicardium as described earlier by Reimer et al. (60) using a simple model of coronary occlusion. The only difference between the two investigations was that in the early study by Eng et al. the dogs did not have a transmural gradient of coronary blood flow.

The results of Eng et al. (23) could have been caused by a heightened metabolic state in the subendocardium. Nienaber et al. (53) suggest that the metabolic state *at the time of the onset of ischemia* is a major determinant of the amount of cell death which will be experienced. In the Eng study, the subendocardium would have had a heightened metabolism due to its mechanical load at the time the ischemia was begun. Lowe et al. (44) overcame this problem by excising a portion of the ventricle and incubating it *in vitro*. In this preparation, not only was blood flow zero but the tissue was also mechanically uncoupled. Nevertheless, ATP was still found to fall more rapidly in the subendocardium, and ultrastructural changes associated with cell death were first seen in the subendocardium. *Thus, a wavefront of infarction, starting at the inner layers, occurred even when both the blood flow gradients and the development of wall stress were prevented.*

*In light of this recent evidence, it would seem that despite all of its biochemical adaptations, the subendocardium is less resistant to ischemia than the rest of the ventricle.*

## CONCLUDING COMMENTS

In summary, and as illustrated in Fig. 4, *the subendocardium of experimental animals seems to be faced with (a) a reduced blood flow reserve due to mechanical compression of the coronary vessels; (b) an elevated metabolic demand due to the augmented wall tension in that region; and (c) an inherently lower tolerance for ischemic challenge. There is no reason not to assume that these conditions also occur in the ischemic patient. Thus, when the coronary vessels become narrowed or occluded, it is of little surprise that damage will first involve the subendocardial tissue and then spread to overlying tissue as the process continues.*

Protection of the subendocardium in the clinical setting has been a frustrating challenge. The most effective way to augment the blood flow reserve would be to prophylactically cause collateral vessels in the heart to develop. Unfortunately, *no really effective means of stimulating significant collateral growth in healthy hearts has been identified.* Several mechanisms have been introduced for restoring patency to narrowed and occluded coronary arteries. Unfortunately, these can seldom be

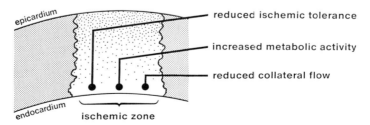

**FIG. 4.** Subendocardial Vulnerability to Ischemic Injury: The Triple Threat. The proclivity of the subendocardium to ischemic injury is the result of three unrelated phenomena: (a) reduced residual blood flow, (b) augmented metabolic need, and (c) reduced tolerance to ischemia.

instituted early enough to prevent a significant amount of cell death in the acute myocardial infarction patient.

How about the stresses in the heart wall which augment subendocardial metabolic requirements and compress the coronary vessels to cause a blood flow deficit? Most of the evidence would indicate that stresses in the heart wall are already at a theoretical minimum, and little could be done to further reduce them and still allow the heart to pump blood. Perhaps the most encouraging developments in recent years have been related to the possibility of raising the threshold of cell death in the heart. Current evidence, as outlined in the other chapters of this book, supports the idea that ischemic cells do not just starve to death but, rather, events occur such that these tissues are damaged by deleterious reactions in and around the cardiac cell. These events might include evolution of free radicals, the activation of phospholipase, the accumulation of toxic intermediates of metabolism, and the loss of purines. Intense investigation is currently under way to try to identify these unfavorable events and find interventions which will counter them. Thus, it is my opinion that studies in this area should provide the greatest opportunity for improving our ability to protect the ischemic myocardium.

## REFERENCES

1. Allison, T. B., and Holsinger, J. W., Jr. (1977): Transmural metabolic gradients in the normal dog left ventricle: effect of right atrial pacing. *Am. J. Physiol.*, 233:H217–H221.
2. Allison, T. B., and Holsinger, J. W., Jr. (1977): Transmural gradients of left ventricular tissue metabolites after circumflex artery ligation in dogs. *J. Mol. Cell. Cardiol.*, 9:837–852.
3. Armour, J. R., and Randall, W. C. (1971): Canine left ventricular intramyocardial pressures. *Am. J. Physiol.*, 270:1833–1839.
4. Bagger, H. (1977): Distribution of coronary blood flow in the left ventricular wall of dogs evaluated by the uptake of Xe-133. *Acta Physiol. Scand.*, 99:421–431.
5. Bassenge, E., Schoot, A., and Walter, P. (1968): Effect of coronary underperfusion on the energy metabolism in different layers of cardiac muscle. *Proceedings of the 5th European Congress of Cardiology, Athens*, pp. 189–195.
6. Boatwright, R. B., Downey, H. F., Bashour, F. A., and Crystal, G. J. (1980): Transmural variation in autoregulation of coronary blood flow in hyperperfused canine myocardium. *Circ. Res.*, 47:599–609.
7. Brandi, G., and McGregor, M. (1976): Intramural pressure in the left ventricle of the dog. *Cardiovasc. Res.*, 39:53–57.
8. Brown, G., Gundel, W. D., Gott, V. L., and Covell, J. W. (1974): Coronary collateral flow following acute coronary occlusion: a diastolic phenomenon. *Cardiovasc. Res.*, 8:621–631.
9. Buckberg, G. D., Fixler, D. E., Archie, J. P., and Hoffman, J. I. E. (1972): Experimental subendocardial ischemia in dogs with normal coronary arteries. *Circ. Res.*, 30:67–81.
10. Cutarelli, R., and Levy, M. N. (1963): Intraventricular pressure and the distribution of coronary blood flow. *Circ. Res.*, 12:322–327.
11. DeBoer, L. W. V., Strauss, H. W., Kloner, R. A., Rude, R. E., Davis, R. F., Moroko, P. R., and Braumwald, E. (1980): Autoradiographic method for measuring the ischemic myocardium at risk; effects of verapamil on infarct size after experimental coronary artery occlusion. *Proc. Natl. Acad. Sci.*, 77:6119–6123.
12. Downey, H. F., Bashour, F. A., Parker, P. E., Bashour, C. A, and Rutherford, C. S. (1975): Myocardial and total body extractions of radiopotassium in anesthetized dogs. *J. Appl. Physiol.*, 38:31–32.
13. Downey, H. F., Bashour, F. A., Stephens, A. J., Kechejian, S. J., and Underwood, R. H. (1973): Transmural gradients of retrograde collateral blood flow from acutely ischemic canine myocardium. *Circ. Res.*, 35:365–371.

14. Downey, J. M. (1976): Myocardial contractile force as a function of coronary blood flow. *Am. J. Physiol.*, 230:1–6.

15. Downey, J. M., and Chagrasulis, R. W. (1976): The effect of cardiac contraction on collateral resistance in the canine heart. *Circ. Res.*, 39:797–800.

16. Downey, J. M., Downey, H. F., and Kirk, E. S. (1974): Effects of myocardial strains on coronary blood flow. *Circ. Res.*, 34:286–292.

17. Downey, J. M., and Kirk, E. S. (1974): Distribution of coronary blood flow across the canine heart wall during systole. *Circ. Res.*, 34:251–257.

18. Downey, J. M., and Kirk, E. S. (1975): Inhibition of coronary blood flow by a vascular water fall mechanism. *Circ. Res.*, 36:753–760.

19. Downey, J. M., and Kirk, E. S. (1975): The transmural distribution of coronary blood flow during maximal vasodilation. *Proc. Soc. Exp. Biol. Med.*, 150:189–193.

20. Dunn, R. B., and Griggs, D. M., Jr. (1975): Transmural gradients in ventricular tissue metabolites produced by stopping coronary blood flow in the dog. *Circ. Res.*, 37:438–445.

21. Dunn, R. B., Hickey, K. M., and Griggs, D. M., Jr. (1975): Effect of loading conditions on transmural lactate gradient in the ischemic left ventricle. *Physiologist*, 18:200 (abstract).

22. Ehrlich, J. C., and Shinohara, Y. (1962): Low incidence of recent thrombotic coronary occlusion in hearts with myocardial infarction studied by serial block technique. *Circulation*, 26:710–715.

23. Eng, C., Cho, S., and Kirk, E. S. (1982): The wavefront pattern of necrosis occurs despite uniform blood flow conditions. *Circulation*, 66:II66 (abstract).

24. Feigl, E. O. (1983): Coronary physiology. *Physiol. Rev.*, 63:1–205.

25. Forman, R., Kirk, E. S., Downey, J. M., and Sonnenblick, E. H. (1973): Nitroglycerine and heterogeneity of myocardial blood flow. *J. Clin. Invest.*, 52:905–911.

26. Gamble, W. J., LaFarge, C. G., Fyler, D. C., Weisul, J., and Monroe, R. G. (1974): Regional coronary venous oxygen saturation and myocardial oxygen tension following abrupt changes in ventricular pressure in the isolated dog heart. *Circ. Res.*, 34:672–681.

27. Goodlett, M., Dowling, K., Eddy, L. J., and Downey, J. M. (1980): Direct metabolic effects of isoproterenol and propranolol in ischemic myocardium of the dog. *Am. J. Physiol.*, 239:H469–H476.

28. Griggs, D. M., Jr., and Nakamura, Y. (1968): Effect of coronary constriction on myocardial distribution of iodoantipyrine-131 I. *Am. J. Physiol.*, 215:1082–1088.

29. Griggs, D. M., Jr., Tchokoer, V. V., and DeClue, J. W. (1971): Effect of beta-adrenergic receptor stimulation on regional myocardial metabolism: importance of coronary vessel patency. *Am. Heart J.*, 82:492–502.

30. Heineman, F., Grayson, J., and Bayless, C. E. (1979): Intramyocardial pressure distribution in the left ventricular wall. *Fed. Proc.*, 38:1038.

31. Hickey, K. M., Dunn, R. B., and Griggs, D. M., Jr. (1975): Transmural differences in cellular constituents of the normal canine myocardium. *Physiologist*, 18:247 (abstract).

32. Hirzel, H. O., Sonnenblick, E. H., and Kirk, E. S. (1977): Absence of a lateral border zone of intermediate creatine phosphokinase depletion surrounding a central infarct 24 hours after acute coronary occlusions in the dog. *Circ. Res.*, 41:673–683.

33. Holtz, J., Grunewald, W. A., Manz, R., Restorff, W. V., and Bassenge, E. (1977): Intracapillary hemoglobin oxygen saturation and oxygen consumption in different layers of the left ventricular myocardium. *Pfluegers Arch.*, 370:253–258.

34. Horn, H., Field, L. E., Dack, S., and Master, A. M. (1950): Acute coronary insufficiency: Pathological and physiological aspects analysis of twenty-five cases of subendocardial necrosis. *Am. Heart J.*, 40:63–80.

35. Ichihara, K., and Abiko, Y. (1975): Difference between endocardial and epicardial utilization of glycogen in the ischemic heart. *Am. J. Physiol.*, 229:1585–1589.

36. Jedeikin, L. A. (1964): Regional distribution of glycogen and phosphorylase in the ventricles of the heart. *Circ. Res.*, 14:202–211.

37. Johnson, J. R., and DiPalma, J. R. (1939): Intramyocardial pressure and its relation to aortic pressure. *Am. J. Physiol.*, 125:234–243.

38. Kirk, E. S., (1980): Equivalence of retrograde blood flow and collateral flow following acute coronary occlusion. *Circulation*, 52(Suppl. III):66 (abstract).

39. Kirk, E. S., and Honig, C. R. (1964): An experimental and theoretical analysis of myocardial tissue pressure. *Am. J. Physiol.*, 207:361–367.

40. Lee, J. T., Ideker, R. E., and Reimer, K. A. (1981): Myocardial infarct size and location in relation to the coronary vascular bed at risk in man. *Circulation*, 64:526–631.
41. Long, J. W., Jr., Martin, A. P., Griggs, D. M., Jr., Dunn, R. B., and Vorbeck, M. L. (1978): Transmural mitochondrial respiration of canine left ventricular tissue. *Fed. Proc.*, 37:230 (abstract).
42. Love, W. D., and Burch, G. E. (1957): A study in dogs of methods suitable for estimating the rate of myocardial uptake of Rb[86] in man and the effect of 1-norepinephine and pitressin on Rb[86] uptake. *J. Clin. Invest.*, 36:468–478.
43. Love, W. D., and Burch, G. E. (1959): Influence of the rate of coronary plasma flow on the extraction of Rb[86] from coronary blood. *Circ. Res.*, 74:24–30.
44. Lowe, J. E., Cummings, R. G., Adams, D. H., and Hull-Ryde, E. A. (1983): Evidence that ischemic cell death begins in the subendocardium independent of variations in collateral flow or wall tension. *Circulation*, 68:190–202.
45. Lowe, J. E., Reimer, K. A., and Jennings, R. B. (1978): Experimental infarct size as a function of the amount of myocardium at risk. *Am. J. Pathol.*, 90:363–376.
46. Marcus, M. L., Kerber, R. E., Ehrhardt, J., and Abboud, F. J. (1976): Effects of time on volume and distribution of collateral flow. *Am. J. Physiol.*, 230:297–285.
47. Mathes, R., and Rival, J. (1971): Effect of nitroglycerine on total and regional coronary blood flow in the normal and ischemic canine myocardium. *Cardiovasc. Res.*, 5:54–61.
48. Mirsky, I. (1969): Left ventricular stresses in the intact human heart. *Biophys. J.*, 9:189–208.
49. Moir, T. W., and DeBra, D. W. (1967): Effect of left ventricular hypertension, ischemia and vasoactive drugs on the myocardial distribution of coronary flow. *Circ. Res.*, 21:65–74.
50. Moss, A. J. (1968): Intramyocardial oxygen tension. *Cardiovasc. Res.*, 2:314–318.
51. Mosher, P., Ross, J., Jr., McFate, P. A., and Shaw, R. F. (1964): Control of coronary blood flow by an autoregulatory mechanism. *Circ. Res.*, 14:250–259.
52. Munch, D. F., and Downey, J. M. (1980): Prediction of regional myocardial blood flow in dogs. *Am. J. Physiol.*, 239:H308–H315.
53. Neinaber, C. H., Gottwik, M., Winklen, B., and Schaper, W. (1983): The relationship between the perfusion deficit, infarct size and time after experimental coronary artery occlusion. *Basic Res. Cardiol.*, 78:210–226.
54. Okun, E. M., Factor, S. M., and Kirk, E. S. (1979): End capillary loops in the heart: an explanation for discrete myocardial infarctions without border zones. *Science*, 206:565–567.
55. Opie, L. H. (1976): Effects of ischemia on metabolism of glucose and fatty acids. *Circ. Res.*, 38(Suppl. II):52–86.
56. Paradise, N. F., Tripp, M. R., Burchell, H. B., Gerasch, D. A., Swayze, C. R., and Fox, I. J. (1976): Effect of nitroglycerine with and without systemic hypotension on canine regional myocardial tritiated water deposition. *Cardiovasc. Res.*, 10:182–191.
57. Permutt, S., Bromberger-Barnea, B., and Bane, H. N. (1962): Alveolar pressure, pulmonary venous pressure and vascular waterfall. *Med. Thoracalis*, 19:239–260.
58. Permutt, S., and Riley, R. L. (1963): Hemodynamics of collapsible vessels with tone: vascular waterfall. *J. Appl. Physiol.*, 18:924–932.
59. Prokop, E. K., Strauss, H. W., Shaw, J., Pitt, B., and Wagner, H. N., Jr. (1974): Comparison of regional myocardial perfusion determined by ionic potassium-43 to that determined by microspheres. *Circulation*, 50:978–984.
60. Reimer, K. A., Lowe, J. E., Rasmussen, M. M., and Jennings, R. B. (1977): The wavefront phenomenon of ischemic cell death: myocardial infarct size vs. duration of coronary occlusion. *Circulation*, 56:786–792.
61. Rabb, W. (1963): The non-vascular metabolic myocardial vulnerability factor in coronary artery disease. *Am. Heart J.*, 66:685–706.
62. Rivas, F., Cobb, F. R., Bache, R. J., and Greenfield, J. C. (1976): Relationship between blood flow to ischemic regions and extent of myocardial infarction: serial measurements of blood flow to ischemic regions in dogs. *Circ. Res.*, 38:439–447.
63. Rudolph, A. M., and Heymann, M. A. (1967): The circulation of the fetus in utero methods for studying distribution of blood flow, cardiac output and organ blood flow. *Circ. Res.*, 21:163–184.
64. Russell, R. E., Chagrasulis, R. W., and Downey, J. M. (1977): Inhibitory effect of cardiac contraction on coronary collateral blood flow. *Am. J. Physiol.*, 233:H541–H546.
65. Sabbah, H. N., Marzilli, M., and Stein, P. D. (1981): The relative role of epicardium and subendocardium in left ventricular mechanics. *Am. J. Physiol.*, 240:H920–H926.

66. Schaper, W. (1971): *The Collateral Circulation of the Heart*. North-Holland, Amsterdam.
67. Schaper, W., Hofmann, M., Muller, K. D., Genth, K., and Carl, M. (1979): Experimental occlusion of two small coronary arteries in the same heart. A new validation method for infarct size manipulation. *Basic Res. Cardiol.*, 74:224–229.
68. Simson, M. B., Harden, W., Barlow, C., and Harken, A. H. (1979): Visualization of the distance between perfusion and anoxia along an ischemic border. *Circulation*, 60:1151–1155.
69. Spaan, J. A. E., Breuls, N. P. W., and Laird, J. D. (1981): Diastolic-systolic coronary flow differences are caused by intramyocardial pump action in the anesthetized dog. *Circ. Res.*, 49:584–593.
70. Stein, P. D., Marzilli, M., Sabbah, H. N., and Lee, T. (1980): Systolic and diastolic pressure gradients within the left ventricular wall. *Am. J. Physiol.*, 238:H625–H630.
71. Weiss, H. R., Neubauer, J. A., Lipp, J. A., and Sinha, A. K. (1978): Quantitative determination of regional oxygen consumption in the dog heart. *Circ. Res.*, 42:394–401.
72. Whalen, W. J., Nair, P., and Buerk, D. (1973): Oxygen tension in the beating cat heart *in situ*. In: *Oxygen Supply*, edited by M. Kessler et al., pp. 199–201. University Park Press, Baltimore, Maryland.
73. Wichmann, J., Losa, R., Diemer, H. P., and Lochner, W. (1978): Pharmacological alterations of coronary collateral circulation. *Pfluegers Arch.*, 373:219–224.
74. Windbury, M. M., Howe, B. B., and Weiss, H. R. (1971): Effect of nitroglycerine and dipyridimole on epicardial and endocardial oxgyen tension—further evidence for redistribution of myocardial blood flow. *Pharmacol. Exp. Ther.*, 176:184–199.
75. Wyatt, D., Lee, J., and Downey, J. M. (1982): Determination of coronary collateral flow by a load line analysis. *Circ. Res.*, 50:663–670.
76. Yellon, D. M., Hearse, D. J., Crome, R., Grannell, J., and Wyse, R. K. H. (1981): Characterization of the lateral interface between normal and ischemic tissue in canine heart during evolving myocardial infarction. *Am. J. Cardiol.*, 47:1233–1239.
77. Yellon, D. M., Hearse, D. J., Maxwell, M. P., Chambers, D. E., and Downey, J. M. (1981): Sustained limitation of myocardial necrosis 24 hours after coronary occlusion: Verapamil infusion in dogs with small myocardial infarcts. *Am. J. Cardiol.*, 51:1409–1413.

*Therapeutic Approaches to Myocardial Infarct Size Limitation*, edited by D. J. Hearse and D. M. Yellon. Raven Press, New York © 1984.

# 9

# How Well Can We Measure Coronary Flow, Risk Zones, and Infarct Size?

Sanford P. Bishop

*Department of Pathology, University of Alabama in Birmingham, Birmingham, Alabama 35294*

The notion that it may be possible to limit the eventual size of an infarct depends on the well-established fact that there is a specific time course involved in the evolution of myocardial necrosis following an ischemic insult. *Evaluation of the amount of tissue saved as a consequence of an intervention depends on our ability to predict the size of an infarct during the early stages of ischemia before irreversible damage has occurred.* This, in turn, is dependent on our ability to measure those variables which can influence the ultimate size of the evolving infarct. These

*139*

factors include: the rate of development of necrosis, the size of the occluded bed or area at risk, and the amount of collateral flow.

The rate of development of necrosis during ischemia has been extensively studied in recent years, but the process remains incompletely understood. It is known, however, that in the anesthetized open chest dog (a commonly used model for studies of infarct size reduction) with a rapid heart rate, at least 20 min of complete coronary occlusion is required for the development of irreversible injury. At slower heart rates, with the chest closed and with the animal fully conscious, this time period is longer. In other species, the time course will also be different; for example, in the rat we have found that irreversible damage occurs with less than 10 min of coronary occlusion. *Unfortunately, the length of time required for irreversible injury to occur in man is not yet known.*

The rate of development of necrosis is not uniform within the ischemic area, and it also varies considerably between individuals. Thus, as discussed in Chapters 2 and 8, it is now well recognized that there is a progressive spread of irreversible injury starting at the endocardium and extending toward the epicardium (30). Development of irreversible ischemic damage is dependent on the length of time involved, functional state of tissue, mass of tissue affected, and the severity of the reduction of blood flow to the tissue. It is the presence of these variables which provides the possibility for preservation of some tissue which eventually would become necrotic.

Just as it is clear that the loss of blood flow to tissue will result in the development of ischemic necrosis, it is also clear that the early return of flow to tissue will result in preservation or the prevention of irreversible changes. *It is this loss or reduction in blood flow to an identifiable vascular bed, and the attendant changes in the tissue, which provide the basis of techniques to identify the extent of tissue at risk in both man and experimental animals.* In this chapter, I explore some of the available methods to identify the tissue at risk, the extent of collateral flow, and eventual size of an infarct in both experimental and clinical circumstances.

## DETERMINANTS OF INFARCT SIZE

### Collateral Flow

From early studies of experimental myocardial infarction it became clear that even when vessels were occluded at the same site there was a great deal of variability in the size of the ultimate infarct. In my laboratory, for example, we observed that proximal occlusion of the left circumflex coronary artery in the conscious dog produced infarcts ranging in size from zero to 35% of the left ventricular mass (4). *The size of the infarct was found to be inversely related to the blood flow to the ischemic tissue, indicating firstly that collateral flow was highly variable between animals, and, secondly, that it was an important determinant of the size of the eventual infarct (see Fig. 1).* Schaper (34) had previously demonstrated that collateral development could be stimulated in the dog by the gradual occlusion of

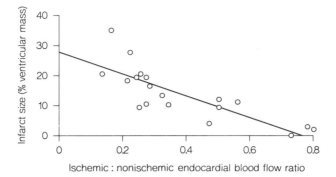

**FIG. 1.** Effect of Collateral Blood Flow on Infarct Size. Infarct size as a percent of left ventricular mass is plotted against ischemic to nonischemic blood flow in subendocardial tissue from the left ventricle 24 hr after occlusion of the proximal left circumflex or left anterior descending coronary artery in the conscious dog. Infarct size is inversely related to blood flow in the center of the ischemic region. (From ref. 4, with permission.)

a coronary artery and that infarction was completely prevented when ameroid constrictors, requiring 1 to 2 weeks for complete vessel occlusion, were used. This observation is of particular interest since it had long been recognized that patients with chronic coronary artery disease often have a very well-developed collateral circulation, and that complete occlusion of one or more coronary arteries can occur without necessarily producing myocardial necrosis (5). *These studies, and others, serve to stress that an ability to measure collateral flow is necessary if we are to be able to predict the outcome of sudden coronary artery occlusion.*

## Area at Risk

In addition to the extent of collateral flow, the size of the vascular bed previously supplied by the occluded vessel is also important in determining the ultimate size of an evolving infarct. *An ability to determine the risk area, or the region of jeopardized tissue, is essential if we are to predict infarct size.* In the dog heart very good correlations have been demonstrated (17,20) between the size of the occluded vascular bed and the size of the resulting infarct (see Fig. 2). In these particular studies, vascular bed sizes, or risk regions, amounting to less than about 20% of the left ventricular mass, did not result in myocardial infarction. However, observations in my own laboratory, and studies by others including Yellon et al. (44) and Schaper (35), have shown that necrosis often does occur in cases where the risk zone is considerably less than 20% of the left ventricular mass. Although the reason for the failure of small risk regions to infarct in some models is not well understood, one explanation may be that with decreasing risk region size there is increasing peripheral surface relative to mass, thus providing greater opportunity for collateral circulation to penetrate the region (35). Another explanation may be related to the size of the heart. Thus, in studies like those of Yellon et al. (44), large hearts were used; under such circumstances, a small percentage of the left

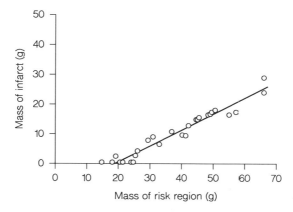

**FIG. 2.** Effect of Risk Region Size on Infarct Size. The mass of the infarct following left cir-cumflex coronary artery occlusion in conscious dogs is directly proportional to the size of the risk region. Risk region was determined from radiograms of barium-gel injected hearts. It is apparent that the infarct mass, as a percentage of the risk region, decreases with decreasing size of risk region, and that for small risk regions, less than approximately 20 g in this model, the amount of necrosis is very small or nonexistent. (From ref. 17, with permission.)

ventricle may well represent a relatively large amount of tissue exceeding the mass associated with 20% of a small heart. However, although there may be some disagreement over the last issue, it is unanimous that it is clearly *essential to be able to determine the risk area as well as the amount of collateral flow if an accurate prediction of infarct size is to be made.*

## Consideration of "Border Zones" and Ischemic Interfaces

The concept of preferential tissue salvage through the timely application of protective interventions depends on the fact that not all tissue becomes irreversibly damaged at the same time. A number of early studies suggested that regional differences in residual blood flow existed within an ischemic region, and it was proposed that "border zones" of tissue with intermediate blood flow occurred and that they provided targets for therapeutic salvage (2,17,23,38).

As has been discussed in Chapter 2, the border zone concept has led to much confusion such that, at present, the very existence of border zones is the subject of controversy (13). There appears to be no doubt that irreversible damage occurs at the endocardium first, and spreads toward the epicardium with time (30). Restoration of blood flow prior to the time that maximal tissue has undergone irreversible damage undeniably results in prevention of necrosis of some tissue. *This observation may be used to provide a strong argument for the existence of a transmural border zone. Whether, however, there is also a lateral border zone is still contested. Most investigators, however, appear to believe that the lateral limits* of necrotic tissue are established very early in the development of an infarct (8,13,24,25,30).

The question of a lateral border zone has been examined by several investigators and is pertinent to the consideration of factors that determine eventual infarct size, as well as the amount of salvable tissue available. Early studies using radioactive microspheres suggested that the lateral borders of an infarct were characterized by a level of blood flow intermediate between that in the center of the ischemic region and that of the surrounding normal tissue (2,17). However, histologic studies of the borders of necrotic tissue revealed a sharp delineation between normal and necrotic tissue. Detailed serial sections of the border zone regions revealed that what had originally been interpreted as islands of normal tissue within the area of necrosis was in fact not islands, but extensions or peninsulas of normal tissue interdigitating with necrotic tissue (15). Further discrediting the lateral border zone concept, it was subsequently shown that the intramyocardial lateral border regions between two adjacent perfusion beds of different coronary arteries did not have anastomotic connections (28). *In support of this conclusion, recent dog studies (25,45) utilizing microspheres, have shown that there is a very sharp change in flow at the lateral border between normal and ischemic tissue.* In one study (25) 3-mm transmural slices were cut across the junction between normal and ischemic tissue beds, the junction having been identified by radiographic examination of vessels injected postmortem with barium. The location of samples with flow values intermediate between normal and severely ischemic were restricted to a 3-mm wide band at the lateral junction, indicating that any lateral border zone of intermediate perfusion could be no wider than 3 mm, i.e., the limits of resolution of the technique. In studies in my laboratory, we have demonstrated a very good correlation between early ischemic blood flow levels and the amount of viable tissue in histologic sections obtained from samples of border zone tissue 48 hr after left circumflex coronary occlusion *(unpublished observations).* The good correlation between histologic necrosis and blood flow adds further support to the concept that the border zone is very sharp and that intermediate blood flow measured with microspheres is due to an admixture of normal and ischemic tissue. Furthermore, in recent studies (46) by the editors of this book, the interface between normal and ischemic tissue was characterized in the dog heart after various ischemic intervals ranging between 5 min and 2 hr. With the use of multiple radiolabeled microspheres they were able to demonstrate that there was no movement in the position or sharpness of the lateral interface during the critical period of evolving injury.

*If a very sharp border zone at the lateral edges of the risk region exists for other species including man, then it will be important to develop methods to identify the lateral borders of the perfusion bed of an occluded vessel. The concept of a sharp interface of flow does not, however, exclude the possibility that a lateral zone of tissue might be subjected to less severe metabolic disturbances that are not flow-*

*related and that could be altered in a way to provide salvage of tissue. However, such flow-independent regional metabolic disturbances have not yet been identified.*

## INFARCT SIZE: IDENTIFICATION AND QUANTIFICATION

*The positive identification of irreversibly damaged tissue early in the course of an ischemic insult, in other words within 12 to 24 hr, has plagued pathologists and experimentalists for years.* In experimental animals a number of techniques using special dyes or stains such as the tetrazolium stains have been utilized to aid in this identification, and the limitations of these techniques have been discussed elsewhere (11,12,47). At later stages, for example after 24 hr or more of ischemia, necrotic tissue is easily recognized in experimental infarcts by gross inspection and this can be confirmed readily by histologic examination. Several methods have been developed utilizing gross or histologic identification of necrosis in necropsy tissue together with computerized planimetry to determine the total mass of necrotic tissue in acute infarction (16,37).

*Identification of regions of necrotic tissue in living patients is of prognostic interest* and several methods have been developed to identify the location and extent of necrosis. The use of various serum enzymes such as the isoenzymes of creatine kinase or the specific uptake of radioactive substances such as technetium-99m pyrophosphate allows at least a semiquantitative assessment of infarct size and an approximate localization of necrotic tissue. But, however useful these methods might be for the clinical assessment of patients, they are of little use in the evaluation of individual patients or animals with regard to the identification of potentially salvable tissue. This is because by the time these techniques are applicable, the previously jeopardized tissue is already dead, and thus there appears to be no tissue left to salvage. Despite their limitation for the detection of tissue salvage, serial determinations of markers such as creatine kinase leakage have proven useful in the identification of myocardial infarct extension. It is my belief that if used in combination with other methods to predict infarct size prior to development, the above methods to measure infarct size could eventually be of value in determining the effectiveness of any intervention, provided that sufficient quantitative reliability can be achieved.

## RADIOACTIVE TRACER MICROSPHERES

Radiolabeled particles injected into the blood stream of animals have been used for many years to study distribution of blood flow to various organs, and with the introduction of uniform-size microspheres, the methodology has been adapted for use in blood flow measurement in many laboratories. The methodology for use of carbonized microspheres was introduced by Rudolph and Heymann in 1967 (33), and problems associated with use of this method have been thoroughly reviewed by Heymann et al. (14). Commonly used radiolabels are listed in Table 1. *Radioactive tracer microspheres have become accepted, perhaps optimistically, by many investigators to be the "gold standard" for measurement of regional myocardial*

TABLE 1. *Commonly used radionuclides for labeling microspheres*

| Nuclide | Photon peak keV | Half-life (days) |
|---------|-----------------|------------------|
| Iodine-125 | 27-35 | 60 |
| Gadolinium-153 | 41, 97-103 | 242 |
| Cobalt-57 | 122-136 | 271 |
| Cerium-141 | 145 | 32.5 |
| Chromium-51 | 320 | 27.8 |
| Tin-113 | 255, 393 | 115 |
| Ruthenium-103 | 497 | 39.8 |
| Strontium-85 | 514 | 64.7 |
| Niobium-95 | 765 | 35 |
| Manganese-54 | 835 | 313 |
| Scandium-46 | 889, 1,120 | 84 |
| Iron-59 | 1,095, 1,292 | 45 |

*blood flow. Although the methodology has many pitfalls that may trap the unwary, in the hands of experienced and vigilant investigators, reproducible information may be obtained in experimental animals.*

## General Principles

The successful use of tracer microspheres requires that several basic principles be adhered to as closely as possible. There are several assumptions that are made in the use of microspheres including: (a) microspheres are thoroughly mixed within the blood stream and uniformly distributed throughout the body according to distribution of blood flow; (b) the introduction of microspheres into the blood stream does not result in abnormal functional changes in the circulation; (c) microspheres are trapped on the first circulation through an organ and that, once localized in that organ, do not move; and that (d) microspheres have rheologic properties similar to that of the formed elements within the blood and are distributed throughout the tissues in a similar manner to whole blood.

## Specific Problems of Microspheres in Studies of Ischemic Myocardium

Among factors that must be given special consideration in the study of blood flow alterations during studies of acute myocardial ischemia are: (a) effect of microsphere size on endocardial:epicardial flow distribution; (b) number of microspheres to administer to insure adequate counting rates in low flow areas; (c) effect of thoracotomy on flow distribution; (d) number of time periods to be studied during the experiment; and, (e) consideration of microsphere loss from tissue and factors affecting microsphere density in tissue. Each of these considerations is briefly discussed below.

### Microsphere Size

The use of microspheres larger than 15-$\mu$m diameter has been shown to result in marked distortion in endocardial to epicardial flow ratios in canine myocardium, and is not recommended for determination of regional myocardial blood flow (14). The use of 15-μm diameter spheres ensures that very little immediate loss from tissue will occur; we have found that fewer than 0.5% of microspheres present in arterial blood are present in coronary sinus blood during the postinjection period when 15-μm diameter spheres are used. With 9-μm spheres, we have found 1 to 4% of arterial spheres in coronary sinus blood. Crystal et al. (9) demonstrated a linear relationship of 9-μm microspheres shunting across the coronary circulation in the coronary pressure range of 100 to 200 mm Hg. We have noted a 50 to 75% loss of 9-μm microspheres over a 6-week period in dogs with systemic mean arterial pressures of 180 to 200 mm Hg induced by uninephrectomy and perine-phritis. Therefore, if coronary pressures will be elevated by the protocol, 9-μm microspheres must be avoided.

The size of microspheres used will affect the endocardial to epicardial flow ratio as mentioned above, since the larger-sized spheres appear to be preferentially carried in the center of the blood stream and distributed to the peripheral areas of the vascular bed (14). In my laboratory, a series of 7 lightly anesthetized but closed chest dogs were given a simultaneous injection of 9- and 15-μm diameter microspheres. Microspheres were injected into the left atrium through a transseptally placed catheter to insure adequate mixing. Left ventricular myocardium was divided into transmural thirds and the right ventricle into transmural halves. Endocardial to epicardial mean flow ratios for the 7 dogs for 9-μm and 15-μm microspheres were 1.15 and 1.38 for the left ventricle and 1.27 and 1.41 for the right ventricle, respectively. Which of these flow ratios more accurately represents true flow is unresolved. However, carefully conducted studies with 9-μm spheres and the diffusible indicator thallium-201 (26) have found a correlation coefficient of better than $r = 0.98$ in canine myocardium over a wide range of flows. *It would appear reasonable to me to use 15-μm microspheres in experiments where loss or shunting might be expected as long as it is recognized that a slight overestimation of subendocardial flow may be made.*

## *Number of Microspheres to Administer*

The number of microspheres that must be administered for each study will depend on the accuracy required for blood flow determination, the size of tissue sample to be measured, the extremes in blood flow to be measured, and other factors related to nuclide counting efficiency. *It has been shown that to attain a 95% confidence limit with the coefficient of variation less than 10%, at least 400 microspheres must be counted in each sample (6).* If $1 \times 10^6$ microspheres are injected into the left atrium of a 15-kg dog with a 100-g heart, approximately 40,000 spheres (4% of cardiac output) will be delivered to the normally functioning heart at rest and each 1-g sample will contain the minimum 400 spheres. If blood flow is reduced as with coronary occlusion, if sample size is reduced to improve resolution, if animal size is increased, or if a variety of hemodynamic changes are induced, it is obvious that the number of microspheres injected must be increased.

Many investigators are routinely administering 6 to $8 \times 10^6$ microspheres to 20-kg dogs at each blood flow study, and others have administered more than twice this number with very little apparent permanent effect on the animal. This number will ensure that samples with less than 20% of normal flow will have adequate counting efficiency even when samples are 0.5 g or less in size. *How many microspheres can be given without causing significant plugging of capillaries and interference with blood flow to tissue?* This question has not been answered in detail, but some simple calculations may help put the question into perspective. Capillary density in dog myocardium is approximately 3,000/mm². Therefore, one face of a 1-g cube of myocardium has approximately 300,000 capillaries. When this number is extrapolated to the entire volume of the 1-g sample, it is apparent that even five separate injections of $8 \times 10^6$ microspheres results in rather insignificant mechanical blockage of blood flow. [Using the above example, $5 \times (8 \times 10^6) \times 4\%$ to heart/100-g heart = 16,000 spheres/g tissue.] Although transient effects on blood pressure and coronary flow are sometimes encountered with administration of large numbers of spheres they do not appear to persist.

### Effect of Thoracotomy on Blood Flow Distribution

The use of fully conscious, chronically instrumented animals has been adopted by many investigators. The closed chest experimental preparation provides many advantages and may more closely approximate conditions in man than the anesthetized open chest animal with artificial respiration. Endocardial:epicardial flow ratios are altered by thoracotomy. In a previous study (4) in which 15-μm microspheres were injected into the left atrium of 27 chronically instrumented conscious dogs, endocardial to epicardial flow ratios were $1.28 \pm 0.04$ and $1.30 \pm 0.04$ for anterior and posterior wall left ventricle, respectively. In 5 separate open chest dogs anesthetized with fentanyl citrate-droperidol-pentobarbital, endocardial:epicardial ratios were $1.04 \pm 0.04$ and $1.12 \pm 0.03$ in the anterior and posterior wall regions. In another study, 9-μm spheres were injected into the left atrium of 7 closed chest but anesthetized dogs (fentanyl citrate-droperidol-halothane), and then the chest opened and a second injection given to the same animals. Mean left ventricular endocardial:epicardial flow ratios decreased from 1.15 in the closed chest condition to 0.90 with the chest open. Heart rates were less than 100/min. *These experiments serve to illustrate the importance of thoracotomy on interpretation of microsphere blood flow data.*

### Number of Blood Flow Determinations

A serious limitation for many experiments is the number of blood flow determinations that can be performed in an individual animal without loss of accuracy. With the traditional method of blood flow analysis using sodium iodide gamma detectors and the "stripping" technique (33), the practical limitation is five or six different determinations, although some investigators claim more. As may be seen in Fig. 3, with sodium iodide crystals, nuclides have photoactivity due to Compton

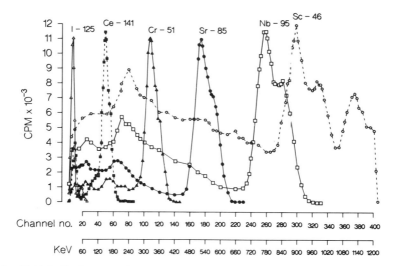

**FIG. 3.** Multiple Radionuclide Spectra. The spectra of the six different radionuclides were obtained from a 3-inch well-type sodium iodide crystal and redrawn to have equivalent height photo peaks. The Compton and X-ray peaks are correspondingly exaggerated, illustrating the portions of the spectra which must be removed by the analysis program.

and X-ray effects in channels other than the one of interest, and this must be subtracted, or "stripped," from other regions of interest. The energy resolution is about 75 keV, thus further limiting the number of nuclides that may be evaluated. The most serious problem with the "stripping" techniques is that errors in the matrix calculation, including effects due to geometry and tissue density differences, are compounded. With the addition of more nuclides, those at the lower end of the keV range are the most severely affected due to repeated "stripping."

Blood flow analysis using sodium iodide crystal detectors and the "stripping" technique requires calculation of a matrix for "spillover" activity of each radionuclide into the other regions of interest. In our laboratory, this matrix is recalculated from pure nuclide samples with each batch of samples analyzed. The total radioactivity in each region of interest, the matrix, tissue weight, and the reference blood flow data are calculated with a computer program to determine blood flow/ g tissue/min. (See Fig. 4 for example of isotope spectra and matrix for an experiment with five separately labeled microspheres).

Improvement in the number of nuclides that may be counted with a sodium iodide crystal is obtained by use of a least squares best fit mathematical analysis of the spectral data obtained with a 500 or more channel pulse height analyzer. Nuclide spectra within the sample are compared to stored reference spectra. *Theoretically, a large number of different nuclides could be separately and accurately counted with this system, but, in practice, eight or nine isotopes have been a practical limit in our hands.*

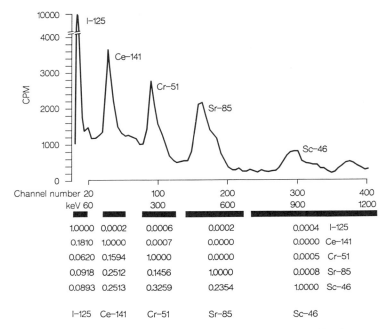

| I-125 | Ce-141 | Cr-51 | Sr-85 | Sc-46 | |
|---|---|---|---|---|---|
| 1.0000 | 0.0002 | 0.0006 | 0.0002 | 0.0004 | I-125 |
| 0.1810 | 1.0000 | 0.0007 | 0.0000 | 0.0000 | Ce-141 |
| 0.0620 | 0.1594 | 1.0000 | 0.0000 | 0.0005 | Cr-51 |
| 0.0918 | 0.2512 | 0.1456 | 1.0000 | 0.0008 | Sr-85 |
| 0.0893 | 0.2513 | 0.3259 | 0.2354 | 1.0000 | Sc-46 |
| I-125 | Ce-141 | Cr-51 | Sr-85 | Sc-46 | |

**FIG. 4.** Matrix Used for Multiple Radiolabeled Microspheres. The combined spectrum for a tissue sample with five differently labeled microspheres collected with a sodium iodide crystal is illustrated. The matrix was calculated from assay of each nuclide individually, and represents the contribution of each nuclide to other regions of interest as a ratio of activity in the peak region of interest for that nuclide. The *heavy bars* under each photon peak define the region of interest.

*A major advancement is the counting efficiency and the number of differently labeled microspheres that can be separated in the germanium (lithium) crystal as used by Schaper's laboratory (43).* With this system, energy resolution is about 3 keV, thus allowing separation of nuclides with closely situated energy photo peaks which could not be separated with sodium iodide crystals. Additionally, there is very little Compton effect, greatly simplifying the calculation procedure (see Fig. 5).

## Problem of Microsphere Loss and Tissue Density Change

In addition to the shunting problems that may occur with 9-μm microspheres mentioned above, it has also been suggested (7) that there is a loss of microspheres from chronically ischemic myocardium. However, Reimer and Jennings (30) have suggested that edema and inflammatory cell infiltration may account for a major portion of this apparent loss. These changes occurring early in the course of an acute ischemic insult would tend to increase the tissue mass, thus giving the false impression that microspheres were lost from the tissue. In later stages of an infarct when scar tissue has formed, there is contraction of tissue with an apparent increase

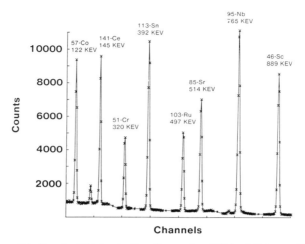

**FIG. 5.** Radionuclide Spectra Obtained with a Germanium (Lithium) Detector. The very narrow photon peaks detected with this type of crystal are readily visible in this sample containing multiple differently labeled tracer microspheres. (Illustration kindly supplied by Dr. W. Schaper.)

in microsphere density (30). *Nevertheless, there does appear to be some real loss of microspheres from acutely ischemic myocardium during the first 24 to 72 hr. However, Murdock and Cobb (24) have demonstrated that even if microsphere loss from ischemic tissue is real, the sharp reduction of blood flow observed during acute ischemia is so great that it essentially renders the effects of microsphere loss biologically unimportant.*

## Application of Microsphere Technique to Follow Sequential Blood Flow Changes

As an example of the use of radiolabeled microspheres to follow blood flow changes in an experimental animal, the following study, performed in my laboratory, is presented. The dog discussed is from a larger series in which the effects on myocardial structure as a result of reflow to previously ischemic tissue were studied. The dog was anesthetized with fentanyl citrate-droperidol-halothane-nitrous oxide and studied with the chest open. A major marginal branch and diagonal branch of the left circumflex and anterior descending coronary arteries were sequentially occluded 30 min apart with reflow after 60 min of ischemia to the first occluded artery. Differently labeled 9-μm microspheres were injected into the left atrium prior to occlusion, during occlusion, and during the immediate postrelease period, reference blood flow collected from the terminal aorta, and blood flow determined by gamma spectrometry using the "stripping" technique. Regional myocardial blood flow from three layers of a single slice from the left ventricle including the ischemic areas is shown in Fig. 6. This method of blood flow presentation, popularized by Schaper (35), illustrates the similarity of flow from different circumferential positions and the same transmural layer, the sharp change in blood flow at the margins

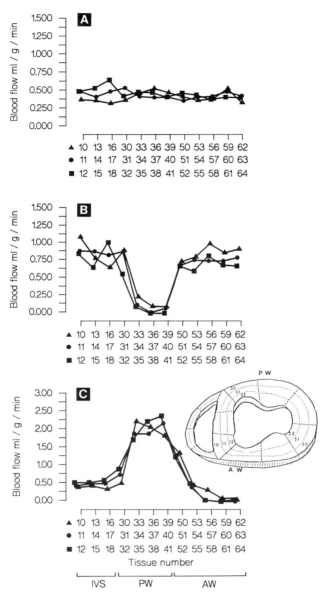

**FIG. 6.** Regional Myocardial Blood Flow During Experimental Myocardial Ischemia. Blood flow in a midregion slice of the left ventricle is illustrated. The dog was prepared as described in the text. Location of numbered tissue samples is as shown in the diagram. **A:** Blood flow during basal state prior to occlusion; **B:** 10 min after first major marginal branch of circumflex coronary artery occluded; **C:** immediately after marginal artery reflow established and first major diagonal of left anterior descending coronary artery occluded. Reactive hyperemia is evident. Note change of scale in **C.** IVS: intraventricular septum; PW: posterior wall; AW: anterior wall; *triangle:* subepicardial samples; *circle:* midwall samples; *square:* subendocardial samples.

of the ischemic area, and the changes in blood flow such as induced by reactive hyperemia.

## RISK AREA: IDENTIFICATION AND QUANTIFICATION IN EXPERIMENTAL ANIMALS

The two major determinants of infarct size in an individual animal are the size of the perfusion bed of the occluded artery, i.e., the risk area, and the amount of collateral flow to this area. As discussed, the amount of collateral flow delivered to the ischemic myocardium is highly variable but, in general, it is inversely related to the size of the vascular bed (35).

Several studies have now confirmed the earlier results of Jugdutt et al. (17) and Rivas et al. (32) both of which demonstrated a very good correlation between infarct size and the risk size. These two groups of investigators used different methods to delineate the region at risk (a factor which may account for the different percentage of risk area which became infarcted in the two studies) but the tight association between infarct size and risk zone was clearly evident in both studies. *It is now abundantly clear that any study endeavoring to evaluate the potential effects of a surgical or therapeutic intervention on infarct size must consider the size of the perfusion bed of the occluded artery.* The anatomic limits of the perfusion beds of the coronary arteries in the dog have been studied by a variety of methods.

### Barium Radiography

Schaper (34) injected canine coronary vessels with a fluid barium-gel that was then allowed to harden during the fixation of the tissue in formalin. The fixed hearts were then sliced into horizontal sections of approximately 1.0 cm thickness, and radiographs were then prepared from the slices (see Fig. 7). By visual inspection of the different coronary arteries on the radiographs, the junction between adjacent vascular beds could be identified. This technique has been used by other investigators (17,25) and *is certainly an acceptable and reproducible method of determining the perfusion bed of an occluded artery.*

### Dyes and Colored Resins

A number of other investigators have outlined perfusion beds by injecting occluded coronary arteries with colored dyes (see Fig. 8) or vinyl (20,32). Although this method is useful, *it is likely that even with relatively short periods of ischemia, and particularly with extended periods of ischemia lasting more than several hours, that flow through the ischemic vessels will be impaired and the size of the occluded vascular bed will be underestimated.* Scheel and colleagues have undertaken a detailed study of the entire coronary vascular bed of the dog using Microfil injection techniques (36), and in this study a sharp demarcation between various vascular beds was demonstrated and a strong correlation was revealed between the size of the bed and flow to the bed under conditions of maximal vasodilation.

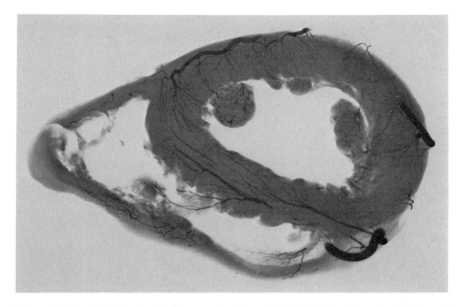

**FIG. 7.** Barium-Gel Injection Radiogram of a Human Heart. The heart was fixed in formalin after injecting the coronary arteries with a barium-gel mixture. The vascular beds of each coronary artery are easily visualized in this type of preparation with the aid of stereoscopic examination.

## Radioactive Microspheres

Radioactive microspheres are an established technique in the study of regional blood flow (6,14,33) and they have been used extensively in a variety of manners to demonstrate the perfusion limits of a coronary bed. Hirzel et al (15) have, for example, utilized a shadow technique in which the perfusion bed under investigation is perfused at normal pressure with microsphere-free blood while at the same time microspheres are circulated to the rest of the myocardium. This method is useful for determining collateral blood flow to tissue under conditions of normal perfusion pressure in both vascular beds.

Hirzel et al. (15) have also demonstrated the important point that *when used in the absence of perfusion pressure in the occluded bed, the microsphere technique slightly underestimates the extent of the perfusion bed*. Recent studies by Murdock et al. (25) have confirmed this conclusion. However, as discussed in the next section, quantification of microspheres in the risk area does provide a measure of collateral flow to that area during occlusion.

## Autoradiography

Several investigators (10,21,44,47) have used autoradiography to define the normally perfused myocardium in experiments where microspheres or other radioactive substances are injected during the occlusion period. After fixation or freezing of the heart, autoradiograms are prepared from sequential tissue slices so as to outline

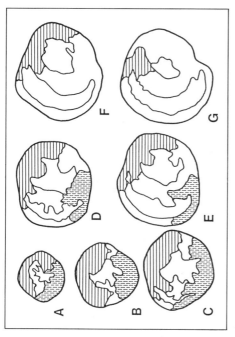

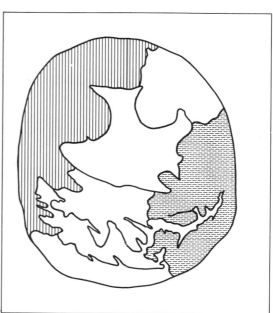

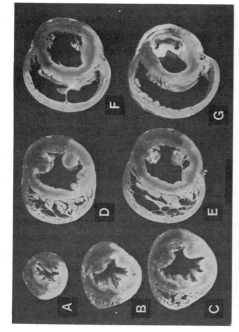

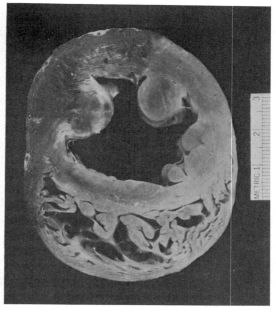

the area served by the occluded artery (see Fig. 9). The mass of an occluded vascular bed can also be determined in hearts given microspheres during the occlusion period, by summing the weights of all tissues with less than 50% (or some other arbitrary value) of the nonischemic tissue radioactivity. Such a method is useful in studies in which, for technical reasons, injection of the coronary vascular system with dyes or barium is not possible, but, as mentioned earlier, *use of radioactive microspheres injected during the occlusion period may result in an underestimation of the true risk region due to entry of microspheres by collateral flow.*

## COLLATERAL FLOW: QUANTIFICATION IN EXPERIMENTAL ANIMALS

As stressed earlier, the extent of collateral circulation to an ischemic zone is a major determinant of tissue survival. This collateral supply can vary greatly between species and between individuals and can be influenced by a number of factors. Schaper (35), for example, demonstrated an inverse relationship between the extent of collateral circulation and the size of the perfusion bed. *Any prediction of infarct size reduction must be based on a knowledge of the residual or collateral flow to the tissue,* and a number of methods exist for the measurement of this flow in experimental animals.

### Radioactive Microspheres

The most readily available and widely used method for determination of collateral flow to an occluded vascular bed involves the use of radioactive microspheres (1,2,4,8,17,32,35,44,46). Although this method is reliable in demonstrating the presence of flow, the method does suffer several important disadvantages as discussed previously (6,7,9). Counting efficiency is less reliable at low flows, thus making even minor contamination with normally perfused tissue a significant problem. A further disadvantage is that only relatively few separate measurements can be conducted in a single heart. Therefore, the method is of limited usefulness in the evaluation of flow changes occurring sequentially during changing experimental conditions. *In spite of these deficiencies, the microsphere method is likely to remain a valuable and reliable method for definition of risk region and the measurement of collateral flow.*

---

**FIG. 8.** Dye Injection Method to Identify Risk Area in a Dog Heart. A 10% dextran solution containing 1% either Monastral blue dye (dark area, posterior wall at top of sections: *horizontal, solid lines*) or Monastral yellow dye (light, poorly defined area in black and white photograph, anterior wall: *vertical, hashed lines*) was injected into the circumflex or anterior descending branches of the left coronary artery respectively at the point of occlusion. Single section is an enlargement of slice D. Heart was immersion fixed in 10% formalin after dye injection. Perfusion bed limits are sharply outlined in color photographs and the mass may be readily quantified with standard digitizer methods. The method works equally well by injecting the nonoccluded vascular bed and leaving the occlusive tie in place to prevent staining of the perfusion bed, thus avoiding possible perfusion defect artifacts induced by prolonged ischemia or reflow.

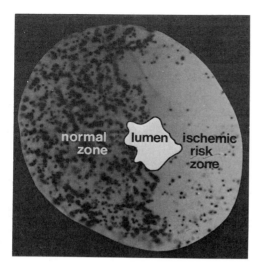

**FIG. 9.** Autoradiogram of Canine Heart with Left Anterior Descending Coronary Artery Occlusion. Cerium-141 microspheres were injected during occlusion of the anterior descending coronary artery. The heart was removed from the dog at the end of the experiment, frozen, and an autoradiogram prepared from a slice through the midregion of the left ventricle. (Illustration kindly supplied by Dr. D. Yellon.)

### Retrograde Flow and Peripheral Coronary Pressure

The traditional method of studying collateral flow to an obstructed vascular bed is to measure the pressure in a coronary artery distal to the occlusion, i.e., peripheral coronary pressure, or to measure the flow from the distal end of a transected artery occluded proximally. Both methods have been criticized because of differences in opposing resistance present in the open chest experimental animal with a transected coronary artery open to air rather than to a closed vascular bed. Furthermore, collateral flow may be diverted from the cannula by the distal vasculature of the occluded vessels. Nevertheless, the methods do provide a measure of flow to an occluded vascular bed via collaterals, which may be monitored constantly over several hours to evaluate changes due to alterations in experimental conditions.

To circumvent the disadvantages of the microsphere method, Wyatt et al. (42) have recently proposed a method allowing repeated measurement of collateral flow in the open chest dog. In this method collateral flow is calculated from measured peripheral coronary pressure and aortic pressure. This system offers the additional advantage of economy.

## METHODS FOR MEASURING REGIONAL MYOCARDIAL BLOOD FLOW, RISK ZONES, AND INFARCT SIZE IN MAN

### Myocardial Blood Flow

Myocardial blood flow has been evaluated in man and animals by many different techniques. The use of inert gases and diffusible substances such as helium, hydrogen, nitrogen, antipyrene, and xenon has provided important information relating to myocardial blood flow under normal and pathologic conditions. By the selective placement of catheters in various positions in the coronary sinus, estimates of flow from the anterior wall or total left ventricle may be obtained. The methods for determination of myocardial blood flow with diffusible indicators have been reviewed by Klocke (18). Other methods have been applied to the measurement of myocardial blood flow in man which provide estimates of flow to the entire heart or a vascular bed of a single coronary artery. These include: (a) specially designed ultrasonic flowmeters applied to epicardial coronary arteries during open chest surgical procedures, (b) videodensitometry in which videographically recorded density of injected radiographic contrast media is quantified over time in selected coronary vessels, (c) thermodilution following coronary vein injection of cooled fluid and thermistor measurement in the coronary sinus, and (d) use of positron emission tomography. The latter method is basically a diffusible indicator technique employing short-lived positron emitting radionuclides; the method holds considerable promise of providing accurate blood flow measurement in man. *These methods are useful for identification of major abnormalities in flow from different regions of the myocardium, but, at present do not provide sufficient sensitivity to be useful in the quantitation of the amount of ischemic myocardium.*

### Methods that Identify Ischemic or Necrotic Myocardium

#### Infarct-Avid Agents

Imaging of myocardial infarction has progressed remarkably over the past two decades [for recent review see Marcus et al. (22)]. Several infarct-avid imaging agents have been developed which are selectively localized in ischemic myocardium and, as such, they are useful to identify the location of necrotic myocardium accurately. The most useful of these is technetium-99m-pyrophosphate, which, following intravenous administration, can provide detailed scintigrams. Other agents, including radiolabeled anticardiac myosin antibodies and polymorphonuclear leukocytes, have also been recently proposed. *However, although these agents are undoubtedly useful in identifying the location of an infarct, at present they are of less value in the quantification of the amount of infarction. However, with the development of newer techniques for computerized tomography, these infarct-avid agents should eventually provide the means for very accurate measurement of the amount of tissue necrosis.* When used in combination with methods to predict the amount of infarction during early stages of acute myocardial infarction, these techniques are also likely to prove useful adjuncts for evaluation of methods to limit infarct size in man.

#### Agents Taken Up by Normal Tissue

Agents selectively removed from the blood by normal myocardium have been very useful in the identification of regional areas of poor perfusion, and thallium-201 has been the most useful of these (27,39). Thallium-201 is rapidly removed from the blood by viable myocardial cells and is concentrated intracellularly in much the same manner as potassium. After its administration, thallium-201 is distributed in myocardial tissue in a very similar manner to radioactive microspheres (26), and in the closed chest dog, it exhibits an increasing accumulation from epicardium to endocardium. When thallium-201 is given intravenously to patients with acute coronary occlusion, the poorly perfused areas of myocardium are readily visualized on scintigrams. Wackers and associates (40) were able to demonstrate that when thallium-201 was given within the first 6 hr of acute myocardial infarction, very good correlation existed between images obtained during life and the distribution of lesion and thallium-201 in the myocardium of patients who died within 2 to 5 days following the study. The relatively rapid equilibration of thallium-201 between the tissues and the blood has provided a useful tool for the study of regions of temporary ischemia induced by exercise (3,31). Thus, this agent provides a useful means to identify both chronic myocardial ischemia and the acute lesion. However, it must be remembered that the detection of a focal area of myocardium that does not accumulate thallium-201 may well indicate old scar tissue, which could easily be confused with recent areas of acute ischemia. The use of thallium-201 holds much promise for the future, since with improvements in resolution, it may be possible to identify accurately and to quantitate the area at risk early in the course of acute myocardial infarction in man. *Combined with methods to evaluate the extent of collateral blood flow to the ischemic region, the method may thus prove highly valuable for evaluating revascularization or therapeutic treatments designed to salvage jeopardized myocardium.*

### Degradable Microspheres

Another method used to identify focal perfusion defects in the myocardium involves the injection of macroaggregated albumin spheres labeled with indium-133, technetium-99m, or iodine-131. These biodegradable particles are injected into the left atrium or directly into a coronary artery and, like radioactive microspheres, are trapped in the capillaries in proportion to blood flow. *Unfortunately, quantitation of blood flow with this method has been difficult* due to: inaccuracies in determining the amount of material injected, inhomogeneities in the images obtained, and streaming defects due to coronary artery injection which can lead to a selective distribution of the particles. In addition, the method requires invasive techniques and is not able to be repeated at frequent intervals.

### Newer Techniques for Measurement of Risk Zones and Infarct Size in Man

There are several new methods holding great promise for the more precise localization and quantitation of risk zones and infarct size. These include positron emission tomography (PET), computerized tomography with fast scanners (fast CT), and nuclear magnetic resonance (NMR). Some of these methods do not require injection of foreign substances into the body, whereas in others it is possible to rely on the administration of markers with very short half-lives which may be repeatedly injected after relatively short intervals, thus allowing repeated examination.

Edema is an early change in ischemic myocardium and it precedes the development of irreversible damage. Both CT and NMR techniques are able to recognize a variety of edema-induced physical or biochemical alterations including changes in density, thus providing a means for the identification of tissue at risk very early in the ischemic course. At present, the resolving power of these techniques is insufficient for the precision in quantitation needed for the evaluation of tissue salvage. However, there is a tremendous amount of current interest in these methods and their improvement; advanced equipment is now becoming available, and *it can be expected that, despite their high cost, these techniques will find considerable application in the near future.* (For reviews of the current status of these procedures see refs. 19, 27, 29, and 41.)

## CONCLUDING COMMENTS

The many studies related to the salvage of ischemic myocardium, which have been conducted over the past few years, have provided considerable information that will aid in the design of future studies aimed at identifying factors which reduce the size of an infarct. Utilizing our knowledge that a good correlation exists between the predicted size of an infarct and the size of the occluded vascular bed, or area at risk, coupled with our ability to measure collateral flow, it should now be possible to predict infarct size in individual animals and detect deviations from this prediction. This should allow investigators to reduce the number of animals required to evaluate a particular intervention.

In experimental animals the use of radioactive tracer microspheres provides us with a means for measuring collateral flow as well as a means of defining the perfusion limits of tissue. Barium-gel injections of the vascular system and microsphere autoradiographic techniques can now be routinely used and reproducible methods exist for the identification of the boundaries of nonperfused tissue, all of which should enable us to define relatively precise locations for regions of perfused and nonperfused tissue.

Studies in man are of course more difficult since, at present, there are no readily available methods that allow accurate identification and quantification of the risk region and collateral flow in patients at an early stage of an acute myocardial infarction. *I would stress yet again, that until we are able to measure the size of a perfusion bed of an occluded artery in man accurately, we cannot quantitatively predict or evaluate the effects of agents that purport to reduce infarct size.* However, several new methodologies are appearing on the horizon and should be available in the near future. These techniques include PET, fast CT scans, and NMR. With active research with these new techniques, *it is my belief that methods will soon be available to predict accurately infarct size in individual patients prior to the development of irreversible injury.* The development of these new techniques will, therefore, finally allow the evaluation of interventions designed to limit the extent of myocardial infarction in man. However, until that time, we remain reliant on carefully executed experimental studies designed to assess the likely efficacy of antiinfarct agents.

## REFERENCES

1. Becker, L. C., Fortuin, N. J., and Pitt, B. (1971): Effect of ischemia and antianginal drugs on the distribution of radioactive microspheres in the canine left ventricle. *Circ. Res.*, 28:263–269.
2. Becker, L. C., Ferreira, R., and Thomas, M. (1973): Mapping of left ventricular blood flow with radioactive microspheres in experimental coronary artery occlusion. *Cardiovasc. Res.*, 7:391–400.
3. Beller, G. A., Watson, D. D., Ackell, P., and Pohost, G. M. (1980): Time course of Thallium-201 redistribution after transient myocardial ischemia. *Circulation*, 61:791–797.
4. Bishop, S. P., White, F. C., and Bloor, C. M. (1976): Regional myocardial blood flow during acute myocardial infarction in the conscious dog. *Circ. Res.*, 38:429–438.
5. Blumgart, H. L., Schlesinger, M. J., and Davis, D. (1940): Studies on the relation of the clinical manifestations of angina pectoris, coronary thrombosis and myocardial infarction to the pathologic findings, with particular reference to the significance of collateral circulation. *Am. Heart J.*, 19:1–91.
6. Buckberg, G. D., Luck, J. C., Payne, D. B., Hoffman, J. I. E., Archie, J. P., and Fixler, D. E. (1971): Some sources of error in measuring regional blood flow with radioactive microspheres. *J. Appl. Physiol.*, 31:598–604.
7. Capurro, N. L., Goldstein, R. E., Aamodt, R., Smith, H. J., and Epstein, S. E. (1979): Loss of microspheres from ischemic canine cardiac tissue: An important technical limitation. *Circ. Res.*, 44:223–227.
8. Cobb, F. R., Murdock, R. H., Jr., and Morris, K. G. (1982): Regional myocardial blood flow: A model for assessing intervention therapy in the conscious animal. In: *Myocardial Infarction: Measurement and Intervention*, edited by G. S. Wagner, pp. 273–293. Martinus Nijhoff, The Hague.
9. Crystal, G. J., Boatwright, R. B., Downey, H. F., and Bashour, F. A. (1979): Shunting of microspheres across the canine coronary circulation. *Am. J. Physiol.*, 236:H7–H12.
10. DeBoer, L. W. V., Strauss, H. W., Kloner, R. A., Rude, R. E., Davis, R. F., Moroko, P. R., and Braunwald, E. (1980): Autoradiographic method for measuring the ischemic myocardium at risk; effects of verapamil on infarct size after experimental coronary artery occlusion. *Proc. Natl. Acad. Sci.*, 77:6119–6123.
11. Fallon, J. T. (1982): Postmortem: Histochemical techniques. In: *Myocardial Infarction: Measurement and Intervention*, edited by G. S. Wagner, pp. 373–384. Martinus Nijhoff, The Hague.
12. Fishbein, M. C., Meerbaum, S., Rit, J., Lando, U., Kanmatsuse, K., Mercier, J. C., Corday, E., and Ganz, W. (1981): Early phase acute myocardial infarct size quantification: Validation of the triphenyl tetrazolium chloride tissue enzyme staining techniques. *Am. Heart J.*, 101:593–600.
13. Hearse, D. J., and Yellon, D. M. (1981): The "Border Zone" in evolving myocardial infarction: Controversy or confusion? *Am. J. Cardiol.*, 47:1321–1334.
14. Heymann, M. A., Payne, D. B., Hoffman, J. I. E., and Rudolph, A. M. (1977): Blood flow measurements with radionuclide-labelled particles. *Prog. Cardiovasc. Dis.*, 20:55.
15. Hirzel, H. O., Sonnenblick, E. H., and Kirk, E. S. (1977): Absence of a lateral border zone of intermediate creatine phosphokinase depletion surrounding a central infarct 24 hours after acute coronary occlusion in the dog. *Circ. Res.*, 41:673–683.
16. Ideker, R. E., Hackel, D. B., and McClees, E. C. (1982): Postmortem: Anatomic quantitation. In: *Myocardial Infarction: Measurement and Intervention*, edited by G. S. Wagner, pp. 347–371. Martinus Nijhoff, The Hague.
17. Jugdutt, B. I., Hutchins, G. M., Bulkley, B. H., and Becker, L. C (1979): Myocardial infarction in the conscious dog: Three-dimensional mapping of infarct, collateral flow and region at risk. *Circulation*, 60:1141–1150.
18. Klocke, F. J. (1976): Coronary blood flow in man. In: *Progress in Cardiovascular Diseases*, pp. 117–166. Grune & Stratton, New York.
19. Lerch, R. A., Ambos, H. D., Bergmann, S. R., Welch, M. J., Ter-Pogossian, M. M., and Sobel,

B. E. (1981): Localization of viable, ischemic myocardium by positron-emission tomography with [11]C-palmitate. *Circulation*, 64:689–698.

20. Lowe, J. E., Reimer, K. A., and Jennings, R. B. (1978): Experimental infarct size as a function of the amount of myocardium at risk. *Am. J. Pathol.*, 90:363–380.

21. Malsky, P. M., Vokonas, P. S., Paul, S. J., Robbins, S. L., Hood, W. B., Jr. (1977): Autoradiographic measurement of regional blood flow in normal and ischemic myocardium. *Am. J. Physiol.*, 232:H576–H583.

22. Marcus, M. L., Go, R. T., and Ehrhardt, J. C. (1982): Infarct-avid imaging techniques. In: *Myocardial Infarction: Measurement and Intervention*, edited by G. S. Wagner, pp. 325–346. Martinus Nijhoff, The Hague.

23. Maroko, P. R., Kjekshus, J. K., Sobel, B. E., Watanabe, T., Lovell, J. W., Ross, J., and Braunwald, E. (1971): Factors influencing infarct size following experimental coronary artery occlusions. *Circulation*, 43:67–82.

24. Murdock, R. H., Jr., and Cobb, F. R. (1980): Effects of infarcted myocardium on regional blood flow measurements to ischemic regions in canine hearts. *Circ. Res.*, 47:701–709.

25. Murdock, R. H., Jr., Harlan, D. M., Morris, J. J., III, Pryor, W. W., Jr., and Cobb, F. R. (1983): Transitional blood flow zones between ischemic and nonischemic myocardium in the awake dog. [analysis based on distribution of the intramural vasculature] *Circ. Res.*, 52:451–459.

26. Nielsen, A. P., Morris, K. G., Murdock, R., Bruno, F. P., and Cobb, F. R. (1980): Linear relationship between the distribution of Thallium-201 and blood flow in ischemic and nonischemic myocardium during exercise. *Circulation*, 61:797–801.

27. Okada, R. D., Boucher, C. A., and Pohost, G. M. (1982): Radionuclide perfusion techniques. In: *Myocardial Infarction: Measurement and Intervention*, edited by G. S. Wagner, pp. 295–324. Martinus Nijhoff, The Hague.

28. Okun, E. M., Factor, S. M., and Kirk, E. S. (1979): End-capillary loops in the heart: An explanation for discrete myocardial infarctions without border zones. *Science*, 206:565–572.

29. Pohost, G. M., and Ratner, A. V. (1984): Nuclear magnetic resonance. *JAMA*, 251:1304–1309.

30. Reimer, K. A., and Jennings, R. B. (1979): The changing anatomic reference base of evolving myocardial infarction: underestimation of myocardial collateral blood flow and overestimation of experimental anatomic infarct size due to tissue edema, hemorrhage and acute inflammation. *Circulation*, 60:866–876.

31. Ritchie, J. L., Trobaugh, G. B., Hamilton, G. W., Gould, K. L., Narahara, K. A., Murray, J. A., and Williams, D. L. (1977): Myocardial imaging with Thallium-201 at rest and during exercise: Comparison with coronary arteriography and resting and stress electrocardiography. *Circulation*, 56:66–71.

32. Rivas, F., Cobb, F. R., Bache, R. J., and Greenfield, J. C. (1976): Relationship between blood flow to ischemic regions and extent of myocardial infarction. Serial measurement of blood flow to ischemic regions in dogs. *Circ. Res.*, 38:439–447.

33. Rudolph, A. M., and Heymann, M. A. (1967): The circulation of the fetus in utero. [Methods for studying distribution of blood flow, cardiac output and organ blood flow.] *Circ. Res.*, 21:163–184.

34. Schaper, W. (1971): *The Collateral Circulation of the Heart.* North-Holland, Amsterdam.

35. Schaper, W. (1978): Experimental coronary artery occlusion. III. The determinants of collateral blood flow in acute coronary occlusion. *Basic Res. Cardiol.*, 73:584–594.

36. Scheel, K. W., Ingram, L. A., and Gordey, R. L. (1982): Relationship of coronary flow and perfusion territory in dogs. *Am. J. Physiol.*, 243:H738–H747.

37. Smith, L. R., Zissermann, D., Cunningham, W., Wixson, S. E., Bishop, S. P., Hood, W. P., Jr., Mantle, J. A., Rogers, W. J., Russell, R. O., Jr., Logic, J. R., and Rackley, C. E. (1976): Measurement of cardiac parameters from cardiovascular images. In: *Computers in Cardiology*, edited by H. G. Ostrow. Institute of Electrical and Electronics Engineering, New York.

38. Sobel, B. E., and Shell, W. E. (1973): Jeopardized, blighted and necrotic myocardium. *Circulation*, 47:215–216.

39. Strauss, H. W., Harrison, K., Langan, J. K., Lebowitz, E., and Pitt, B. (1975): Thallium-201 for myocardial imaging [Relation of Thallium-201 to regional myocardial perfusion] *Circulation*, 51:641–645.

40. Wackers, F. J. T., Becker, A. E., Samson, G., Sokole, E. B., van der Schoot, J. B., Vet, A. J. T. M., Lie, K. I., Durrer, D., and Wellens, H. (1977): Location and size of acute transmural myocardial

infarction estimated from Thallium-201 scintiscans: A clinicopathological study. *Circulation*, 56:72–78.

41. Whitaker, J. W., and Ritman, E. L. (1982): Computerized tomography. In: *Myocardial Infarction: Measurement and Intervention*, edited by G. S. Wagner, pp. 261–276. Martinus Nijhoff, The Hague.
42. Wyatt, D., Lee, J., and Downey, J. M. (1982): Determination of coronary collateral flow by a load line analysis. *Circ. Res.*, 50:663–670.
43. Winkler, B. (1979): The tracer microsphere method. In: *The Pathophysiology of Myocardial Perfusion*, edited by W. Schaper, pp. 13–42. Elsevier/North Holland, Amsterdam.
44. Yellon, D. M., Hearse, D. J., Maxwell, M. P., Chambers, D. E., and Downey, J. M. (1983): Sustained limitation of myocardial necrosis 24 hours after coronary artery occlusion: Verapamil infusion in dogs with small myocardial infarcts. *Am. J. Cardiol.*, 51:1409–1413.
45. Yellon, D. M., Hearse, D. J., Crome, R., Grannell, J., and Wyse, R. K. H. (1981): Characterisation of the lateral interface between normal and ischemic tissue in the canine heart during evolving myocardial infarction. *Am. J. Cardiol.*, 47:1233–1239.
46. Yellon, D. M., Hearse, D. J., Crome, R., and Wyse, R. K. H. (1983): Temporal and spatial characteristics of evolving cell injury during regional myocardial ischemia in the dog: The "border zone" controversy. *J. Am. Coll. Cardiol.*, 2:661–670.
47. Yellon, D. M., Maxwell, M. P., Hearse, D. J., Yoshida, S., Eddy, L., and Downey, J. M. (1984): Flurbiprofen causes an apparent but not real delay of necrosis in the dog. *Advances in Myocardiology*, Vol. 6, edited by N. S. Dhalla and D. J. Hearse. Plenum, New York.

*Therapeutic Approaches to Myocardial Infarct
Size Limitation*, edited by D. J. Hearse and
D. M. Yellon. Raven Press, New York © 1984.

# 10

# Can We Really Quantitate Myocardial Cell Injury?

## Keith A. Reimer and Robert B. Jennings

*Department of Pathology, Duke University Medical Center,
Durham, North Carolina 27710*

During the last 15 years, many laboratories have become interested in the idea of protecting ischemic myocardium. The hypotheses underlying this idea are as follows: (a) Following acute myocardial infarction, cardiac function and patient morbidity and mortality are related to infarct size. (b) Ischemic myocytes are reversibly injured for a period of time, during which an intervention might be applied which would prevent or slow a key step in the ischemic process, preventing the death of some of the myocytes destined to die in a zone of ischemia and thereby limit infarct size. (c) Such therapy should minimize loss of cardiac function and reduce patient morbidity and mortality.

*Although the concepts are seemingly simple, testing the hypotheses has been extraordinarily costly and fraught with difficulties.* In our opinion the following have been the major problems.

*First, it is difficult to estimate and virtually impossible to measure infarct size in living patients precisely.* Furthermore, infarct size is highly variable among patients. While estimates of the final size of an infarct in a treated patient may be difficult to obtain with precision, it is even more difficult to predict how big an infarct would have been had one not intervened with therapy. Thus, it is difficult to detect an effect of a therapy in a small group of patients with evolving infarction.

*Second, in order to select potential therapies for study in man, it is necessary to have reliable experimental models to assess the efficacy of interventions.* At the present time, well over fifty different pharmacologic interventions have been tested, often in several different experimental models. The medical literature contains a preponderance of positive, often highly positive, results with many of these interventions. *And yet, few of these agents have undergone clinical trial and none have been accepted for general use among practicing cardiologists.* Why? We believe the answer is twofold. First, the imprecision of clinical indices of infarct size, which make interpretation of clinical studies difficult and, second, a growing mistrust of the validity of the experimental models and/or endpoints used in the published experimental reports.

In this chapter, we review the general features of the clinical assessment of the effects of intervention on infarct size briefly, and discuss in greater detail various experimental models designed to detect the effect of an intervention on infarct size.

## CLINICAL EVALUATION OF INTERVENTIONS DESIGNED TO LIMIT INFARCT SIZE

We shall not attempt to review the many important considerations that enter into the proper design of clinical trials such as patient selection, randomization, and blinding of therapy and statistical methodology. In the clinical evaluation of therapy designed to limit myocardial infarct size, a variety of potential methodological pitfalls obviously must be avoided. Such clinical trials have, in addition, the very difficult problem of selecting reliable and meaningful endpoints.

The ultimate goal of patient therapy is clearly the reduction of mortality and morbidity; mortality and various indices of morbidity are readily measured endpoints. However, these endpoints provide no information about the validity of the underlying hypothesis that intervention limits infarct size and thereby improves prognosis. The causes of mortality and morbidity are legion; consequently it may require extraordinarily large numbers of patients to distinguish a specific therapeutic effect from the many other factors contributing to such endpoints. *Furthermore, a positive effect on mortality does not prove the underlying hypothesis. For example, antiarrhythmic drugs may reduce mortality without having any effect on infarct size. Similarly, indices of cardiac function may be good predictors of patient morbidity but, for the following reasons, may have little if any relationship to the effect of therapy on infarct size:* (a) Many other factors influence cardiac function, such as the presence or absence of prior infarcts, the severity of atherosclerosis in noninfarcted regions, the presence or absence of anatomic complications of infarction such as aneurysms, the inotropic state of nonischemic regions of myocardium, and the complex interplay between peripheral vascular and cardiac functions. (b) A number of studies have shown that myocardium that has been reversibly injured by ischemia may require several days to recover normal function even though the myocytes are viable and blood flow has been restored (18,55,56).

## Biologic Basis

In order to understand the potential value of a variety of indices used to estimate infarct size in man, it is necessary to understand the spatial and temporal development of a myocardial infarct and to understand how limitation of infarct size might occur. In the dog, and most likely in man, coronary occlusion results in myocardial ischemia throughout the anatomic region supplied by the occluded vessel (the anatomic area at risk) (35,43). However, in both the dog and man, the entire area at risk seldom undergoes infarction. In both species, the lateral boundaries of an infarct coincide (within 1–2 mm) with the margins of the ischemic vascular bed (9,35,43,51). However, there usually is sparing of some myocardium in the subepicardial zone of the ischemic region. In both species, there is seldom significant sparing at the lateral margins of the subendocardial zone of ischemia but the transmural extent of infarction varies considerably among dogs (43) and among patients studied at autopsy (35). *In dogs, the amount of subepicardial sparing is related to the amount of collateral flow which persists in this zone after coronary occlusion (Fig. 1) (43).* The same relationship probably exists in man, but cannot be measured. In addition, whereas the final infarct size is related in part to the initial area at risk and to subepicardial collateral flow, *not all of the ischemic myocardium destined for infarction dies simultaneously.* This has been demonstrated in dogs by comparing nonreperfused infarcts versus infarcts that were reperfused at 40 min or 3 hr after occlusion (43). Early reperfusion at 40 min usually results in a subendocardial infarct, with salvage of the subepicardial region, obviously indicating that the subepicardial zone was still viable at that time. Reperfusion at 3 hr results in lesser subepicardial ischemic injury (Fig. 2). The reason for this transmural progression may be partly related to the gradient of collateral flow (Fig. 3) (43). However, as discussed in Chapter 8, several investigators have shown that a similar progression of injury occurs even in the absence of coronary flow, and

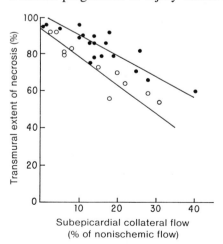

**FIG. 1.** Relation Between Transmural Necrosis and Subepicardial Collateral Flow in the Dog. Permanent infarcts and infarcts reperfused at 6 hr formed the same line and were combined *(solid circles)*. Infarcts reperfused at 3 hr are indicated by the *open circles*. In both groups, the transmural extent of necrosis was inversely related to subepicardial flow measured at 20 min after left circumflex coronary occlusion. However, in the 3-hr reperfusion group the regression line was shifted downward, indicating that reperfusion at 3 hr limited infarct size. (From ref. 43, with permission.)

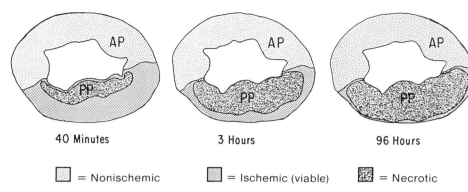

**40 Minutes**    **3 Hours**    **96 Hours**

☐ = Nonischemic    ▨ = Ischemic (viable)    ▨ = Necrotic

**FIG. 2.** Progression of Cell Death Versus Time After Left Circumflex Coronary Artery Occlusion in the Dog. Necrosis occurs first in the subendocardial myocardium. With longer occlusions, a wavefront of cell death moves from the subendocardial zone across the wall to involve progressively more of the transmural thickness of the ischemic zone. In contrast, the lateral margins in the subendocardial region of the infarct are established as early as 40 min after occlusion and are sharply defined by the anatomic boundaries of the ischemic bed. AP: anterior papillary muscle; PP: posterior papillary muscle. (From ref. 43, with permission.)

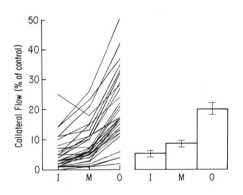

**FIG. 3.** Transmural Distribution of Collateral Flow After Circumflex Occlusion in 31 Dogs. Flow was measured with $9 \pm 1$ μm microspheres before and 20 min after coronary occlusion. Collateral flow is expressed as a percentage of preocclusion flow to the same samples. The individual dogs ($n = 31$) are illustrated on the *left* and the group means $\pm$ SEM are shown on the *right*. I, M, and O: inner, middle, and outer thirds of the transmural wall in the circumflex bed. Subendocardial flow was almost always severely depressed ($< 15\%$) and averaged 4.5% of control. Subepicardial flow was greater (averaged 20% of control) and much more variable than subendocardial flow. (From ref. 25, with permission.)

this is perhaps attributable to an intrinsic metabolic difference across the wall of the ventricle (7,8,13,14,37). *How does this relate to the concept of limiting infarct size? The ideal goal to be achieved with therapy, instituted immediately after coronary occlusion, is to prevent infarction. However, this goal is not likely to be achievable in most clinical circumstances. Thus, a more realistic clinical goal, based on the above temporal and spatial biology of infarction, must be the conversion of a potentially transmural infarct to one which is subendocardial, or at least nontransmural (35).*

## Methods of Measurement

We can now return to the clinical problems of (a) estimating the size of a myocardial infarct, and (b) determining whether infarct size has been limited by therapy. Of the clinical tests that have been used to estimate "infarct size" several measure, with variable degrees of precision, the size of the region of ischemic myocardial dysfunction or infarction. The indices in this category include estimates of segmental wall motion abnormalities, whether assessed by echocardiography (2) or radionuclide ventriculography (22), and myocardial imaging using gamma-emitting or positron-emitting agents, or NMR (11,15,19,57). Continued improvement in electronics and development of new imaging agents have gradually improved the resolution of such methods. *Because these methods measure the size of the involved region, and to date have not been capable of estimating the transmural extent of infarction in patients, these estimates of "infarct size" should more properly be regarded as estimates of the area at risk.* This is not meant to deprecate the value of such measurements. Larger areas at risk usually mean larger infarcts and larger areas of myocardial dysfunction (irrespective of whether myocytes in the nonfunctional region are still viable) may be associated with worse overall cardiac function. *Thus, these clinical indicators have prognostic value. However, because they measure primarily area at risk and not transmural extent of involvement, these methods are not likely to be capable of detecting therapeutic efficacy.* The reason, as noted above, is that the goal of therapeutic intervention is the conversion of a potentially transmural infarct into a nontransmural or subendocardial infarct (35). *Indeed, if in a clinical trial, treated and control groups of patients were found to have different "infarct sizes" based on methods of this type, the results might be more indicative of differences in a baseline characteristic (area at risk) than of any therapeutic effect.*

Other clinical indicators have been developed to estimate myocardial infarct size, and some of these do reflect the total amount of myocardial necrosis rather than the area involved. Such indices include enzymatic estimates (53) based on time-activity curves of total creatine kinase (CK) or the MB isoenzyme fraction of CK (MBCK), and electrocardiographic indices based on changes in the QRS complex (1,23,49). [ST-segment mapping techniques also have been used but their validity has been seriously questioned and it is not certain what such maps really measure (21).] The precision of enzymatic techniques for estimating infarct size depends in small part on the accuracy of enzyme assays, but in larger part on the validity of assumptions that must be made to calculate the estimate. Active enzyme entering the plasma is estimated from the time-activity curve which depends not only on the rate of entry of CK from the infarct into the general circulation, but also on the rate of removal of the enzyme from the plasma. In addition, the amount of active enzyme entering the plasma must be assumed to be directly proportional to the number of myocytes dying and releasing enzyme. However, local denaturation and/or degradation of the enzyme contributes variability to this assumed proportionality. For example, the amount of residual collateral perfusion and/or the presence or absence of reperfusion may alter the fraction of active enzyme that reaches the systemic circulation. Thus, enzymatic estimates of infarct size have been shown to be flow-dependent in some studies (54). Electrocardiographic indices are similarly influenced by a variety of confounding factors such as the presence of left ventricular hypertrophy or conduction abnormalities, variation in activation sequence, and the presence of prior myocardial infarcts.

*Despite their limitations, both enzymatic and QRS point score estimates of myocardial infarct size have shown reasonable correlations with infarct size measured anatomically at autopsy (3,16,17,23,49). In contrast to the previously mentioned indices, these estimates of infarct size relate to total myocardial necrosis and not to area at risk. Thus, these estimates are potentially able to detect a therapeutic limitation of infarct size as long as sufficiently large groups of patients are compared. However, the comparison would still be difficult because the area at risk is highly variable between patients and great within-group variation of infarct size would be expected even under the ideal circumstances of having reasonably precise estimates of infarct size and a strongly positive therapeutic effect.*

*Thus, what is most needed for the clinical assessment of therapies designed to limit infarct size is not only a precise way of estimating infarct size but also a way to normalize such estimates for variation in baseline parameters such as the area at risk.* For example, an enzymatic estimate of infarct size might be evaluated in terms of the area at risk estimated from coronary angiograms (if done in conjunction with therapy such as intracoronary thrombolytic therapy) or from less invasive indices of "infarct size" such as those based on regional wall motion abnormalities (as discussed earlier). The continued refinement of clinical markers to estimate infarct size and describe important baseline parameters such as the area at risk and the degree of collateral perfusion remains a challenge for future investigation.

## EXPERIMENTAL EVALUATION OF INTERVENTIONS DESIGNED TO PRESERVE ISCHEMIC MYOCARDIUM

### Biologic Basis

It seems appropriate to review briefly the nature of this very complex dynamic process we call myocardial infarction. Indeed, specific animal models and experimental endpoints used to evaluate the effect of therapies on ischemic injury or infarct size must be selected with regard to one or more aspects of this process (25,41,45).

In myocardial infarction, ischemia causes cardiac myocytes to undergo necrosis and eventually to be replaced by scar. The major aspects of this process are illustrated in Fig. 4. As discussed in Chapter 2, ischemia has been defined as the reduction in blood flow to a level at which the oxygen supply is insufficient to provide enough energy to meet the demands of the tissue for high energy phosphates (HEP). The inequality of oxygen supply versus metabolic demand is hypoxia. From the point of view of functional effects, hypoxia is the most important component of ischemia. However, the reduction in blood flow causes, in addition to hypoxia, the accumulation in the tissue of numerous metabolites such as lactate, protons, inosine, and inorganic phosphate; it also limits the supply of various substrates.

## Determinants of Cell Death

An initial prompt consequence of myocardial ischemia is the inhibition of a number of cellular functions including oxidative metabolism and contractile function. The loss of contractile function, which may not recover quickly even if blood flow is restored, is of obvious importance to the well-being of the experimental animal or the patient. *However, the loss of contractile function must not be equated with the death of the ischemic myocytes. Although dead myocytes are, by definition, noncontractile, loss of contractility is neither a cause nor an indicator of cell death.*

In considering determinants of cell death, one or more specific cellular function(s) must be crucial for cell survival. The failure of such a function must at some point result, not simply in altered activity of the cellular machinery, but in the destruction of that machinery. *This is the transition to irreversibility (27). The precise cause of this irreversible injury remains unknown.* However, some of the well-known metabolic consequences and consequences of ischemia, which could eventually result in irreversible cell injury, are listed in Table 1. These include: (a) depletion of high energy phosphate reserves; (b) end-product accumulation of, for example, lactate, protons, and fatty acyl derivatives; and (c) altered ionic gradients leading, in particular, to calcium overload. Just a few of the potential consequences of severe high energy phosphate depletion include: activation of endogenous phospholipases; inhibition of anaerobic glycolysis, thereby eliminating any further production of ATP; loss of purine nucleotides; and continued catabolism without resynthesis of enzymes, cofactors, or structural components of the cell. Inhibition of ATP production could occur because ATP is required at an early stage of the glycolytic pathway to phosphorylate fructose-6-phosphate to fructose-1,6-diphosphate. It is of note that glycolytic ATP, while inadequate to support contractile function, may be critical for homeostatic activities such as maintenance of ionic gradients.

TABLE 1. *Some potential causes and consequences of irreversible myocardial ischemic cell injury*

Depletion of high energy phosphates
  Activation of phospholipases
  Inhibition of anaerobic glycolysis
  Loss of purine nucleotides
  Catabolism without resynthesis
End-product accumulation
  Enzyme denaturation
  Membrane damage
Altered ionic gradients and osmolarity
  Cell swelling
  Calcium overload
    Activation of phospholipases and proteases
    Impaired mitochrondrial function
    Activation of ATPases

Accumulation of certain catabolites may have toxic effects on the cell. For example, cellular acidosis is associated with inhibition or denaturation of certain enzymes. Fatty acyl derivatives such as acyl CoA or acyl carnitine may act as detergents and so disrupt cell membranes. Lysolipids, produced by the action of phospholipases on cell membranes, may affect the electrical activity of myocytes (4).

Ischemia results in modest changes in ionic transport and this can be detected even before a marked loss of tissue ATP has occurred (20). Loss of cell volume regulation, and perhaps production of small molecular weight catabolites, cause cell swelling with possible structural disruption. Increased sarcoplasmic calcium also has widespread deleterious effects that include activation of various phospholipases and proteases, impaired mitochondrial function, and the activation of ATPases, which would then act to accelerate the loss of the high energy phosphate pool (24,40).

### Site of Irreversible Injury

*There are a number of lines of evidence favoring the hypothesis that sarcolemmal damage occurs early and is the lethal event for the ischemic myocyte (27). However, whether plasmalemmal damage is the cause of irreversible injury remains an unproven hypothesis and the mechanism of membrane damage remains unknown (30).* Furthermore, the process of infarction may involve more than the direct consequence of ischemia on the affected myocytes. For example, as indicated in Fig. 4, the microvasculature is also injured by ischemia (28) and, in turn, this could cause more severe ischemia than could be attributed to the initial coronary obstruction. As discussed in Chapter 7, it is now clear that ischemia causes endothelial damage, which may result in white cell trapping, platelet aggregation, microthrombi, or intramyocardial hemorrhage. Whether such events ever contribute to the death of additional myocytes remains open to question. In our studies, and those of some other investigators, these changes have been observed only within the confines of an evolving infarct, not at the periphery. *This localization of vascular pathology suggests that endothelial cells undergo ischemic injury more slowly than the highly differentiated myocytes, and that severe microvascular damage is a later event occurring in areas in which myocytes have already been lethally injured (43). However, as is apparent from Chapter 2, this view is not universally accepted.*

Another aspect of the process of myocardial infarction is the inflammatory response to either injured myocytes or microvasculature (see Chapter 13). Whereas the inflammatory response is essential for the repair of the infarct, there is evidence that one or more components of this process may also cause additional myocyte injury (50). For example, it is well known that polymorphonuclear leukocytes are rich in a variety of lysosomal proteases and lipases, which are released into the interstitial milieu of an infarct. Moreover, the inflammatory response is most pronounced at the periphery of the infarct where the microvasculature is intact.

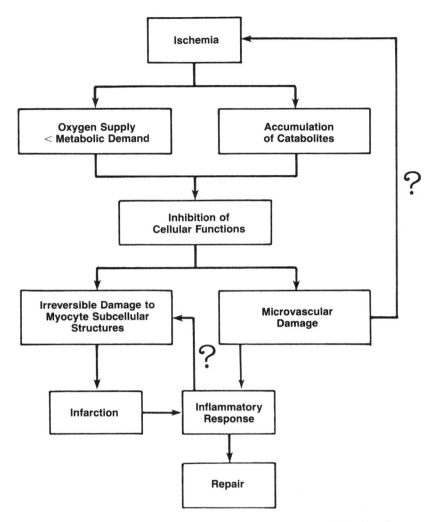

**FIG. 4.** Key Steps Contributing to the Evolution of a Myocardial Infarct. Selection of an appropriate experimental model and of appropriate experimental endpoints depends on which aspect of this dynamic process is under study. (See text for a more detailed explanation.)

*However, whether the inflammatory response does, in fact, cause additional myocyte necrosis is, in our view, open to question.*

## Selection of an Appropriate Animal Model and Primary Endpoint(s)

During the past decade and a half, investigators in many laboratories have been interested in assessing the effects of a variety of different interventions on acutely ischemic myocardium. It seems likely that the widespread interest in this problem has led to the development of more experimental models to study myocardial ischemia than there are laboratories conducting the studies.

Major variables among these various animal models include: (a) species, breed, and sex of the experimental animal; (b) whether the studies are carried out using the intact animal, using isolated whole hearts or portions of heart muscle, or using isolated myocytes in culture; (c) if carried out in intact animals, whether the animal is in a conscious or an anesthetized state; (d) whether myocardial injury is caused by ischemia as opposed to hypoxia; (e) whether the ischemic insult involves the entire heart (global ischemia) or only part of the intact heart (regional ischemia); (f) the duration and severity of the insult; (g) whether or not reperfusion is employed; and (h) the dose, the time of initiation of treatment (pre- versus postocclusion) and the duration of the therapeutic intervention.

For every model used, there must be one or more primary endpoints used to assess the effect of an intervention. The number of possible primary endpoints are perhaps even larger than the number of animal models available (Table 2).

Many experimental models and endpoints are valid for particular applications; however, there are right and wrong models and endpoints, depending on the specific question posed for experimental study. Some general considerations that must go into the selection of a particular model are listed in Table 3.

Simple models of myocardial ischemic injury may be used (a) to evaluate the role of specific metabolic pathways or organelle function in the pathogenesis of ischemic injury, and (b) to screen a variety of interventions to identify those with sufficient promise to merit testing in a more complex model. More complex models

TABLE 2. *Endpoints commonly used to identify potentially beneficial effects of an intervention*

Infarct size
  Histologic assessments
  Gross measurement (with or without dehydrogenase staining)
Indirect indices of infarct size *in vivo*
  Enzyme release curves, ST segment and QRS mapping
  Various imaging techniques
  Echocardiography
Collateral blood flow
Myocardial contractile function
Ultrastructural changes
Function of subcellular organelles
  Intact cells
  Mitochondria
  Sarcoplasmic reticulum
  Sarcolemma
  Lysosomes
Biochemical changes
  High energy phosphates,
  Ion gradients,
  Catabolites
  pH

TABLE 3. *Criteria for selecting animal models and endpoints*

---

Experimental model
  Simple screening models
  Complex models to reproduce clinical conditions
Primary endpoint(s)
  Question under investigation
  Accuracy versus simplicity
Secondary variables
  Controls for the variation of primary endpoints

---

are necessary to more closely reproduce myocardial infarction as it occurs clinically and to provide a more reliable analysis of the likelihood of clinical efficacy.

*As a basis for limiting infarct size, one could intervene at any one of the general steps illustrated in Fig. 4. However, an appropriate endpoint might measure only that step in the process.* For example, one might ask whether a calcium antagonist would reduce the metabolic demand of ischemic myocardium. An appropriate endpoint would be myocardial high energy phosphate content after a given period of ischemia and the model could be either simple (e.g., an isolated rat heart) or complex. As another example, one might question whether a particular cardioplegic solution improved postischemic contractile function (a question of particular relevance to the preservation of ischemic myocardium during cardiac surgery). In this case, a model of global ischemia might be more appropriate than coronary occlusion with regional ischemia. The appropriate endpoint would be a measure of contractile function, for example, contractile force at constant preload. Such studies could be done either with isolated hearts or in intact animals. However, if one were to pose the additional question: "Is the postischemic survival of the animal improved?", then the answer only could be obtained in an intact and much more complex, whole animal model. If one wanted to know whether a calcium antagonist prevented mitochondrial calcification following ischemia and reperfusion, an analysis of tissue calcium content and electron microscopic evaluation of the injured mitochondria would be appropriate endpoints.

*When the question is: "Does this therapy limit infarct size?", then there can only be one appropriate endpoint, and that is infarct size itself. Measurement of the indices such as myocardial contractile function or high energy phosphate content cannot directly answer this question.*

## Selection of Secondary Endpoints

In the preceding section, we defined "primary endpoints" as those variables which provide the direct answer to the question posed. In many studies of myocardial ischemic injury, there will be natural variation among animals for any primary endpoint selected for study and this variation will be unrelated to therapy. For example, there is considerable variation in infarct size among untreated control dogs. This variation exists even though details of the experimental procedures, such as site of coronary occlusion, may be precisely controlled. *Given this basic characteristic of any biological system, it is essential to identify those variables within the experimental model that are most responsible for the variation in the primary endpoint. These variables should be included in the experimental design and measured as "baseline variables" or "secondary endpoints."* For example, in dogs subjected to coronary occlusion, two variables, (a) the size of the occluded vascular bed (anatomic area at risk of infarction) (31,38,43,52), and (b) the collateral blood flow to the subepicardial zone of this area at risk (43,51), account for the majority of the variation in infarct size (in the absence of therapy to limit infarct size). Additional factors influencing infarct size but accounting for a relatively small fraction of the natural variation in infarct size include those factors which determine myocardial metabolic demand (29,51) (hemodynamic parameters which influence myocardial oxygen requirements include heart rate, developed myocardial wall tension, and inotropic state).

Measurement of these baseline variables is essential for at least three reasons. *First, when these variables are measured and used to normalize the primary endpoint, it becomes possible to detect a therapeutic effect with greater confidence* than is possible when only the primary endpoints are compared; this is illustrated in Fig. 1. In this study, a simple comparison of infarct size (without reference to baseline collateral blood flow) in the group of dogs with reperfusion at 3 hr versus the groups with 6 or more hours of coronary occlusion revealed a slight and barely significant ($p < 0.05$) limitation of infarct size with reperfusion. However, when the transmural extent of infarction is plotted against coronary collateral blood flow in the subepicardial zone of the ischemic region, it is clearly evident (with or without statistics) that for any level of collateral flow, infarct size was limited by reperfusion (43). The second reason to measure these baseline variables is that failure to do so may result in an inability to detect random selection differences among animals that could lead to erroneous positive conclusions. *This may be a particular problem if a significant fraction of animals are lost from study because of premature mortality.* For example, we believe that this has occurred in our own studies with propranolol. In our early studies (46,47), propranolol delayed ischemic injury and thereby reduced myocardial necrosis following 40 min of ischemia and reperfusion. However, in subsequent studies, with lower mortality and control of baseline variables, no protective effect could be demonstrated (26). The third reason is that if baseline variables, measured before and after initiation of therapy, are altered by therapy, then information about the mechanism of myocardial preservation may possibly be gained. This concept is illustrated in Fig. 5. The contribution of the area at risk to the variation in infarct size can be dealt with by normalizing infarct size as a fraction of the area at risk. This normalized infarct size can then be plotted in relation to collateral blood flow in the subepicardial region of the ischemic zone. Limitation of infarct size by any mechanism would alter the relationship between infarct size and baseline collateral flow. Figure 5 illustrates a hypothetical relationship between infarct size and collateral flow using a posttherapy measure of collateral flow for control infarcts (refer again to Fig. 1

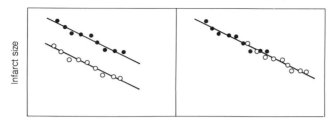

Collateral flow (post therapy)

**FIG. 5.** Possible Effects of Interventions That Limit Infarct Size, on the Regression of Infarct Size Versus Collateral Blood Flow. Theoretical results with protection which is flow-independent versus protection which is flow-dependent. *Solid circle:* control; *open circle:* treated. (See text for details reproduced from ref. 44.)

for an actual example) and an intervention that limits infarct size. An intervention that limits infarct size without improving collateral flow would alter the relationship *(left panel)* when either baseline or a posttherapy measure of collateral flow was used. Conversely, an intervention that improved collateral flow would shift points down the curve when posttreatment collateral flow was considered *(right panel)*. *Thus, by measuring and using the baseline variables, area at risk and collateral flow, as well as posttreatment collateral flow, it can be possible not only to detect a positive effect with greater precision but also to establish whether the observed protection is independent of blood flow or is related to improved collateral perfusion.*

## Methods of Measuring Selected Endpoints

It this brief chapter, it is impossible to discuss in detail all methods that can be employed for measuring the many primary and secondary experimental endpoints which have been used in the various models of myocardial ischemic injury. We, therefore, restrict our consideration to two important endpoints—namely infarct size and area at risk.

### Infarct Size

Essentially there are two ways to measure infarct size. One is based on histologic evaluation (43,48) and the other is based on gross macroscopic evaluation. *There are many other methods that have been used in papers, which by their titles claim to be studies of infarct size. In reality, however, these methods do not measure infarct size. For example, it is not possible, without prohibitive expense, to measure infarct size using electron microscopy.* To measure infarct size, it is necessary to evaluate a much larger representative sample of the myocardium than is feasible with electron microscopy. Despite this limitation, electron microscopy, is of course, an extraordinarily valuable tool for identifying the qualitative nature of the cellular response to injury.

*Electrocardiographic ST-segment maps, measurements of cardiac enzymes in plasma, cardiac radionuclide images, echocardiograms, and other methods of estimating infarct size in the living patient also do not provide direct measurements of infarct size. These techniques are measurements of one or another consequence of myocardial infarction that can be used to estimate infarct size indirectly. Indirect techniques of this type may be essential for the clinical evaluation of the effect of a therapy on infarct size; however, the use of these indirect techniques in experimental animals, as primary endpoints for the evaluation of infarct size, is simply unacceptable. At present there is no justification for the use of an indirect estimate of a primary endpoint when a direct and simple measurement is readily available.*

In the following sections we discuss various aspects of the two direct methods for infarct size measurement, namely microscopic and macroscopic assessment.

*Microscopic methods.* The only absolute criteria for the diagnosis of myocardial infarction are the microscopic criteria of myocardial necrosis. *Thus, histologic evaluation is, in our view, the definitive way to measure infarct size.* However, histologic evaluation does have certain disadvantages. For example, animals generally must survive 24 hr and preferably 3 to 4 days for necrotic and viable myocardium to be readily distinguishable at low magnification. This is a necessary feature if histologic sizing is to be done efficiently. A second problem is that infarct sizing by histologic techniques is costly, time consuming, and requires expertise in the recognition of the features of myocardial necrosis. Multiple histologic slides (minimum of eight in dog studies) must be prepared and analyzed in order to achieve sufficiently representative sampling of the infarct region.

*Macroscopic methods.* Infarct size can also be quantitated from macroscopic evaluation. At the macroscopic level, the interface between viable and infarcted myocardium may not be sharply defined, particularly during the first 2 or 3 days after onset. In order to enhance the macroscopic distinction between viable and necrotic regions, special staining techniques are often used. As discussed in Chapter 5, the most commonly used methods involve the use of dyes [para-nitro blue tetrazolium (pNBT) or triphenyl tetrazolium chloride (TTC)], which are colorless when oxidized but are colored blue (pNBT) or red (TTC) when reduced (10,12,34,36,39). These dyes are applied to the myocardium in the oxidized state and if dehydrogenase enzyme activity and appropriate cofactors (for example NADH) are present, then the dyes will be reduced. The absence of blue or red staining indicates lack of enzyme activity and/or cofactors and implies that the myocardium has undergone necrosis. TTC is employed more commonly than pNBT primarily because the former is much less expensive than the latter. TTC can be applied either directly to the surface of myocardial slices or can be perfused into the myocardium via the coronary arteries. In contrast, pNBT can only be applied to slices because transcapillary and/or transsarcolemmal movement of the dye is slow.

Coronary perfusion with TTC, either *in vivo* or postmortem, is used by some investigators. After initial coronary perfusion and incubation of the heart the resulting distribution of oxidized and reduced forms of the dye are stable and the heart can be formalin-fixed (which destroys the enzyme activity). Later, the fixed heart can be sliced for quantitative analysis. Using such methods, more uniform slices can be cut and histologic confirmation of infarct boundaries can be undertaken. Alternatively, in order to cut reasonably uniform slices prior to formalin fixation, some investigators partially freeze the heart. This, however, creates freezing artifacts at the cellular level making subsequent histologic evaluation more difficult. The principal limitation to coronary perfusion with TTC is that perfusion defects (which may occur when postmortem coronary perfusion is carried out *in vitro*) will result in absence of red staining and this may be difficult to distinguish from infarct.

By comparison with histologic methods of infarct sizing, the advantage of the TTC method is simplicity. The limitations of this technique are: (a) the retention of some dehydrogenase activity may not mean that ischemic myocytes are viable; this applies particularly to very early infarcts; and (b) in infarcts having many interdigitations of viable and necrotic myocytes, staining viable cells may provide sufficient stain to the entire region so that it masks the presence of necrosis. Even infarcts that are solid in their centers often have highly irregular convoluted interfaces with viable myocardium where staining of viable cells may mask necrosis. *In our experience, when TTC staining and histologic evaluation have been used in the same hearts, the TTC technique consistently underestimates histologic infarct size* (unpublished observations). *In our view, TTC sizing of myocardial infarcts should therefore not be used without at least some direct histologic confirmation in each infarct studied.*

### Area at Risk

Throughout this chapter, we have used the term "area at risk" to refer to the anatomic region normally supplied by an occluded coronary artery. We have stated earlier that myocardial infarcts seldom occupy this entire area at risk in the dog or in man because collateral blood flow permits survival of myocytes in the subepicardial region. *Because of the usual survival of mildly ischemic myocytes in the subepicardium, some investigators have preferred to consider a "physiologic" rather than an "anatomic" area at risk, the physiologic risk region being the region that is "severely" ischemic and thus truly at risk of undergoing infarction.*

*Physiologic risk region.* This type of risk region is measured by injecting dyes, or isotope-labeled microspheres, or aggregated albumin into the systemic circulation during life and identifying the risk region as the region devoid of perfusion (5,6,33,58). Identification of this "physiologic" risk region can be highly useful if, for example, one desires to study the metabolism, subcellular function, or ultrastructure of severely ischemic myocardium which is destined to undergo necrosis, because identification of the zone of severe ischemia will permit exclusion of mildly ischemic and less injured regions when myocardial samples are obtained (42).

*As a baseline variable for normalizing infarct size in studies of the effect of therapy on infarct size, we prefer a measure of the anatomic area at risk (31,35,43) because we think that physiologic risk regions have two major limitations. The first*

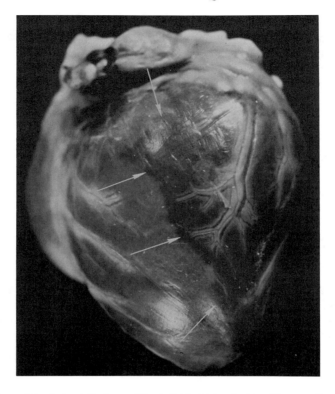

**FIG. 6.** View of the Lateral Surface of the Left Ventricle of a Dog Heart to Show the Sharp Junction Between Myocardium Supplied by the Circumflex and Anterior Descending Coronary Arteries. The animal was heparinized before excision of the heart. Both vessels were perfused simultaneously at 100 mm Hg pressure with dyes suspended in 6% dextran-70 in normal saline. The ischemic vascular bed distal to a circumflex occlusion is delineated by blue dye *(dark areas arrowed)* and includes the posterolateral wall of the left ventricle. (From ref. 25, with permission.)

problem is that if there is not a sharp boundary between "severely ischemic" and "mildly ischemic" myocardium within the ischemic region, the boundary of the physiologic risk region measured with pre-terminal dye injections may be arbitrary and be determined as much by the concentration of marker in the blood, the duration of perfusion time, and the limits of dye visibility, as it is by the absolute rate of local collateral perfusion. The second limitation is that any spontaneous or therapeutically induced change in collateral blood flow could alter the boundary of the physiologic risk region. In this event, a physiologic risk zone measured any time after the initiation of therapy would not be suitable as a baseline variable.

*Anatomic area at risk.* Two general methods of identifying the anatomic area at risk are considered. The first method involves postmortem coronary injection with two different colored dyes, one being injected into the occluded artery at the site of occlusion, and the other into the remaining nonoccluded vasculature. The area at risk is then identified by the boundary between the two different colors

(43). The second method involves postmortem coronary injection with radioopaque material and the identification of the boundaries of the vascular beds on the basis of radiographs of serial slices of the ventricle (32,35).

The dye injection method requires that dyes be injected simultaneously, at identical pressure, into all ischemic and nonischemic regions. When this is done, the boundaries between vascular regions are sharply defined (Fig. 6). The primary limitation to this method involves the fact that dye may readily cross the anatomic boundary between vascular regions if collateral connections are extensive, or if a pressure gradient exists between the two vascular beds. A pressure gradient may arise, even with simultaneous coronary perfusion, if, for example, arterial branches are partially or completely obstructed by the catheter tip or by microthrombi. This dye injection method is most suited for use with a reperfusion model, where excessive collateral growth has not been induced. The advantages of this method are, first, that X-ray equipment is not required and the technique is relatively simple and, second, that because vascular boundaries are seen directly on the ventricular slices, the technique provides an aid to precise sampling of ischemic and nonischemic areas for blood flow analysis.

The radiographic technique (Fig. 7) depends on the visualization of the arterial tree. Measurement of the area at risk requires identification of the origin of arterial branches on radiographs of heart slices and the identification of the boundary between arteriolar beds. The latter is facilitated by the different orientation of vessels originating from the left versus the right side of the ischemic to nonischemic interface. Since the development of collaterals does not alter the basic vascular anatomy of the heart, this method is not limited by extensive collateralization and is preferred over the dye technique when collaterals have been induced. The limitations of this technique include: the need for X-ray equipment; the greater difficulty in precisely defining vascular boundaries because of vascular overlap if slices are not sufficiently thin; and the imprecision of using X-rays to determine the precise sampling of ischemic and nonischemic myocardium, for blood flow or other analysis.

## CONCLUDING COMMENTS

Because myocardial infarct size is related to patient prognosis following myocardial infarction, much effort has been devoted to developing methods to measure and therapeutically modify infarct size in patients. In addition, many experimental models have been developed to study the pathogenesis of ischemic cell injury and to identify therapies that might protect ischemic myocardium, and thereby limit infarct size in man. Several methods have been developed to estimate infarct size in man. Some of these, such as measurement of regional wall function, may reflect the total area of ischemia rather than the size of the actual infarct. Other methods, such as enzymatic estimates, reflect total tissue necrosis but do not permit normalization of infarct size to area at risk. None of the clinical methods currently in use can accurately distinguish nontransmural from transmural infarcts. The latter

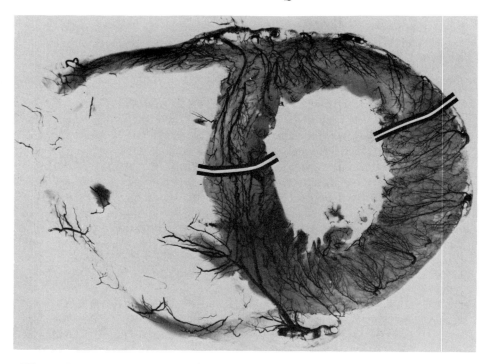

**FIG. 7.** Radiograph of a Cross Section of the Ventricles of a Human Heart. This section was obtained following postmortem coronary injection of a suspension of barium sulfate in gelatin (micropaque). The view is from the base of the heart with posterior wall of the heart at the *top* of the photograph. In this heart, an infarct involving the posteroseptal region of the left ventricle was present. The anatomic area at risk of infarction was the region supplied by an occluded right coronary artery. The boundaries of this vascular region *(lines)* were identified by following the epicardial arteries on radiographs of sequential ventricular slices. Identification of this boundary was also aided by the fact that branches of the right and circumflex arteries penetrated the myocardium in different directions. (From ref. 35, with permission.)

distinction is desirable because the realistic clinical goal for therapy to limit infarct size must be to produce a subendocardial or nontransmural infarct where a transmural infarct might otherwise have occurred.

Many different experimental models and a variety of experimental endpoints have been used to study myocardial ischemic injury. The appropriate selection of an experimental model should be based on the hypothesis under test, thus, simple models are useful for screening potential therapies. The relatively few that show sufficient promise can then be selected for study in complex and costly experimental settings. Simple models may also be the best choice if one wishes to study the role of specific mechanisms in the pathogenesis of ischemic cell injury. More complex animal models of myocardial infarction have the advantage of mimicking clinical conditions and are useful for evaluating interventions prior to development of clinical trials.

In any experimental study, the primary endpoint must be selected on the basis of the hypothesis under test. In addition, secondary experimental endpoints should be selected, first, to act as controls for baseline variables that produce the biologic variation of the primary endpoint and, second, to elucidate the mechanism of a therapeutic effect on the primary endpoint. In experimental studies of the effect of therapy on infarct size, a direct measurement of infarct size is the appropriate primary endpoint. The two most important baseline variables that determine infarct size in dogs are, first, the size of the occluded vascular bed (anatomic area at risk) and, second, the collateral blood flow to the subepicardial zone of this ischemic region. These two variables should be measured as secondary endpoints. Additional baseline variables which are readily measurable include hemodynamic determinants of myocardial metabolic demand such as heart rate and systolic blood pressure.

*It is our opinion that if the guidelines put forth in this chapter are adhered to, it may be possible to finally resolve the question: "Is infarct size limitation possible in man?"*

## REFERENCES

1. Abildskov, J. A. (1980): The relation of localized myocardial lesion size to the QRS complex of vectorcardiographic leads. *J. Electrocardiol.*, 13:307–310.
2. Armstrong, W. F., West, S. R., Mueller, T. M., Dillon, J. C., and Feigenbaum, H. (1983): Assessment of location and size of myocardial infarction with contrast-enhanced echocardiography. *J. Am. Coll. Cardiol.*, 2:63–69.
3. Bleifeld, W., Mathey, D., Hanrath, P., Buss, H., and Effert, S. (1977): Infarct size estimated from serial serum creatine phosphokinase in relation to left ventricular hemodynamics. *Circulation*, 55:303–311.
4. Corr, P. B., Cain, M. E., Witkowski, F. X., Price, D. A., and Sobel, B. E. (1979): Potential arrhythmogenic electrophysiological derangements in canine Purkinje fibers induced by lysophosphoglycerides. *Circ. Res.*, 44:822–832.
5. Darsee, J. R., Kloner, R. A., and Braunwald, E. (1981): Demonstration of lateral and epicardial border zone salvage by flurbiprofen using an *in vivo* method for assessing myocardium at risk. *Circulation*, 63:29–35.
6. DeBoer, L. W. V., Strauss, H. W., Kloner, R. A., Rude, R. E., Davis, R. E., Maroko, P. R., and Braunwald, E. B. (1980): Autoradiographic method for measuring the ischemic myocardium at risk: Effects of verapamil on infarct size after experimental coronary artery occlusion. *Proc. Natl. Acad. Sci. USA*, 77:6119–6123.
7. Dunn, R. B., and Griggs, D. M., Jr. (1975): Transmural gradients in ventricular tissue metabolites produced by stopping coronary blood flow in the dog. *Circ. Res.*, 37:438–445.
8. Eng, C., Cho, S., and Kirk, E. S. (1982): The wavefront pattern of necrosis occurs despite uniform blood flow conditions. *Circulation*, 66:II–66 (abstract).
9. Factor, S. M., and Kirk, E. S. (1982): Microcirculatory determinants of infarct dimensions. In: *Microcirculation of the Heart, Theoretical and Clinical Problems*, edited by H. Tillmanns, W. Kübler, and H. Zebe, pp. 141–148. Springer-Verlag, Heidelberg.
10. Fallon, J. T. (1979): Simplified method for histochemical demonstration of experimental myocardial infarct. *Circulation*, 60(Suppl. 2):11–42.
11. Falsetti, H. L., Marcus, M. L., Kerber, R. E., and Skorton, D. J. (1981): Quantification of myocardial ischemia and infarction by left ventricular imaging. *Circulation*, 63:747–751 (editorial).
12. Fishbein, M. C., Meerbaum, S., Rit, J., Lando, U., Kanmatsuse, K., Mercier, J. C., Corday, E., and Ganz, W. (1981): Early phase acute myocardial infarct size quantification: Validation of the triphenyl tetrazolium chloride tissue enzyme staining technique. *Am. Heart J.*, 101:593–600.
13. Fujiwara, H., Ashraf, M., Sato, S., and Millard, R. W. (1982): Transmural cellular damage and blood flow distribution in early ischemia in pig hearts. *Circ. Res.*, 51:683–693.

14. Geary, G. G., Smith, G. T., and McNamara, J. J. (1982): Quantitative effect of early coronary artery reperfusion in baboons. Extent of salvage of the perfusion bed of an occluded artery. *Circulation*, 66:391–396.

15. Goldman, M. R., Brady, T. J., Pykett, I. L., Burt, C. T., Buonanno, F. S., Kistler, J. P., Newhouse, J. H., Hinshaw, W. S., and Pohost, G. M. (1982): Quantification of experimental myocardial infarction using nuclear magnetic resonance imaging and paramagnetic ion contrast enhancement in excised canine hearts. *Circulation*, 66:1012–1016.

16. Grande, P., Hansen, B. F., Christiansen, C., and Naestoft, J. (1982): Estimation of acute myocardial infarct size in man by serum CK-MB measurements. *Circulation*, 65:756–764.

17. Hackel, D. B., Reimer, K. A., Ideker, R. E., Mikat, E. M., Hartwell, T. D., Parker, C. B., Braunwald, E. B., Gold, H. K., Raabe, D. S., Rude, R. E., Sobel, B. E., Stone, P. H., Buja, M., Muller, J. E., Roberts, R., and the MILIS Study Group (1984): Comparison of enzymatic and anatomic estimates of myocardial infarct size in man. *Circulation (in press)*.

18. Heyndrickx, G. R., Baig, H., Nellens, P., Leusen, I., Fishbein, M. C., and Vatner, S. F. (1978): Depression of regional blood flow and wall thickening after brief coronary occlusions. *Am. J. Physiol.*, 234:H653–H659.

19. Higgins, C. B., Hagen, P. L., Newell, J. D., Schmidt, W. S., and Haigler, F. H. (1982): Contrast enhancement of myocardial infarction: Dependence on necrosis and residual blood flow and the relationship to distribution of scintigraphic imaging agents. *Circulation*, 65:739–746.

20. Hill, J. L., and Gettes, L. S. (1980): Effect of acute coronary artery occlusion on local myocardial extracellular $K^+$ activity in swine. *Circulation*, 61:68–78.

21. Holland, R. P., and Brooks, H. (1977): TQ-ST segment mapping: critical review and analysis of current concepts. *Am. J. Cardiol.*, 40:110–129.

22. Ideker, R. E., Behar, V. S., Wagner, G. S., Starr, J. W., Starmer, C. F., Lee, K. L., and Hackel, D. B. (1978): Evaluation of asynergy as an indicator of myocardial fibrosis. *Circulation*, 57:715–725.

23. Ideker, R. E., Wagner, G. S., Ruth, W. K., Alonson, D. R., Bishop, S. P., Bloor, C. M., Fallon, J. T., Gottlieb, G. J., Hackel, D. B., Phillips, H. R., Reimer, K. A., Roark, S. F., Rogers, W. J., Savage, R. M., White, R. D., and Selvester, R. H. (1982): Evaluation of a QRS scoring system for estimating myocardial infarct size. II. Correlation with quantitative anatomic findings for anterior infarcts. *Am. J. Cardiol.*, 49:1604–1614.

24. Jennings, R. B. (1984): Calcium ions in ischemia. In: *Calcium Antagonists and Cardiovascular Disease*, edited by L. H. Opie, pp. 85–95. Raven Press, New York.

25. Jennings, R. B., and Reimer, K. A. (1979): Biology of experimental acute myocardial ischaemia and infarction. In: *Enzymes in Cardiology. Diagnosis and Research*, edited by D. J. Hearse and J. DeLeiris, pp. 21–57. John Wiley, New York.

26. Jennings, R. B., and Reimer, K. A. (1979): Effect of beta-adrenergic blockade on acute myocardial ischaemic injury. In: *Modulation of Sympathetic Tone in the Treatment of Cardiovascular Diseases*, edited by F. Gross, pp. 103–116. Hans Huber, Berne.

27. Jennings, R. B., and Reimer, K. A. (1981): Lethal myocardial ischemic injury. *Am. J. Pathol.*, 102:241–255.

28. Jennings, R. B., Kloner, R. A., Ganote, C. E., Hawkins, H. K., and Reimer, K. A. (1982): Changes in capillary fine structure and function in acute myocardial ischemic injury. In: *Microcirculation of the Heart*, edited by H. Tillmanns, W. Kübler, and H. Zebe, pp. 87–97. Springer-Verlag, Berlin.

29. Jennings, R. B., and Reimer, K. A. (1983): Factors involved in salvaging ischemic myocardium: effect of reperfusion of arterial blood. *Circulation*, 68(Suppl.I):I-25-I-36.

30. Jennings, R. B., Steenbergen, C., Kinney, R. B., Hill, M. L., and Reimer, K. A. (1983): Comparison of the effect of ischaemia and anoxia on the sarcolemma of the dog heart. *Eur. Heart J.*, 4(Suppl.H):123–137.

31. Jugdutt, B. I., Hutchins, G. M., Bulkley, B. H., and Becker, L. C. (1979): Myocardial infarction in the conscious dog. Three-dimensional mapping of infarct, collateral flow and region at risk. *Circulation*, 60:1141–1150.

32. Jugdutt, B. I., Hutchins, G. M., Bulkley, B. H., Pitt, B., and Becker, L. C. (1979): Effect of indomethacin on collateral blood flow and infarct size in the conscious dog. *Circulation*, 59:734–743.

33. Kloner, R. A., Ganote, C. E., Reimer, K. A., and Jennings, R. B. (1975): Distribution of coronary arterial flow in acute myocardial ischemia. *Arch. Pathol.*, 99:86–94.

34. Kloner, R. A., Darsee, J. R., DeBoer, L. W. V., and Carlson, N. (1981): Early pathologic detection of acute myocardial infarction. *Arch. Pathol. Lab. Med.*, 105:403–406.
35. Lee, J. T., Ideker, R. E., and Reimer, K. A. (1981): Myocardial infarct size and location in relation to the coronary vascular bed at risk in man. *Circulation*, 64:526–534.
36. Lie, J. T., Pairolero, P. C., Holley, K. E., and Titus, J. L. (1975): Macroscopic enzyme-mapping: Verification of large, homogeneous, experimental myocardial infarcts of predictable size and location in dogs. *J. Thor. Cardiovasc. Surg.*, 69:599–604.
37. Lowe, J. E., Cummings R. G., Adams, D. H., and Hull-Ryde, E. A. (1983): Evidence that ischemic cell death begins in the subendocardium independent of variations in collateral flow or wall tension. *Circulation*, 68:190–202.
38. Lowe, J. E., Reimer, K. A., and Jennings, R. B. (1978): Experimental infarct size as a function of the amount of myocardium at risk. *Am. J. Pathol.*, 90:363–379.
39. Nachlas, M. M., and Shnitka, T. K. (1963): Macroscopic identification of early myocardial infarcts by alterations in dehydrogenase activity. *Am. J. Pathol.*, 42:379–405.
40. Nayler, W. G. (1981): The role of calcium in the ischemic myocardium. *Am. J. Pathol.*, 102:262–270.
41. Reimer, K. A. (1982): Overview of potential mechanisms for limiting infarct size with emphasis on decreasing myocardial energy utilization. In: *Quantitation of Ischemic and Infarcted Myocardium*, edited by G. S. Wagner, pp. 387–395. Martinus Nijhoff, Boston.
42. Reimer, K. A., Hill, M. L., and Jennings, R. B. (1981): Prolonged depletion of ATP and of the adenine nucleotide pool due to delayed resynthesis of adenine nucleotides following reversible myocardial ischemic injury in dogs. *J. Mol. Cell. Cardiol.*, 13:229–239.
43. Reimer, K. A., and Jennings, R. B. (1979): The "Wavefront Phenomenon" of myocardial ischemic cell death. II. Transmural progression of necrosis within the framework of ischemic bed size (myocardium at risk) and collateral flow. *Lab. Invest.*, 40:633–644.
44. Reimer, K. A., and Jennings, R. B. (1984): Effects of calcium channel blockers on myocardial preservation during experimental acute myocardial infarction. *Am. J. Cardiol. (in press)*.
45. Reimer, K. A., Jennings, R. B., and Tatum, A. H. (1983): Pathobiology of acute myocardial ischemia: metabolic, functional, and ultrastructural studies. *Am. J. Cardiol.*, 52(Suppl.2):72a–81a.
46. Reimer, K. A., Rasmussen, M. M., and Jennings, R. B. (1973): Reduction by propranolol of myocardial necrosis following temporary coronary artery occlusion in dogs. *Circ. Res.*, 33:353–363.
47. Reimer, K. A., Rasmussen, M. M., and Jennings, R. B. (1976): On the nature of protection by propranolol against myocardial necrosis after temporary coronary occlusion in dogs. *Am. J. Cardiol.*, 37:520–527.
48. Rivas, F., Cobb, F. R., Bache, R. J., and Greenfield, J. C., Jr. (1976): Relationship between blood flow to ischemic regions and extent of myocardial infarction. *Circ. Res.*, 38:439–447.
49. Roark, S. F., Ideker, R. E., Wagner, G. S., Alonso, D. R., Bishop, S. P., Bloor, C. M., Bramlet, D. A., Edwards, J. E., Fallon, J. T., Gottlieb, G. J., Hackel, D. B., Phillips, H. R., Reimer, K. A., Rogers, W. J., Ruth, W. K., Savage, R. M., White, R. D., and Selvester, R. H. (1983): Evaluation of a QRS scoring system for estimating myocardial infarct size. III. Correlation with quantitative anatomic findings for inferior infarcts. *Am. J. Cardiol.*, 51:382–389.
50. Romson, J. L., Hook, B. G., Kunkel, S. L., Abrams, G. D., Schork, M. A., and Lucchesi, B. R. (1983): Reduction of the extent of ischemic myocardial injury by neutrophil depletion in the dog. *Circulation*, 67:1016–1023.
51. Schaper, W. (1979): Residual perfusion of acutely ischemic heart muscle. In: *The Pathophysiology of Myocardial Perfusion*, edited by W. Schaper, pp. 345–378. Elsevier/North Holland, New York.
52. Schaper, W., Frenzel, H., Hort, W., and Winkler, B. (1979): Experimental coronary artery occlusion. II. Spatial and temporal evolution of infarcts in the dog heart. *Basic Res. Cardiol.*, 74:233–239.
53. Sobel, B. E., and Shell, W. E. (1972): Serum enzyme determinations in the diagnosis and assessment of myocardial infarction. *Circulation*, 45:471–482.
54. Swain, J. L., Cobb, F. R., McHale, P. A., and Roe, C. R. (1980): Non-linear relationship between creatine kinase estimates and histologic extent of infarction in conscious dogs: Effects of regional myocardial blood flow. *Circulation*, 62:1239–1247.
55. Wackers, F. J., Berger, H. J., Weinberg, M. A., and Zaret, B. L. (1982): Spontaneous changes in

left ventricular function over the first 24 hours of acute myocardial infarction: Implications for evaluating early therapeutic intervention. *Circulation*, 66:748–754.

56. Weiner, J. M., Apstein, C. S., Arthur, J. H., Pirzada, F. A., and Hood, W. B. (1976): Persistence of myocardial injury following brief periods of coronary occlusion. *Cardiovasc. Res.*, 10:678–686.

57. Weiss, E. S., Ahmed, S. A., Welch, M. J., Williamson, J. R., Ter-Pogossian, M. M., and Sobel, B. E. (1977): Quantification of infarction in cross sections of canine myocardium *in vivo* with positron emission transaxial tomography and $^{11}$C-Palmitate. *Circulation*, 55:66–73.

58. Yellon, D. M., Hearse, D. J., Maxwell, M. P., Chambers, D. E., and Downey, J. M. (1983): Sustained limitation of myocardial necrosis 24 hours after coronary artery occlusion: Verapamil infusion in dogs wihh small myocardial infarcts. *Am. J. Cardiol.*, 51:1409–1413.

*Therapeutic Approaches to Myocardial Infarct
Size Limitation*, edited by D. J. Hearse and
D. M. Yellon. Raven Press, New York © 1984.

# 11

# Can Drugs Really Limit Infarct Size?

## Robert J. Bache

*Department of Medicine, Cardiovascular Section, University of Minnesota Medical
School, Minneapolis, Minnesota 55455*

*Therapeutic interventions in patients with myocardial infarction may exert different effects at differing times during the evolution of the ischemic process.* Different therapeutic strategies may be appropriate in the setting of unstable angina (18), evolving acute myocardial infarction (75), or following completion of the infarction process (10). Substantial clinical data indicate that medical therapy with vasodilators and β-adrenergic blocking drugs may cause symptomatic improvement in patients with unstable angina, and may potentially reduce the incidence of unstable angina culminating in acute myocardial infarction (18,75). Long-term β-adrenergic blocking therapy has been demonstrated to reduce the incidence of sudden death and myocardial infarction in patients during the months following hospital discharge for treatment of acute myocardial infarction (10,36,59). These represent important therapeutic achievements that have had substantial impact on the treatment of patients with unstable angina and following recovery from the acute phase of myocardial infarction. However, I confine this discussion to a consideration of the process of acute myocardial infarction with emphasis on therapeutic attempts to reduce infarct size. Before undertaking such a discussion it will be necessary to consider a number of important factors and complications that affect the interpretation of both clinical and experimental studies. These include the design and relevance of models; the influence of some complex and variable interacting factors which determine the ultimate size of an evolving infarct; the difficulty of measuring infarct size, particularly under clinical conditions; and the fact that induced or spontaneous reperfusion might complicate the interpretation of studies.

## FACTORS AND COMPLICATIONS IN THE INTERPRETATION OF STUDIES

### Design and Relevance of Models

The design of various models of myocardial infarction and the validity of various indices of injury and protection are discussed fully in Chapters 2 and 10. The importance of an appreciation of the relevance and the disadvantages of various models cannot be overestimated. Such assessments are, however, not always easy to make when, for example, basic aspects of the natural history of myocardial infarction remain controversial; an example of such a situation is the debate over the possibility that infarction can arise without necessarily involving thrombotic occlusion.

### Is Thrombotic Occlusion a Prerequisite for Myocardial Infarction?

Pathologic studies of hearts from patients dying of acute myocardial infarction have demonstrated a variable relationship between acute coronary thrombosis and the infarction process. Substantial numbers of hearts can be shown to have occlusive high-grade chronic atherosclerotic disease but without demonstrable acute thrombotic coronary artery occlusion (72). However, angiographic studies of patients with electrocardiographic evidence of acute transmural myocardial infarction have demonstrated a very high incidence of total coronary artery occlusion (70). The failure of some pathologic studies to document a similarly high incidence of acute coronary artery occlusion in patients dying from myocardial infarction (especially those in whom death has occurred early in the course of the infarction process) may be related to postmortem dissolution of thrombus or dislodgement of the thrombotic occlusion during manipulation of the heart (19). Thus, it is my opinion that, *in most patients, the syndrome of acute transmural myocardial infarction appears to develop secondary to thrombotic occlusion of a previously diseased but patent epicardial coronary artery.* This pathophysiologic mechanism is further supported by the finding that, in a large proportion of these patients, thrombolytic therapy results in recanalization of the artery and restoration of blood flow, implying a causal relationship between recent thrombotic coronary occlusion and initiation of the infarction process (70,83).

### Difficulties in Extrapolation from Animal Models

*It is unclear to what extent these experimental findings may be extrapolated to the clinical situation of acute myocardial infarction.* Whereas, in the animal model, infarction is generally initiated by abrupt total coronary occlusion, the rate of onset of coronary occlusion is less clear and likely to be variable in patients who develop myocardial infarction. Occlusion of a coronary artery in patients may be of more gradual onset, or could be heralded by waxing and waning thrombotic obstruction, which might require several hours to result in total occlusion. The range of clinical descriptions (Chapter 1) provided by patients suffering acute myocardial infarction, from abrupt onset of severe chest pain to "stuttering" and cumulative symptoms developing over many hours suggests that *the mechanism of infarction and rapidity of coronary occlusion may vary substantially between patients.* In addition, precise timing of the onset of the clinical syndrome of myocardial infarction is dependent on the patient's perception and description of his symptoms. Because of these vagaries in the mechanisms responsible for initiation of clinical myocardial infarction, as well as the not infrequent difficulties in ascertaining the exact timing of the event, it is difficult to use data from the animal laboratory to ascertain the optimal or permissable time for therapeutic intervention in patients with acute myocardial infarction. Nevertheless, as discussed in the next section, it is clear from the laboratory data that time is a *critical variable* in the development of irreversible injury following coronary occlusion, so that for a given pathophysiology (which may be variable from patient to patient) an earlier intervention will have greater potential for benefit than if that same intervention is delayed.

## Determinants of Infarct Size

*Experimental studies have demonstrated several variables that importantly influence infarct size* following acute coronary artery occlusion. These include the metabolic requirements of the myocardium during the period of coronary occlusion (9,55,71) and the time of onset of irreversible injury; the volume of myocardium denied perfusion (9,71) following acute coronary artery occlusion ("risk region"), and the rate of collateral blood flow into the area of ischemic myocardium (71).

### Time: The Critical Factor

*The timing of a potentially useful intervention for salvage of ischemic myocardium after the onset of ischemia is of great importance. The rate of evolution from severely ischemic myocardium to irreversibly injured tissue will determine when a potentially useful intervention could no longer exert a beneficial effect.* In experimental canine models of myocardial infarction in which abrupt coronary artery occlusion is used to produce myocardial ischemia, potentially salvable tissue may be demonstrated by reduction of infarct size as a result of reperfusion for approximately 3 hr after the onset of ischemia (8,52,67). If arterial inflow is reestablished more than 3 hr after coronary occlusion, the resultant infarct is not different in size from that occurring in response to permanent coronary occlusion (77). Thus, a *relatively narrow window in time exists during which a potentially useful therapeutic agent might salvage ischemic myocardium.* The progression from severely ischemic to irreversibly injured myocardium proceeds rapidly during the first 2 to 3 hr following coronary occlusion, so that salvage of tissue would be most likely during this time interval, while later interventions would have potential for less benefit, and the processes resulting in tissue death would be nearly completed within 3 hr.

### Volume of Myocardium Denied Perfusion

Since the volume of myocardium jeopardized by acute coronary occlusion is determined by the level in the arterial system at which occlusion occurs, no intervention short of reperfusion would be likely to affect this variable. Consequently, interventions to modify infarct size have concentrated on the use of therapeutic agents which may increase intercoronary collateral blood flow, or which may decrease metabolic requirements of the ischemic myocardium. In addition, several interventions have been proposed that might alter components of the local, or systemic, inflammatory response to ischemia, or during reperfusion following relief of coronary occlusion (Chapter 13).

### Collateral Blood Flow: The Major Determinant of the Extent of Infarction

Although abrupt permanent occlusion of a major coronary artery in the experimental laboratory consistently leads to acute myocardial infarction, the resultant infarct generally is smaller than the area of myocardium normally perfused by the occluded artery. Thus, Schaper and associates (78) found that occlusion at the midpoint of the left anterior descending coronary artery in dogs resulted in myocardial infarction involving about 10% of the left ventricular mass, while injection techniques showed that this artery supplied more than 20% of the left ventricular muscle. Pathologic data obtained from patients dying with acute myocardial infarction similarly demonstrate that a portion of the acutely ischemic myocardium is preserved from infarction (47). Survival of a portion of the myocardium normally perfused by an occluded artery is dependent on delivery of a limited inflow of arterial blood by preexisting intercoronary collateral vasculature; *the proportion of myocardium surviving acute coronary occlusion is related quantitatively to the volume of collateral flow available to the acutely ischemic myocardium early after coronary occlusion* (71). Studies of coronary occlusion in both experimental laboratory models and in human pathologic studies demonstrate that the area of preserved myocardium tends to be subepicardial in location, overlying the region of infarct (Chapter 8), whereas a relatively sharply delineated lateral boundary corresponds to the anatomic limits of the perfusion bed of the occluded artery (23,47,71,78).

*It is clear that patients with occlusive coronary artery disease have potential for development of substantial intercoronary collateral vasculature.* Thus, total coronary artery occlusion without gross morphologic or histologic evidence of myocardial infarction is a well-documented finding, occurring in over 20% of hearts with total coronary occlusion examined by Baroldi and Scomazzoni (7). Although it is thus clear that human coronary collateral vessels have the capacity to undergo substantial growth in response to regional myocardial ischemia, *the rate of collat-*

*eral growth in the human heart is less clear.* In necropsy studies of hearts from patients with a history of angina pectoris, Fulton (27) found that the intercoronary collateral vasculature tended to increase with the duration of angina, with few substantial collateral channels being found in patients with angina of less than 3 months duration. In pathologic studies of hearts from patients dying subsequent to acute myocardial infarction, Jones (43) did not find substantial collateral vessels until approximately 2 months after acute infarction. *These data suggest that the growth of collateral channels proceeds fairly slowly in the human, but that collateral vessels may attain sufficient size to adequately perfuse myocardium distal to a totally occluded major coronary artery.* However, there appears to be substantial variability in the capacity for collateral vessel development in the human heart exposed to myocardial ischemia. Thus, Baroldi and Scomazzoni (7) found marked variability in the diameter of the intercoronary collateral channels in patients dying with occlusive coronary artery disease, so that only a weak relationship existed between the extent of occlusive coronary disease and the degree of collateralization. For this reason, *it is not possible to predict the extent and functional significance of the intercoronary collateral vasculature in individual patients suffering acute myocardial infarction. Since preservation of ischemic myocardium presumably requires a certain minimum collateral inflow, the efficacy of any potentially useful agent for limitation of infarct size would likely be dependent on collateral flow (Chapter 5).*

*Responsiveness to vasoactive agents.* The ability of a vasoactive agent to act on the coronary collateral vessels may depend on the degree of development of the collateral channels. Thus, the small intrinsic collateral vessels which exist in the absence of occlusive coronary artery disease contain little smooth muscle, and consequently would be unlikely to have substantial ability to undergo active vasomotor activity (76). In contrast, well developed collateral channels have characteristics similar to a normal artery, including a substantial smooth muscle coat (76); such collateral vessels may have considerable potential for active vasomotion in response to pharmacologic interventions. It has been suggested that collateral vessels may not be vasodilated in the presence of regional myocardial ischemia, since the smooth muscle of the collateral vessels would be exposed to the high oxygen content of the arterial blood contained within the lumen (17). If this is true, then pharmacologic vasodilators active at the level of the collateral vessels would have potential for increasing collateral blood flow in patients with acute myocardial ischemic syndromes.

*Responsiveness to ischemia. It is not clear that the collateral vessels are actually unresponsive to ischemia occurring downstream in the collateral-dependent myocardium.* Vatner and colleagues (49,88) found that ischemia in the perfusion bed of the left circumflex coronary artery of dogs produces ascending vasodilation which involves the proximal arterial segment. The mechanism of this effect may involve release of a vasoactive messenger by the vascular endothelium in response to increased blood flow rates (28). *If such vasodilation also occurs in the collateral system, the presence of ischemia in the collateral-dependent myocardium could result in maximum vasodilation of the collateral vessels, and thereby render them unresponsive to additional pharmacologic vasodilator stimuli.*

## Clinical Estimation of Infarct Size

In the experimental laboratory animal, infarct size may be directly and precisely measured by pathologic examination of the heart, provided that a sufficient time interval is allowed after coronary occlusion for development of specific histologic changes of infarction to occur. Unfortunately, *clinical evaluation of interventions for limitation of infarct size have been hampered by lack of completely satisfactory techniques for precisely measuring infarct size*, or for predicting the ultimate size of an untreated evolving infarct. Infarct size in patients has been estimated from measurements of plasma creatine kinase released from areas of infarcted myocardium. Shell et al. (80) demonstrated a close linear relationship ($r = 0.96$) between infarct size calculated from serum creatine kinase time-activity curves and the degree of myocardial depletion of creatine kinase in dogs with acute coronary artery occlusion. Subsequently, however, Roe et al. (74) found that although a close linear relationship existed between creatine kinase estimates of infarct size and histologic infarct size for small myocardial infarctions in the dog, this relationship did not hold for larger myocardial infarctions. The inability to accurately predict infarct size for large infarcts appeared to occur because the residual blood flow available to wash creatine kinase out of the area of infarcted myocardium tended to be lower with larger infarcts (15). This suggests that the appearance of creatine kinase in plasma may be influenced by the residual collateral blood flow after coronary occlusion, and that therapeutic manipulations affecting collateral flow may have potential for altering washout of creatine kinase from the infarcted tissue. Grande et al. (33) compared a creatine kinase MB isoenzyme infarct size index with myocardial infarct size, as demonstrated by nitro-blue tetrazolium staining, in 22 patients dying with acute myocardial infarction. These investigators observed a moderately good correlation between observed and predicted infarct size ($r = 0.83$), but they noted that a relatively large standard error of estimate "shows that the estimate is only semi-quantitative." For this reason they suggested that estimates of infarct size from creatine kinase MB isoenzyme curves be used only for comparison of groups of patients, and not for evaluating individual patients. They attributed the imprecision in the estimation of infarct size to unaccounted for variations in the release, distribution, and elimination of enzyme following acute myocardial infarction.

## Effects of Reperfusion

Coronary occlusion of longer than approximately 20 min duration in the anesthetized open chest dog is associated with development of tissue necrosis and morphologic evidence of myocardial infarction (41). Reperfusion prior to this time may be associated with prolonged depression of systolic function and reduction of myocardial adenine nucleotide stores, but complete recovery of these variables eventually occurs (35,84). Although longer durations of occlusion generally result in myocardial infarction, reperfusion up to approximately 3 hr after the onset of coronary occlusion is associated with evidence of myocardial salvage; i.e., infarct size is smaller than predicted had the occlusion been permanent (29). *Despite this evidence for a beneficial effect of coronary reperfusion, it has been suggested that reperfusion of ischemic myocardium may increase the degree of tissue injury (11).* This suggestion has been based, in part, on the finding that reperfusion is often associated with substantial hemorrhage into the ischemic area. The concept of reperfusion injury has been examined by Hofmann et al. (38) in anesthetized open chest dogs. When reperfusion was allowed 3 or 6 hr after coronary occlusion, reperfusion was associated with hemorrhagic infarction, but reperfused and non-perfused myocardium did not differ with regard to infarct size. Since permanent coronary occlusion results in infarction but also produces areas of ischemic myo-cardium which do not go on to infarct, if reperfusion injury occurred, then some of this ischemic, but viable, myocardium should be further injured by reflow. However, reperfusion was not associated with an infarct size greater than that observed following permanent coronary occlusion (38); *these data thus fail to support the concept of reperfusion injury.* Nevertheless, it is possible that at earlier intervals following coronary artery occlusion, the beneficial effect of reperfusion might be compromised by injurious effects resulting from reperfusion. The available data clearly indicate that in the experimental laboratory, reperfusion exerts a beneficial effect within the first 2 to 3 hr after total coronary occlusion. Whether, within this time interval, reperfusion simultaneously exerts a deleterious effect is problematic. Several investigators have presented evidence suggesting that reper-fusion may be associated with production of free radicals, inward migration of leukocytes, or calcium overloading of myocytes which may have potential for causing tissue injury. These topics are discussed in greater detail in other chapters. Nevertheless, data available at present demonstrate that *reperfusion relatively early after the onset of coronary occlusion has potential for salvage of ischemic but not irreversibly injured myocardium.*

## PHARMACOLOGICAL ATTEMPTS TO LIMIT INFARCT SIZE

As discussed in early sections, an important approach to infarct size limitation must be through the promotion of collateral flow or the restoration of preexisting flow. Another approach has been to manipulate cellular metabolism particularly in relation to energy consumption. Numerous methods have been developed and studied, but for the purpose of this chapter I concentrate on three major drug groups: β-blockers, nitrates, and calcium antagonists.

### β-Adrenergic Blocking Drugs

β-Adrenergic blocking agents have been reported to cause reduction in the degree of ST-segment elevation in the precordial electrogram and to cause improvement or relief of chest pain in patients with acute myocardial infarction (30,90). These agents generally cause a significant reduction of heart rate, and ischemic ST-segment elevation is known to be responsive to changes in heart rate (66), although the precise relationship between these rate-related changes in the degree of ST-segment elevation and ultimate infarct size is subject to some controversy. The uncertainty regarding the specificity of ST-segment changes in response to β-adrenergic blockade is illustrated by the finding of Pelides et al. (62) that practolol, 20 mg i.v., resulted in improvement in the degree of ST-segment elevation not only in patients early after the onset of symptoms of acute myocardial infarction, but also for up to 72 hr after the onset of infarction, at a time when there is general agreement that potential for salvage of ischemic myocardium no longer exists.

### Spectrum of Pharmacological Actions

The β-adrenergic blocking drugs exert multiple effects on the cardiovascular system, which may interact to produce differing outcomes, depending on the prevailing degree of adrenergic nervous system activation and the baseline level of cardiac performance. The actions of these agents on the heart may alter each of the three major determinants of myocardial oxygen requirement (heart rate, myocardial contractility, systolic tension), generally producing a reduction in myocardial oxygen need which might be expected to alleviate acute myocardial ischemia (60). Competitive binding of these agents to cardiac β-adrenergic receptors results in a slowing of heart rate and a reduction of cardiac contractility, both of which directly reduce oxygen requirements. The effect of these agents on the third major determinant of myocardial oxygen consumption, systolic tension, is dependent on the interaction between drug-induced changes in arterial pressure and left ventricular volume. The β-adrenergic blocking drugs generally cause a reduction of arterial pressure, which results in a decreased left ventricular afterload. At the same time, these agents cause increased left ventricular volume; the net result of these changes in afterload and ventricular volume is generally an increase in systolic tension which, by itself, would tend to increase the myocardial oxygen requirement. However, because of the favorable effects on heart rate and contractility, the overall effect of β-adrenergic blockade is generally a reduction of myocardial oxygen consumption (60). The magnitude of these effects of β-adrenergic blockade is to a considerable extent dependent on the degree of activation of the sympathetic nervous system. Since sympathetic nervous system activity may be increased in the setting of acute myocardial infarction, the effects of β-blocking drugs may be especially prominent in this situation. However, because patients with acute myocardial infarction and extensive left ventricular wall motion abnormality may be dependent on catecholamine support from the sympathetic nervous system to maintain cardiac compensation, use of these agents is not without hazard.

The effects of β-adrenergic blockade on delivery of arterial blood to the ischemic myocardium are complex and not easily predicted. The reduction of blood pressure produced by these agents, which causes a beneficial decrease of left ventricular afterload may, at the same time, cause reduction of blood flow to collateral-dependent areas of myocardium because of the marked dependence of collateral blood on perfusion pressure (46). The recent demonstration that the severity of coronary stenotic lesions may be influenced by intraarterial distending pressure suggests that reduction of arterial pressure could potentially worsen the degree of coronary stenosis (79). In addition, epicardial coronary arteries have been shown to possess both α-adrenergic vasoconstrictor and β-adrenergic vasodilator activity (61,87,89). Blocking the β-adrenergic vasodilator influence could, at least theoretically, result in unmasking α-adrenergic coronary vasoconstrictor activity. This mechanism may be of importance in patients susceptible to coronary vasospasm, inasmuch as treatment with β-adrenergic blocking drugs may increase the frequency of Prinzmetal's angina in certain susceptible patients (73). It is unclear whether unmasking α-receptor activity by means of β-blockade could also be of significance in patients with critical coronary artery stenoses and acute myocardial ischemia.

In addition to the effects of β-adrenergic blockade on delivery of arterial inflow to collateral-dependent myocardium or to areas served by critically stenotic vessels, β-blockade with propranolol has been shown to produce transmural redistribution of perfusion following acute coronary artery occlusion, with a modest increase in the blood flow to the subendocardium (86). These studies were, however, performed in dogs in which left ventricular diastolic pressures were normal or only mildly elevated. In patients in whom left ventricular filling pressures may be substantially elevated in the setting of acute myocardial infarction, a further increase in left ventricular diastolic pressure produced by administration of a β-adrenergic blocking agent could impede subendocardial blood flow directly. Thus, left ventricular cavity pressure contributes to the intramyocardial tissue pressure which acts to compress the intramural coronary vessels. Since this effect of diastolic left ventricular pressure is most marked in the subendocardium, an increase in left ventricular filling produced by β-adrenergic blockade would act to impede subendocardial blood flow. The net result of β-adrenergic blockade on subendocardial blood flow will thus depend on the relative importance of these two competing mechanisms.

## Animal Studies

Several investigators have examined the effects of β-adrenergic blocking agents on the response to acute coronary artery occlusion in experimental animals. Maroko et al. (51) acutely ligated the left anterior descending or the apical branch of the anterior descending coronary artery in open chest anesthetized dogs. Propranolol was administered in a dosage of 0.5 to 2 mg/kg i.v., followed by 0.5 mg/kg at 4-hr intervals for 12 hr. Twenty-four hours after coronary occlusion, myocardial tissue was analyzed for depletion of creatine kinase as evidence of necrosis. With propranolol treatment, the extent of depression of myocardial creatine kinase activity was significantly less than in control animals, suggesting protection of ischemic myocardium. Pierce et al. (64) examined the effect of propranolol, 1 mg/kg i.v., in anesthetized open chest dogs subjected to occlusion of the distal left anterior descending coronary artery. Infarct size was estimated from nitro-blue tetrazolium staining 6 hr after coronary occlusion. In control animals the unstained area of myocardium corresponded to $11.9 \pm 0.9\%$ of the left ventricle, and was reduced to $7.8 \pm 1.1\%$ of the left ventricle in animals treated with propranolol ($p < 0.01$). Although this finding suggested a decrease in the volume of infarcted tissue, the tetrazolium method may not be entirely reliable when used relatively early after producing coronary occlusion (see Chapters 2, 5, and 10).

Reimer et al. (68) examined the effect of propranolol (5 mg/kg i.v.) in dogs subjected to a 40-min occlusion of the proximal left circumflex coronary artery followed by reperfusion. The animals were killed 2 to 5 days later and infarct size was determined by gross and histologic assessment of the degree of myocardial necrosis. Using this experimental model, myocardial infarction involves the posterior papillary muscle and adjacent subendocardium of the area supplied by the left circumflex coronary artery. Pretreatment with propranolol significantly reduced the area of necrosis in the posterior papillary muscle. When permanent occlusion of the left circumflex coronary artery was produced in dogs, propranolol (5 mg/kg i.v.) 10 min prior to coronary occlusion and an additional 1.0 mg/kg/hr for 24 hr reduced the area of necrosis from $85 \pm 3\%$ of the transmural posterior papillary muscle section to $52 \pm 4\%$ ($p < 0.01$) (65). In a subsequent dose-response study of the effects of propranolol, administered prior to 40-min temporary coronary artery occlusion followed by reperfusion, a significant reduction of infarct size was found only at dosages which were adequate to produce β-adrenergic blockade, whereas smaller dosages were ineffective (65).

In contrast to these initial encouraging results, a later study by Jennings and Reimer (40) failed to reproduce a significant effect of propranolol on infarct size, in dogs subjected to a 40-min occlusion of the proximal left circumflex coronary artery followed by reperfusion. Propranolol was infused at a rate of 0.05 mg/kg/min until β-adrenergic blockade was evidenced by a leveling off of the heart rate response to the drug. The mean dose of propranolol was 0.32 mg/kg of body weight. Infarct size was quantitated histologically 4 days after coronary occlusion. Propranolol significantly decreased heart rate from $166 \pm 9$ to $134 \pm 8$ beats/min ($p < 0.01$), while collateral blood flow into the ischemic area was unchanged. The area at risk was similar in control and treated groups. The percentage of left ventricle which became necrotic, as well as the percentage of the risk region which became necrotic, were similar in treated and control groups. Possible reasons for the failure of this study to demonstrate a significant effect of propranolol on infarct size, in comparison with the encouraging results of earlier studies, were discussed by the investigators (40; Chapter 10). A plausible explanation relates to the high mortality observed in the original studies using this experimental model. Thus, mortality during coronary occlusion and reperfusion was approximately 50%. Coronary occlusion often produced a high left ventricular end-diastolic pressure that would be expected to be further aggravated by administration of propranolol. The investigators postulated that this deleterious effect of propranolol may have caused the death of animals with more severe degrees of myocardial ischemia, thereby causing elimination of those animals destined to have the largest infarcts from the propranolol-treated group. With subsequent refinement of the experimental model, the mortality from left circumflex coronary artery has been reduced to approximately 10%, and a beneficial effect of propranolol on myocardial infarct size could no longer be demonstrated. *This sequence of studies demonstrates the importance of tabulation of all animals entering each treatment group, and not merely those which survive to the termination of study for measurement of infarct size.*

### Patient Studies

Several randomized trials of the effect of β-adrenergic blocker therapy on infarct size have been carried out in patients with acute myocardial infarction. Peter et al. (63) examined the effect of propranolol (0.1 mg/kg i.v., followed by 320 mg orally given over the succeeding 27 hr) on serum creatine kinase in a randomized trial involving 95 patients treated within 12 hr of the onset of symptoms of uncomplicated myocardial infarction. Patients older than 65 years of age or with a heart rate of less than 60 beats/min were excluded, as were patients with contraindications to β-blocker therapy. Only total serum creatine kinase was assayed, without determination of isoenzymes. Propranolol resulted in a modest reduction in heart rate and arterial blood pressure. Patients were divided into 3 groups according to whether chest pain started less than 4 hr, 4 to 8 hr, or 8 to 12 hr before entry into the study. No significant difference in creatine kinase values was observed between control and treated patients in the 2 groups entering the study longer than 4 hr after the onset of symptoms. In the patients with myocardial infarction, treated within 4 hr of the onset of symptoms, peak creatine kinase was reduced by 27% in patients receiving propranolol ($p<0.0125$), while reduction of total calculated creatine kinase appearance was of borderline significance ($p<0.1$ by unpaired *t*-test using the 2-tailed *p*-value). *It should be noted that in this study several unpaired t-tests were performed between treated and control groups without adjustment for performing multiple comparisons; this procedure may inappropriately enhance the significance of the resultant* p-*values.*

Johansson (42) randomized 87 patients with acute myocardial infarction to treatment with practolol (20 mg i.v.) followed by atenolol (50 mg orally twice daily for 7 days), placebo, or diazepam. The median time from the onset of symptoms to beginning treatment was 10 hr in the β-blockade group and 18 hr in the placebo group, with a very large range; a substantial number of patients entered the study later than 24 hr after the onset of symptoms. β-Blockade resulted in a significant reduction of heart rate. Ischemic injury, assessed from the degree of ST-segment elevation on the precordial electrocardiogram, was not different between control and treated patients. However, a relatively small number of patients were included in this trial and a substantial number of patients entered the study relatively late, when the potential for limitation of infarct size may be limited or absent.

Jurgensen et al. (45) randomized 282 patients with acute myocardial infarction to treatment with alprenolol or placebo. Alprenolol was administered in dosages of 5 to 10 mg i.v. followed by 250 mg orally in 3 hr and then twice daily for one year. The median interval from the onset of symptoms to randomization was 6 hr. Total plasma creatine kinase was measured every 4 hr for 2 days; creatine kinase isoenzymes were not determined. Using these measurements, the investigators reported an "infarct size" of 20.6 creatine kinase g-equivalents/m$^2$ in treated patients as compared with 34.4 in patients receiving placebo ($p<0.025$); the fractional rate of disappearance of creatine kinase from blood was not different between the 2 groups. No difference was observed in patients entering the study later than 12 hr after the onset of symptoms. These investigators (1) subsequently reported that of those patients who survived hospitalization for acute myocardial infarction, alprenolol significantly reduced the mortality rate after 1 year of continued treatment in patients less than 65 years of age. *Since a similar reduction of long-term mortality has also been found when treatment with β-blocking agents is begun several weeks after acute myocardial infarction, it is difficult to ascribe this effect on long-term mortality to any specific action of alprenolol during the acute phase of myocardial infarction.*

Yusuf et al. (96) randomized 307 patients with documented myocardial infarction to atenolol or placebo treatment within less than 24 hr of the onset of symptoms. Atenolol, 5 mg i.v., was given immediately; if no undue hypotension or bradycardia occurred, this was followed by an oral dose of 50 mg immediately and 12 hr later, and then 100 mg daily for the next 10 days. Total and creatine kinase MB isoenzyme were determined every 4 hr for the first 48 hr and every 6 hr for the next 24 hr. Mean cumulative creatine kinase MB isoenzyme release was $110 \pm 8.1$ IU/liter in the atenolol group and $157 \pm 13.6$ in the control group ($p<0.002$). R-wave scores were computed as the ratio of the worst R-wave voltage in the region involved with infarct as compared with the prerandomization R-wave voltage in the same electrocardiographic leads. The mean R-wave score was $41.1 \pm 2\%$ in the atenolol-treated group and $30.7 \pm 2.1\%$ in the control group ($p<0.001$). Reduction of plasma creatine kinase and improvement of R-wave score was found both in patients treated early and in patients treated later than 4 hr after the onset of symptoms.

McIlmoyle et al. (53) randomized 391 patients to intravenous metoprolol or placebo within 6 hr after the onset of symptoms of acute myocardial infarction. These investigators observed that the mean log maximum for the creatine kinase MB isoenzyme was significantly lower in patients treated with metoprolol ($2.08 \pm 0.33$ IU) than in placebo-treated patients ($2.17 \pm 0.34$), although mortality during the first 3 months was not different between the 2 groups.

Hjalmarson et al. (36,37) randomly allocated 1,395 patients to double-blind treatment with metoprolol (15 mg i.v. followed by 200 mg/day for 90 days) or placebo. Serum lactate dehydrogenase I and II were measured every 12 hr for the first 3 days. Institution of metoprolol within 12 hr after the onset of pain resulted in significantly lower maximum lactate dehydrogenase I and II values compared with placebo, while no such difference was found in patients entering the study later than 12 hr after the onset of pain. The authors interpreted this finding as evidence of reduced infarct size in metoprolol-treated patients.

## Can β-Blockers Limit Infarct Size?

*The above experimental and clinical studies do not provide a consensus opinion regarding the effects of β-adrenergic blockers on myocardial infarct size. Although early experimental studies appeared to result in infarct size reduction in canine models, these results have not been reproduced when more rigorous methodology has been employed.* Patient studies have relied principally on estimation of infarct size from creatine kinase or creatine kinase MB isoenzyme time-activity curves following myocardial infarction. Although necropsy studies have demonstrated a moderately good correlation between these measurements and actual infarct size determined pathologically in patients dying with myocardial infarction, experimental studies have demonstrated difficulty with this technique in the presence of large infarcts. *Nevertheless, four of six clinical trials of β-adrenergic blockers in patients with acute myocardial infarction demonstrated significant reduction of plasma creatine kinase time-activity curves, peak creatine kinase, or maximum lactate dehydrogenase I and II values compared with placebo. These are encouraging results. However, since improvement in mortality appears no better when β-adrenergic blocking agents are administered during the acute myocardial infarction process or delayed until the time of hospital discharge, and because of the significant side-effects and substantial contraindications to β-blockade in patients with acute myocardial infarction, β-adrenergic blockers cannot be recommended for routine use in patients during the acute phase of myocardial infarction. Nevertheless, β-blocking agents are clearly beneficial in treatment of patients with angina pectoris and for long-term treatment following the acute phase of myocardial infarction.*

## Nitroglycerin

The organic nitrate esters exert hemodynamic effects that are clearly of benefit in patients with angina pectoris or congestive cardiac failure. The pharmacological actions of these drugs are, however, complex.

### Spectrum of Pharmacological Actions

Nitroglycerin causes venodilation with a decrease in left ventricular preload, as well as systemic arteriolar vasodilation which causes a modest reduction in afterload (54,92). The resultant decrease in left ventricular systolic tension is associated with a direct reduction of myocardial oxygen requirements (31). In addition to these systemic hemodynamic effects, the nitrates exert direct effects on the coronary vasculature which may enhance the blood supply to areas of potentially ischemic myocardium. Using a chronically instrumented canine model in which the diameter of the proximal left circumflex coronary artery was continuously measured with ultrasonic crystals, Macho and Vatner (50) demonstrated that nitroglycerin (8 μg/min/kg) resulted in a $29 \pm 5\%$ increase in luminal cross-sectional area. Since atherosclerotic coronary artery lesions are frequently eccentric in location, having a portion of the arterial wall uninvolved, nitroglycerin-induced vasodilation may also result in significant improvement in the degree of coronary artery narrowing at areas of stenotic lesions (12). In addition, nitroglycerin has been demonstrated experimentally to cause vasodilation of intercoronary collateral vessels, which develop in response to gradual chronic occlusion of a major coronary artery in the dog (24). However, the response to nitroglycerin of the small intrinsic collateral vessels that exist at the time of acute coronary artery occlusion has been less clear, with some investigators demonstrating a modest degree of collateral vessel vasodilation while others have been unable to document a significant effect of nitroglycerin on collateral flow (2,20). These data suggest that the response of collateral vessels to nitroglycerin depends on the degree of collateral development, with well developed collateral vessels demonstrating substantial vasodilation while undeveloped collaterals show little response. For this reason, *the effect of nitroglycerin on collateral blood flow in patients with occlusive coronary artery disease might be expected to depend on the degree of collateral vessel development.* In patients undergoing cardiac surgery, Goldstein et al. (32) documented that nitroglycerin produced a variable degree of collateral vessel vasodilation as assessed by retrograde flow from the occluded artery at the time of placement of the vein graft.

*In addition to effects on the epicardial arteries and collateral vessels, nitroglycerin may affect the transmural distribution of myocardial perfusion.* When myocardial perfusion is determined by a proximal flow-limiting coronary artery stenosis, hypoperfusion is most severe in the subendocardium (6). In this situation, nitroglycerin has been demonstrated to favor blood flow to the subendocardium where vulnerability to ischemia is greatest (5). In the presence of left ventricular dysfunction, nitroglycerin may further enhance subendocardial perfusion by decreasing left ventricular filling pressure, since intramyocardial tissue pressure, which impedes subendocardial perfusion during diastole, is directly related to intracavitary pressure (21).

## Animal Studies

Studies of the effects of intravenous nitroglycerin in dogs subjected to acute coronary artery occlusion have generally demonstrated a reduction of electrocardiographic ST-segment elevation from leads overlying the ischemic zone (81) and a modest increase in blood flow to the area of ischemic myocardium (26,44). *Studies of the effect of nitroglycerin on infarct size have yielded conflicting results.*

Jugdutt et al. (44) examined the effect of intravenous nitroglycerin, following permanent occlusion of the mid left circumflex coronary artery, in previously instrumented awake dogs. Nitroglycerin infusion was begun 3 min after the onset of coronary occlusion and continued for 6 hr; the infusion rate was adjusted to reduce mean arterial pressure by 10%, but not below 90 mm Hg. Myocardial infarct size was determined morphologically by postmortem examination 2 days after coronary occlusion. These investigators observed a reduction of mean infarct size from $12.1 \pm 2.2\%$ of the left ventricle in control animals to $6.4 \pm 1.4\%$ in animals treated with nitroglycerin ($p<0.05$). Addition of methoxamine to prevent the nitroglycerin-induced fall in arterial pressure did not result in a significantly different infarct size than was observed with nitroglycerin alone.

In contrast to this study, Fukuyama et al. (26) found no significant effect of nitroglycerin on infarct size in chronically instrumented awake dogs subjected to acute occlusion of the proximal left anterior descending coronary artery. Nitroglycerin infusion was begun 10 min after coronary occlusion and continued for 8 hr; mean arterial pressure in the animals randomized to nitroglycerin was 84 mm Hg as compared with 94 mm Hg in the control group ($p<0.05$). Myocardial infarct size was determined both by gross morphology and by myocardial creatine kinase depletion 24 hr after coronary occlusion. Myocardial infarct size was $25.4 \pm 1\%$ of the left ventricle in the control dogs and $27 \pm 1.3\%$ in the dogs treated with nitroglycerin, an insignificant difference. Infarct size based on myocardial creatine kinase depletion was $23.3 \pm 7.8\%$ of the left ventricle in animals receiving nitroglycerin and $23.6 \pm 7.2\%$ in the control dogs. Although the reason for the disparity between these two studies is unclear, it is possible that the difference in experimentally produced infarct size may have affected the response to nitroglycerin. Thus, occlusion of the mid left circumflex coronary artery by Jugdutt and associates (44) resulted in substantially smaller infarcts than were observed by Fukuyama et al. (26), who occluded the proximal left anterior descending coronary artery.

### Patient Studies

Several clinical studies have attempted to examine the effect of nitroglycerin on infarct size in patients with acute myocardial infarction. Bussmann et al. (13) randomized 60 patients with acute myocardial infarction to treatment with intravenous nitroglycerin or to a control group. Patients were divided into an early intervention group in which therapy was begun within 8 hr (mean = 8.5) of the onset of symptoms, and a late intervention group in which therapy was begun from 8.3 to 23.3 hr (mean = 12.8 hr) after the onset of symptoms. The mean initial infusion rate of nitroglycerin was 2.9 mg/hr for the early intervention group and 2.7 mg/hr for the late intervention group. Nitroglycerin administration resulted in significant reductions of arterial pressure, systemic vascular resistance, and pulmonary artery diastolic pressure. Creatine kinase isoenzymes were determined hourly for the first 12 hr and subsequently for 3-hr intervals during the next 36 hr. Nitroglycerin delayed the time interval from the onset of symptoms to the peak creatine kinase value. Peak creatine kinase values and the creatine kinase MB isoenzyme time-activity curves were significantly lower in patients receiving nitroglycerin than in the control group. Mean "infarct size" computed from the creatine kinase MB time-activity curve was $59 \pm 38$ g-equivalents in the control group, as compared with $36 \pm 28$ g-equivalents in the nitroglycerin-treated group ($p<0.002$). Of interest was the finding that similar results were obtained in a late intervention group when administration of nitroglycerin was not begun until a mean of 12.8 hr after the onset of symptoms. This finding is difficult to understand since the volume of myocardium available for salvage should decrease with the passage of time as ischemic myocardium progressively evolves to irreversibly injured tissue during the infarction process.

Jaffee et al. (39) randomized 85 patients with acute myocardial infarction to either placebo or intravenous nitroglycerin within 10 hr after the onset of symptoms (mean interval = 6.0 hr). Nitroglycerin was infused at a rate that resulted in a 10% reduction of systolic blood pressure, attainment of a systolic blood pressure of 95 mm Hg, or a maximum dosage of 200 μg/min, whichever occurred first. Infusion rates were reduced if the heart rate increased more than 20 beats/min. Mean infusion rate was $57 \pm 21$ μg/min. Creatine kinase isoenzymes were measured every 4 hr during the first 96 hr after admission to the study. For the entire group, analysis of the creatine kinase MB time-activity curve yielded an "infarct size" of $14.9 \pm 2.1$ g-equivalents/m² in the control group and $11.2 \pm 2.1$ g-equivalents/m² in patients receiving nitroglycerin ($p = 0.06$). When patients were subdivided according to the location of the infarct, patients with inferior infarcts had creatine kinase MB time-activity curves yielding a mean value of $19.1 \pm 3.6$ g-equivalents/m² in the control group as compared with $12.0 \pm 1.8$ in the group treated with nitroglycerin ($p < 0.05$), while in patients with anterior infarction the values were $13.9 \pm 2.6$ g-equivalents/m² in the control group as compared with $13.7 \pm 2.8$ in the group treated with nitroglycerin (not significantly different). The mechanism for this difference in behavior of the creatine kinase time-activity curves in patients with anterior and inferior myocardial infarctions was unclear. It is of concern that the enzyme method predicated a larger infarct in untreated patients with inferior infarction as compared with those having anterior infarctions, while pathologic studies generally suggest the reverse.

### Can Nitroglycerin Limit Infarct Size?

The preceding experiments and clinical studies have demonstrated that nitroglycerin can generally be administered safely in the setting of acute myocardial infarction, provided that hypotension or volume depletion is not present. *The venodilating effects of the nitrates may be useful for treatment of cardiac failure in patients with acute myocardial infarction. However, the routine use of these agents with the expectation of reducing infarct size is, at present, not justified.* Experimental studies regarding the ability of nitroglycerin to limit infarct size have produced conflicting results, and although clinical studies have yielded encouraging data, substantial questions regarding the role of nitrates in treatment of acute myocardial infarction remain.

## Calcium Slow Channel Blocking Drugs

### Spectrum of Pharmacological Actions

*The calcium blocking drugs exert systemic and coronary hemodynamic effects which might be expected to alleviate myocardial ischemia.* Peripheral arteriolar vasodilation may directly reduce left ventricular afterload, thereby decreasing left ventricular systolic stress and reducing myocardial oxygen requirements and the need for coronary perfusion (48). Several of the calcium blocking drugs, including verapamil and diltiazem, slow the heart rate and decrease myocardial contractility, both of which would be expected to reduce myocardial oxygen needs (22). In addition to these systemic effects, the calcium blocking drugs exert direct effects on the coronary vasculature, which may enhance perfusion of potentially ischemic myocardium.

## Animal Studies

Using ultrasonic microcrystals to measure epicardial coronary artery diameter directly, Vatner and Hintze (88) demonstrated that nifedipine caused vasodilation of the proximal coronary arteries in chronically instrumented awake dogs. Similarly, using computer-assisted quantitative coronary angiography in patients undergoing diagnostic cardiac catheterization, Chew and associates (16) demonstrated that verapamil and nifedipine caused vasodilation of the epicardial coronary arteries; significant increases in cross-sectional area were observed in both angiographically normal arterial segments as well as in approximately two-thirds of stenotic segments. *Calcium blocker-induced vasodilation of the proximal coronary arteries could assume substantial therapeutic significance in patients with ischemic heart disease in whom atherosclerotic obstruction or spastic occlusion may compromise the lumen of an epicardial coronary artery.*

*Studies of the effects of calcium blocking drugs on collateral blood flow have yielded conflicting results.* Following experimental acute coronary occlusion in the dog, several investigators have reported that calcium blocking drugs increase blood flow to the ischemic "border zone," while blood flow to the most severely hypoperfused central ischemic zone has generally not been demonstrated to increase significantly (34,58). Other investigators have failed to demonstrate a significant effect of the calcium channel blocking agents on collateral blood flow (4,5,82). This disparity may be related to tissue sampling techniques when using the microsphere technique. Thus, Weintraub et al. (91) found that nifedipine (3 μg/kg/min) appeared to increase blood flow in border zones with intermediate reductions of perfusion following acute coronary occlusion in open chest dogs, while no effect was observed in the central ischemic zone. However, when correction was made for overlap between peninsulas of normally perfused myocardium and collateral-dependent myocardium in the border zones, blood flow to truly collateral-dependent myocardial areas actually decreased following administration of nifedipine. Thus, *currently available data suggest little or no effect of the calcium blocking agents on the small intrinsic collateral vessels which exist at the time of acute coronary artery occlusion.*

*Several investigators have examined the effect of calcium blocking agents on collateral vessels which develop in response to chronic gradual coronary artery occlusion in dogs.* Nagao et al. (57) assessed collateral function by measuring retrograde flow 6 weeks after occlusion of the proximal anterior descending coronary arteries with Ameroid constrictors in dogs. Diltiazem (0.1 mg/kg i.v.) resulted in a significant increase in retrograde flow. Franklin et al. (25) measured collateral flow with the microsphere technique 30 days after gradual occlusion of the left circumflex coronary artery in the dogs. Myocardial blood flow and systolic function were normal in the collateral-dependent area during resting conditions, but cardiac pacing resulted in subnormal increases in blood flow with deterioration of systolic function. Diltiazem (20 μg/kg/min i.v.) increased blood flow to the collateral-dependent area during pacing but did not prevent deterioration of myocardial mechanical function. Bache et al. (3) examined coronary collateral flow during treadmill exercise in chronically instrumented dogs 1 month after gradual coronary occlusion. Exercise resulted in worsening hypoperfusion in the collateral-dependent zone, and nifedipine (10 μg/kg i.v.) did not significantly improve blood flow in collateral-dependent myocardium. *Thus, no consensus emerges concerning the effects of calcium blocking agents on coronary collateral vasculature.* Some of the disparities between studies may be related to technical differences between studies, i.e., whether the calcium blocker caused substantial reduction in arterial pressure. This is of considerable importance because of the marked dependence of collateral blood flow on perfusion pressure. In addition, use of the microsphere technique may produce misleading results if care is not taken to eliminate peninsulas of normally perfused tissue from areas of collateral-dependent myocardium. Finally, following acute coronary artery occlusion, the collateral vascular system is poorly developed and may possess little potential for vasomotor activity.

To date, there have been very few studies of the effect of calcium channel blockers on histological infarct size. However, recently Yellon et al. (93,94) have reported that a continuous infusion of either verapamil or nifedipine affected a sustained protective effect in dogs subjected to 24 hr of coronary embolization.

### Patient Studies

Preliminary results of two studies of the effects of calcium blocking agents on myocardial infarct size in patients have been reported. Bussmann et al. (14) performed a randomized trial of verapamil (5–10 mg/hr for 2 days) in 54 patients with acute myocardial infarction. The mean interval from the onset of symptoms to beginning treatment was 8 hr. Patients treated with verapamil had a decrease in the peak creatine kinase MB isoenzyme activity compared with control patients, and a reduction of the myocardial infarct size index from 49 to 31 g-equivalents as determined from the creatine kinase MB isoenzyme time-activity curves ($p<0.005$).

Muller et al. (56) randomized 81 patients with acute myocardial infarction to nifedipine (20 mg orally every 4 hr for 14 days) or placebo. Therapy was begun $5.2 \pm 2.5$ hr after the onset of chest pain. Pain relief was more rapid in nifedipine-treated patients, but infarct size index calculated by the creatine kinase method was similar in patients receiving nifedipine ($15.2 \pm 1.4$ g-equivalents/m²) as compared with placebo-treated patients ($15.1 \pm 1.2$). These investigators observed a significantly greater mortality in patients receiving nifedipine (8%) than in placebo-treated patients (0%) during the first 2 weeks following myocardial infarction ($p<0.05$). Interpretation of this latter finding is complicated by the unexpected finding that no early mortality occurred in the placebo-treated group. Nevertheless, the investigators cautioned that the lack of any beneficial effect, and the excess early mortality, indicate that nifedipine should not be given routinely to patients following acute myocardial infarction.

### Can Calcium Blockers Limit Infarct Size?

Other than recording the preceding note of caution, insufficient data, particularly from patient studies, are available for any considered judgment to be made.

## CONCLUDING COMMENTS

*Infarct size limitation is an attractive concept.* It is reasonable that a smaller infarct should be associated with a lower early mortality and fewer late complications than a larger infarct. This is supported by clinical observations demonstrating that patients sustaining substantial left ventricular dysfunction following myocardial infarction have more disability and greater subsequent mortality than patients with little or no wall motion abnormality (85). It must be admitted, however, that the effect of small differences in infarct size are less clear.

### Situation to Date

*Early enthusiasm for several interventions that appeared to reduce infarct size following coronary occlusion in the experimental laboratory has been dampened by difficulties in reproducing some of these early successes, by the appearance of significant side-effects of therapy, or by the need to exclude a substantial number of subjects in whom contraindications prevent use of the proposed therapy. Clinical studies have been hampered by lack of completely satisfactory methods for assessing the area of myocardium at risk following acute coronary occlusion, for precise quantitation of infarct size, and for prediction of the ultimate size of the untreated infarct in patients undergoing early therapeutic intervention.*

### Is There Now a Need for Antiinfarct Agents?

*The advent of thrombolytic therapy for restoring coronary blood flow has provided an attractive alternative therapy which has been documented experimentally to have potential for reducing infarct size, provided that the intervention is initiated relatively early after coronary occlusion.* Nevertheless, an effective pharmacologic therapy for limiting infarct size, or slowing the progression from acutely ischemic to irreversibly injured myocardium, would have an important therapeutic role for several reasons. First, thrombolytic therapy may not be available to all patients sustaining acute myocardial infarction. Second, thrombolytic therapy does not result in reopening the occluded artery in all patients undergoing treatment. If reperfusion is not achieved, an intervention that could effectively limit infarct size would be of benefit. Third, even in patients in whom reperfusion can be achieved with thrombolytic therapy, there may be significant delay between the time at which the patient first comes to medical attention and the time at which reperfusion occurs. Effective pharmacologic therapy could delay progression of the infarction process, thereby maintaining viability of a greater fraction of the ischemic area until reperfusion is achieved. The concept of the distinction between *reducing* and *delaying* injury, together with the possible protective values of drugs that delay the onset of irreversible injury was illustrated by D. J. Hearse and D. M. Yellon in a recent paper (95). Finally, in patients at high risk for development of myocardial infarction, a safe and effective therapy for reduction of infarct size might be prescribed chronically, so that therapeutic levels of the agent would be present prior to the time that coronary occlusion might occur.

## Future Prospects

*It is my belief that the failure of pharmacologic therapy for reduction of infarct size to meet initial expectations should not cause abandonment of this concept. Techniques that have potential for limitation of infarct size should not be subject to unrealistic expectations.* Such interventions may not be appropriate in every patient, and may not result in universal benefit. However, when certain *a priori* requirements are met (i.e., a certain minimum level of collateral blood flow, the presence of a smaller rather than a larger area at risk, other as yet unidentified conditions), *it is not unreasonable that appropriate therapeutic intervention could have the potential to slow the rate of progression from ischemic to irreversibly injured tissue until reperfusion could be achieved, and perhaps, in some circumstances, to reduce the area of infarcted myocardium even in the absence of early coronary reperfusion.*

## REFERENCES

1. Andersen, M., Bechsgaard, P., Frederiksen, J., Hansen, D. A., Jurgensen, H. J., Nieldsen, B., Pedersen, F., Pedersen-Bjergaard, O., and Rasmussen, S. S. (1979): Effect of alprenolol on mortality among patients with definite or suspected acute myocardial infarction. *Lancet*, 2:865–867.
2. Bache, R. J. (1978): Effect of nitroglycerin and arterial hypertension on myocardial blood flow following acute coronary artery occlusion in the dog. *Circulation*, 57:557–562.
3. Bache, R. J., Dai, X. Z., and Schwartz, J. S. (1984): Effect of nifedipine on myocardial blood flow during exercise in dogs with chronic coronary artery occlusion. *J. Am. Coll. Cardiol.*, 3:143–149.
4. Bache, R. J., and Dymek, D. J. (1982): Effect of diltiazem on myocardial blood flow. *Circulation*, 65:I-19-I-26.
5. Bache, R. J., and Tockman, B. A. (1982): Effect of nitroglycerin and nifedipine on subendocardial perfusion in the presence of a flow-limiting coronary stenosis in the awake dog. *Circ. Res.*, 50:678–687.
6. Ball, R. M., and Bache, R. J. (1976): Distribution of myocardial blood flow in the exercising dog with restricted coronary artery inflow. *Circ. Res.*, 38:60–66.
7. Baroldi, B., and Scomazzoni, G. (1967): *Coronary Circulation in the Normal and the Pathologic Heart*. U.S. Government Printing Office, Washington, D.C.

8. Baughman, K. L., Maroko, P. R., and Vatner, S. F. (1981): Effects of coronary artery reperfusion on myocardial infarct size and survival in conscious dogs. *Circulation*, 63:317–323.
9. Becker, L. C., Schuster, E. H., Jugdutt, B. I., Hutchins, G. M., and Bulkley, B. H. (1983): Relationship between myocardial infarct size and occluded bed size in the dog: Difference between left anterior descending and circumflex coronary artery occlusion. *Circulation*, 67:549–557.
10. Beta-Blocker Heart Attack Trial Research Group (1982): Randomized trial of propranolol in patients with acute myocardial infarction. I. Mortality results. *JAMA*, 247:1707–1714.
11. Bresnahan, G. F., Roberts, R., Shell, W. E., Ross, J., Jr., and Sobel, B. E. (1974): Deleterious effects due to hemorrhage after myocardial reperfusion. *Am. J. Cardiol.*, 33:82–92.
12. Brown, B. G., Petersen, R. B., Pierce, C. D., Bolson, E. L., and Doge, H. G. (1982): Dynamics of human coronary stenoses: Interaction amongst stenosis flow, distending pressure and vasomotor tone. In: *Coronary Artery Disease*, edited by W. P. Stanmore and A. A. Bovee, p. 199. Urban and Schwarzenberg, Munich.
13. Bussmann, W., Passek, D., Seidel, W., and Kaltenbach, M. (1981): Reduction of CK and CK-MB indexes of infarct size by intravenous nitroglycerin. *Circulation*, 63:615–622.
14. Bussmann, W. D., Seher, W., Grungras, M., and Klepzig, H. (1982): Reduktion der CK-und CKMB-Infarktgrosse durch intravenose Gabe von Verapamil. *Z. Kardiol.*, 71:164 (abstract).
15. Cairns, J. A., Missirlis, E., and Fallen, E. L. (1978): Myocardial infarction size from serial CPK: variability of CPK serum entry ratio with size and model of infarction. *Circulation*, 58:1143–1153.
16. Chew, C. Y. C., Brown, B. G., Singh, B. N., Wong, M. M., Pierce, C., and Petersen, R. (1983): Effects of verapamil on coronary hemodynamic function and vasomobility relative to its mechanism of antianginal action. *Am. J. Cardiol.*, 51:699–705.
17. Cohen, M. V., Downey, J. M., Sonnenblick, E. H., and Kirk, E. S. (1973): The effects of nitroglycerin on coronary collaterals and myocardial contractility. *J. Clin. Invest.*, 52:2836–2847.
18. Conti, C. R., and Curry, R. C., Jr., (1979): Therapy of unstable angina pectoris. In: *Diagnosis and Therapy of Coronary Artery Disease*, edited by P. F. Cohn. Little, Brown, Boston.
19. Davies, M. J., Woolf, N., and Robertson, W. B. (1976): Pathology of acute myocardial infarction with particular reference to occlusive coronary thrombi. *Br. Heart J.*, 38:659–664.
20. Diemer, H. P., Wichmann, and Lochner, W. (1977): Coronary collateral flow: Effect of drugs and perfusion pressure. *Basic Res. Cardiol.*, 72:332–343.
21. Domenech, R. J. (1978): Regional diastolic coronary blood flow during diastolic ventricular hypertension. *Cardiovasc. Res.*, 12:639–645.
22. Ellrodt, G., Chew, C. Y. C., and Singh, B. N. (1980): Therapeutic implications of slow-channel blockade in cardiocirculatory disorders. *Circulation*, 62:669–679.
23. Factorr, S. M., Okun, E. M., and Kirk, E. S. (1981): The histological lateral border of acute canine myocardial infarction. A function of microcirculation. *Circ. Res.*, 48:640–649.
24. Fam, W. M., and McGregor, M. (1964): Effect of coronary vasodilator drugs on retrograde flow in areas of chronic myocardial ischemia. *Circ. Res.*, 15:355–365.
25. Franklin, D., Millard, R. W., and Nagao, T. (1980): Responses of coronary collateral flow and dependent myocardial mechanical function on the calcium antagonist diltiazem. *Chest*, 78:(Suppl. I):200–204.
26. Fukuyama, T., Schechtman, K. B., and Roberts, R. (1980): The effects of intravenous nitroglycerin on hemodynamics, coronary blood flow and morphologically and enzymatically estimated infarct size in conscious dogs. *Circulation*, 62:1227–1238.
27. Fulton, W. F. M. (1964): The time factor in enlargement of anastomoses in coronary artery disease. *Scott. Med. J.*, 9:11–23.
28. Furchgott, R. F. (1983): Role of endothelium in responses of vascular smooth muscle. *Circ. Res.*, 53:557–573.
29. Ginks, W. R., Sybers, H. D., Maroko, P. R., Covell, J. W., Sobel, B. E., and Ross, J., Jr. (1972): Coronary artery reperfusion. II. Reduction of myocardial infarct size at 1 week after coronary occlusion. *J. Clin. Invest.*, 51:2717–2723.
30. Gold, H. K., Leinbach, R. C., and Maroko, P. R. (1976): Propranolol-induced reduction of signs of ischemic injury during acute myocardial infarction. *Am. J. Cardiol.*, 38:689–695.
31. Goldstein, R. E., and Epstein, S. E. (1972): Medical management in patients with angina pectoris. *Prog. Cardiovasc. Dis.*, 14:360–398.
32. Goldstein, R. E., Stinson, E. B., Scherer, J. L., Sehingen, R. P., Grehl, T. M., and Epstein, S. E.

(1974): Intraoperative coronary collateral function in patients with occlusive coronary artery disease. Nitroglycerin responsiveness and angiographic correlation. *Circulation*, 49:298–308.

33. Grande, P., Hansen, B. F., Christiansen, C., and Naestoft, J. (1981): Acute myocardial infarct size estimated by serum CK-MB determinations: Clinical accuracy and prognostic relevance utilizing a practical modification of the isoenzyme approach. *Am. Heart J.*, 101:582–586.

34. Henry, P. D., Shuchleib, R., Clark, R. E., and Perez, J. E. (1979): Effect of nifedipine on myocardial ischemia. Analysis of collateral flow, pulsatile heat, and regional muscle shortening. *Am. J. Cardiol.*, 44:817–824.

35. Heyndricks, G. R., Baig, H., Nellens, D., Leusen, I., Fishbein, M. C., and Vatner, S. F. (1978): Depression of regional blood flow and wall thickening after brief coronary occlusion. *Am. J. Physiol.*, 234:H653–H659.

36. Hjalmarson, A., Elmfeldt, D., Hurlitz, J., Homerg, S., Malek, I., Nyberg, G., Ryden, L., Swedbeg, K., Vedin, A., Waagstein, F., Faldenstrom, A., Waldenstrom, J., Wedel, H. Wilhelm-sen, L., and Wilhemsson, C. (1981): Effect on mortality of metroprolol in acute myocardial infarction: A double-blind randomised trial. *Lancet*, 2:823–827.

37. Hjalmarson, A., Herlitz, J., Holmberg, S., Ryden, L., Swedberg, K., Vedin, A., Waagstein, F., Waldenstrom, A., Waldenstrom, J., Wedel, H., Wilhelmsen, L., and Wilhelmsson, C. (1983): The Goteborg metroprolol trial. Effects on mortality and morbidity in acute myocardial infarction. *Circulation*, 67:I-26–32.

38. Hofmann, M., Hofmann, M., Genth, K., and Schaper, W. (1980): The influence of reperfusion on infarct size after experimental coronary artery occlusion. *Basic Res. Cardiol.*, 75:572–582.

39. Jaffee, A. S., Geltman, E. M., Tiefenbrunn, A. J., Ambos, H. D, Strauss, H. D., Sobel, B. E., and Roberts, R. (1983): Reduction of infarct size in patients with inferior infarction with intravenous glyceryl trinirate. A randomized study. *Br. Heart J.*, 49:452–460.

40. Jennings, R. R., and Reimer, K. A. (1979): Effect of beta-adrenergic blockade on acute myocardial ischemic injury. In: *Modulation of Sympathetic Tone in the Treatment of Cardiovascular Diseases*, edited by F. Gross, pp. 103–114. Hans Huber, Berne.

41. Jennings, R. B., Sommers, H. M., Smyth, G. A., Flack, H. A., and Linn, H. (1960): Myocardial necrosis induced by temporary occlusion of the coronary artery in the dog. *Arch. Pathol.*, 70:68–78.

42. Johansson, B. W. (1980): Comparative study of cardio-selective beta-blockade and diazepam in patients with acute myocardial infarction and tachycardia. *Acta Med. Scand.*, 207:47–53.

43. Jones, A. M. (1965): The functional role of intracoronary anastomoses. *Acta Cardiol.*, 11:130–137.

44. Jugdutt, B. E., Becker, L. C., Hutchins, G. M., Bulkley, B. H., Reid, P. R., and Kallman, C. (1981): Effects of intravenous nitroglycerin on collateral blood flow and infarct size in the conscious dog. *Circulation*, 63:17–28.

45. Jurgensen, H. J., Frederiksen, J., Hansen, D. A., and Pedersen-Bjergaard, O. (1981): Limitation of myocardial infarct size in patients less than 66 years treated with alprenolol. *Br. Heart J.*, 45:583–588.

46. Kattus, A. A., and Gregg, D. E. (1959): Some determinants of coronary collateral blood flow in the open chest dog. *Circ. Res.*, 7:628–642.

47. Lee, J. T., Ideker, R. E., and Reimer, K. A. (1981): Myocardial infarct size and location in relation to the coronary vascular bed at risk in man. *Circulation*, 64:526–534.

48. Ludbrook, P. A., Tiefbrunn, A. J., and Sobel, B. E. (1981): Influence of nifedipine on left ventricular systolic and diastolic function. *Am. J. Cardiol.*, 71:683–692.

49. Macho, P., Hintze, T. H., and Vatner, S. E. (1981): Regulation of large coronary arteries by increases in myocardial metabolic demands in conscious dogs. *Circ. Res.*, 49:594–599.

50. Macho, P., and Vatner, S. F. (1981): Effects of nitroglycerin and nitroprusside on large and small coronary vessels in conscious dogs. *Circulation*, 64:1101–1108.

51. Maroko, P. R., Kjeksus, J. K., Sobel, B. E., Watanabe, T., Covell, J. W., Ross, J., Jr., and Braunwald, E. (1971): Factors influencing infarct size following experimental coronary artery occlusions. *Circulation*, 43:67–82.

52. Maroko, P. R., Libby, P., Ginks, W. R., Bloor, C. M., Shell, W. E., Sobel, B. E., and Ross, J., Jr. (1972): Coronary artery reperfusion. I. Early effects on local myocardial function and the extent of myocardial necrosis. *J. Clin. Invest.*, 51:271–272.

53. McIlmoyle, L., Evans, A., McBoyle, D., Cran, G., Barber, J. M., Elwood, H., Salathia, K., and Shanks, R. (1982): Early intervention in myocardial ischaemia. *Br. Heart J.*, 47:189 (abstract).

54. Miller, R. R., Vismara, L. A., Williams, D. O., Amsterdam, E. A., and Mason, D. T. (1976): Pharmacological mechanisms for ventricular unloading in clinical congestive heart failure. Differential effects of nitroprusside, phentolamine and nitroglycerin on cardiac function and the peripheral circulation. *Circ. Res.*, 39:127–133.

55. Muller, K. D., Klein, H., and Schaper, W. (1980): Changes in myocardial oxygen consumption 45 minutes after experimental coronary occlusion do not alter infarct size. *Cardiovasc. Res.*, 14:710–718.

56. Muller, J., Morrison, J., Stone, P., Rude, R., Rosner, B., Roberts, B., Pearle, D., Turi, Z., Schneider, J., Serfas, D., Hennekens, C., and Braunwald, E. (1983): Nifedipine therapy for threatened and acute myocardial infarction: A randomized double-blind comparison. *Circulation*, 68:III–120 (abstract).

57. Nagao, T., Murata, S., and Sato, M. (1975): The effects of diltiazem on developed coronary collaterals in the dog. *Jpn. J. Pharmacol.*, 25:281–288.

58. Nakamura, M., Kikuchi, Y., Senda, Y., Yamada, A., and Koiwaya, Y. (1980): Myocardial blood flow following experimental coronary artery occlusion. *Chest*, 78(Suppl. I):205–209.

59. Norwegian Multicenter Study Group (1981): Timolol-induced reduction in mortality and reinfarction in patients surviving acute myocardial infarction. *N. Engl. J. Med.*, 304:801–807.

60. Opie, L. H. (1980): Drugs and the heart. Beta-blocking agents. *Lancet*, 2:428–429.

61. Parratt, J. R. (1980): Effects of adrenergic antivators and inhibitors on the coronary circulation. In: *Adrenergic Activators and Inhibitors.*, Part I, edited by L. Szekeres, pp. 735–822. Springer-Verlag, Berlin.

62. Pelides, L. J., Reid, D. S., Thomas, M., and Shillingford, J. P. (1971): Inhibition by beta-blockade of the ST-segment elevation after acute myocardial infarction in man. *Circulation*, 43:67–82.

63. Peter, T., Norris, R. M., Clarke, E. D., Heng, M. K., Singh, B. N., Williams, B., Howell, D. R., and Ambler, P. K. (1978): Reduction of enzyme levels by propranolol after acute myocardial infarction. *Circulation*, 57:1091–1095.

64. Pierce, W. S., Carter, D. R., McGavin, M. H., and Waldhausen, J. A. (1973): Modification of myocardial infarct volume: An experimental study in the dog. *Arch. Surg.*, 107:682–686.

65. Rasmussen, M. M., Reimer, K. A., Kloner, R. A., and Jennings, R. B. (1977): Infarct size reduction by propranolol before and after coronary ligation in dogs. *Circulation*, 56:794–798.

66. Redwood, D. R., Smith, E. R., and Epstein, S. E. (1972): Coronary artery occlusion in the conscious dog. Effects of alterations in heart rate and arterial pressure on the degree of myocardial ischemia. *Circulation*, 46:323–332.

67. Reimer, K. A., Lowe, J. E., Rasmussen, M. M., and Jennings, R. B. (1977): The wavefront phenomenon of ischemic cell death. Myocardial infarct size versus duration of coronary occlusion in dogs. *Circulation*, 56:786–794.

68. Reimer, K. A., Rasmussen, M. M., and Jennings, R. B. (1973): Reduction by propranolol of myocardial necrosis following temporary coronary artery occlusion in dogs. *Circ. Res.*, 33:353–363.

69. Reimer, K. A., Rasmussen, M. M., and Jennings, R. B. (1976): On the nature of protection by propranolol against myocardial necrosis following temporary coronary occlusion in dogs. *Am. J. Cardiol.*, 37:520–526.

70. Rentrop, P., Blanke, H., Karsch, K. R., Kaiser, H., Kostering, H., and Leitz, K. (1981): Selective intracoronary thrombolysis in acute myocardial infarction and unstable angina pectoris. *Circulation*, 63:307–317.

71. Rivas, F., Cobb, F. R., Bache, R. J., Greenfield, J. C., Jr. (1976): Relationship between blood flow to ischemic regions and extent of myocardial infarction. *Circ. Res.*, 38:439–447.

72. Roberts, W. C. (1972): Coronary arteries in fatal acute myocardial infarction. *Circulation*, 45:215–230.

73. Robertson, R. M., Wood, A. J. J., Vaughn, W. K., and Robertson, D. (1982): Exacerbation of vasotonic angina by propranolol. *Circulation*, 65:281–285.

74. Roe, C. R., Cobb, F. R., and Starmer, C. F. (1977): The relationship between enzymatic and histologic estimates of the extent of myocardial infarction in conscious dogs with permanent coronary occlusion. *Circulation*, 55:438–449.

75. Russell, R. O., Jr., Moraski, R. E., Kouchowkos, N. et al. (1978): Unstable angina pectoris. National cooperative study group to compare surgical and medical therapy. In hospital experience and initial follow-up results in patients with one, two and three vessel disease. *Am. J. Cardiol.*, 42:839–848.

76. Schaper, W. (1971): *Collateral Circulation of the Heart.* North-Holland, Amsterdam.
77. Schaper, W. (1979): *The Pathophysiology of Myocardial Perfusion,* pp. 359–360. Elsvier/North Holland, Amsterdam.
78. Schaper, W., Remijsen, P., Xhonneux, R. (1969): The size of myocardial infarction after experimental coronary artery ligation. *Z. Kreislaufforsch.,* 58:904–909.
79. Schwartz, J. S., Carlyle, P. F., and Cohn, J. N. (1979): Effect of dilation of the distal coronary bed on flow and resistance in severely stenotic coronary arteries in the dog. *Am. J. Cardiol.,* 43:219–224.
80. Shell, W. E., Kjekshus, J. K., and Sobel, B. E. (1971): Quantitative assessment of the extent of myocardial infarction in the conscious dog by means of analysis of serial changes in serum creatine phosphokinase activity. *J. Clin. Invest.,* 50:2614–2625.
81. Smith, E. R., Redwood, D. R., McCarron, W. E., and Epstein, S. E. (1973): Coronary artery occlusion in the conscious dog. Effects of alterations in arterial pressure produced by nitroglycerin, hemorrhage and alpha-adrenergic agonists on the degree of myocardial ischemia. *Circulation,* 47:51–57.
82. Smith, H. J., Singh, B. N., Norris, R. M., Nisbet, H. D., John, M. B., and Hurley, P. J. (1977): The effect of verapamil on experimental myocardial ischaemia with particular reference to regional myocardial blood flow and metabolism. *Aust. NZ J. Med.,* 7:114–121.
83. Stack, R. S., Phillips, H. R., Grierson, D. S., Beher, V. S., Kong, Y., Peter, R. H., Swain, J. L., and Greenfield, J. C., Jr. (1983): Functional improvement of jeopardized myocardium following intracoronary streptokinase infusion in acute myocardial infarction. *J. Clin. Invest.,* 72:84–95.
84. Swain, J. L., Sabina, R. L., McHale, P. A., Greenfield, J. C., and Holmes, E. W. (1982): Prolonged myocardial nucleotide depletion after brief ischemia in the open chest dog. *Am. J. Physiol.,* 242:H818–H826.
85. Taylor, G. J., Humphries, J. O., Mellitis, E. D., Pitt, B., Schulze, R. A., Griffith, L. S. C., and Achuff, S. C. (1980): Predictors of clinical course, coronary anatomy and left ventricular function after recovery from acute myocardial infarction. *Circulation,* 62:960–970.
86. Vatner, S. F., Baig, H., Manders, W. T., Ocha, H., and Pagani, M. (1977): Effect of propranolol on regional myocardial function, electrogram and blood flow in conscious dogs with myocardial ischemia. *J. Clin. Invest.,* 60:353–360.
87. Vatner, S. F., Pagoni, M., Manders, W. T., and Pasipylarides, A. D. (1980): Alpha-adrenergic vasoconstriction and nitroglycerin vasodilation of large coronary arteries in conscious dogs. *J. Clin. Invest.,* 65:5–14.
88. Vatner, S. F., and Hintze, T. H. (1982): Effects of a calcium-channel antagonist on large and small coronary arteries in conscious dogs. *Circulation,* 66:579–588.
89. Vatner, S. F., Hintze, T., and Macho, P. (1982): Regulation of large coronary arteries by beta-adrenergic mechanisms in the conscious dog. *Circ. Res.,* 51:56–66.
90. Waagstein, F., and Hjalmarson, A. C. (1975): Double-blind study of the effect of cardioselective beta-blockade on chest pain in acute myocardial infarction. *Acta Mea. Scand. (Suppl.),* 201–207.
91. Weintraub, W. S., Hattori, S., Agarwahl, J. B., Bodenheimer, M. M., Banka, V. S., and Helfant, R. H. (1981): The influence of nifedipine on myocardial blood flow in the ischemic and lateral border zone. *Am. J. Cardiol.,* 47:442 (abstract).
92. William, D. O., Amsterdam, E. A., and Mason, D. T. (1975): Hemodynamic effects of nitroglycerin in acute myocardial infarction. Decrease in ventricular preload at the expense of cardiac output. *Circulation,* 51:421–427.
93. Yellon, D. M., Hearse, D. J., Maxwell, M. P., Chambers, D. E., and Downey, J. M. (1983): Sustained limitation of myocardial necrosis 24 hours after coronary artery occlusion: Verapamil infusion in dogs with small myocardial infarcts. *Am. J. Cardiol.,* 51:1409–1413.
94. Yellon, D. M., Downey, J. M., Hearse, D. J., Maxwell, M., and Yoshida, S. (1983): Calcium antagonists limit myocardial infarct size. *Circulation,* 68(Suppl. 3):186.
95. Yellon, D. M., Hearse, D. J., Chambers, D. E., and Downey, J. M. (1983): Effects of flurbiprofen in altering the size of myocardial infarcts in dogs: Reduction or delay? *Am. J. Cardiol.,* 51:884–890.
96. Yusuf, S., Sleight, P., Rossi, P., Ramsdale, D., Peto, R., Furze, L., Sterry, H., Pearson, M., Motwani, R., Parish, S., Gray, R., Bennett, D., and Bray, C. (1983): Reduction in infarct size, arrhythmias and chest pain by early intravenous beta-blockade in suspected acute myocardial infarction. *Circulation,* 67:I–32–I–41.

*Therapeutic Approaches to Myocardial Infarct Size Limitation*, edited by D. J. Hearse and D. M. Yellon. Raven Press, New York © 1984.

# 12

# Are Free Radicals a Major Culprit?

## Joe M. McCord

*Department of Biochemistry, University of South Alabama, Mobile, Alabama 36688*

For about 15 years it has been appreciated that certain biological systems are capable of producing oxygen-derived free radicals especially the superoxide free radical ($O_2^-$), and that *these chemically unstable, generally reactive species are cytotoxic* (3). It is also well appreciated that nature has provided a system of protective or detoxifying enzymes (notably superoxide dismutases, catalases, and glutathione peroxidases), as well as nonenzymatic antioxidants (such as vitamins C and E) that aid in protecting the organism against various kinds of oxidative stress. It has become apparent that several different pathophysiological states give rise to abnormally high rates of production of the superoxide free radical. These states include exposure to hyperoxia, exposure to ionizing irradiation, exposure to various chemical toxicants such as the herbicide paraquat, phagocyte-mediated inflammation, and, most recently, ischemia-induced injury. *The question I address here is: To what extent are superoxide and secondarily-derived free radicals and reduced oxygen metabolites responsible for ischemia-induced tissue injury in the myocardium?*

## WHAT IS A FREE RADICAL?

The normal chemical bond consists of a pair of electrons, opposite in spin, sharing a single molecular orbital. *A free radical is simply a molecule that contains an odd number of electrons.* If, for example, the carbon-carbon bond in ethane, $CH_3CH_3$, is symmetrically broken, the two identical fragments would be methyl radicals ($CH_3^.$). The odd electron is often represented in the formula as a "dot." Because the unpaired electron may be considered to be an "open bond" or a "half bond," the free radical is, in general, a chemically reactive species. If two radicals react, the result may be annihilation (for example, the two methyl radicals could energetically reconstitute ethane). If a radical reacts with a nonradical, one of the products must be another free radical. It is this characteristic that enables free radicals to participate in chain reactions which may be thousands of events long. The peroxidation of unsaturated lipids (LH) by molecular oxygen may be initiated by a free radical ($R^.$) as follows:

$$R^. + LH \rightarrow RH + L^.$$
$$L^. + O_2 \rightarrow LOO^.$$

As the lipid hydroperoxyl radical ($LOO^.$) removes a hydrogen atom from other lipid molecules, it propagates the sequence by producing another $L^.$ radical:

$$LOO^. + LH \rightarrow LOOH + L^.$$

Hence, the cycle may continue thousands of times until a termination reaction occurs. Obviously, this would be a very undesirable reaction sequence to run unchecked *in vivo*. Radicals may also serve as oxidants or reductants. The superoxide radical ($O_2^.$) is a good reductant, a mild oxidant, and is capable of initiating chain reactions as well.

## THE VARIOUS SPECIES OF "ACTIVE OXYGEN"

Molecular oxygen ($O_2$) can maximally accept four electrons to produce two innocuous molecules of $H_2O$. The one, two, and three electron reductions of oxygen, however, give rise to the toxic and reactive intermediates shown in Table 1. The addition of a single electron to oxygen produces superoxide ($O_2^.$), which

TABLE 1. *Reduction products of molecular oxygen*

| Number of electons | Unprotonated | At pH 7.0 | Name | Properties |
|---|---|---|---|---|
| 0 | $O_2$ | $O_2$ | Oxygen | Mild oxidant |
| 1 | $O_2^.$ | $O_2^.$ | Superoxide | Better oxidant<br>Good reductant<br>Free radical |
| 2 | $O_2^=$ | $H_2O_2$ | Hydrogen peroxide | Good oxidant |
| 3 | $O^- + O^=$ | $OH^. + H_2O$ | Hydroxyl radical (+ water) | Potent oxidant<br>Free radical |
| 4 | $O^= + O^=$ | $H_2O + H_2O$ | Water | Innocuous |

via spontaneous or enzyme (superoxide dismutase) catalyzed dismutation gives rise to hydrogen peroxide ($H_2O_2$):

$$O_2^{\tau} + O_2^{\tau} + 2H^+ \rightarrow O_2 + H_2O_2$$

Because, in nature, electrons travel in pairs or singly, the three-electron reduction of molecular oxygen to give the hydroxyl radical($OH^{\cdot}$) does not occur directly, but rather may result via another redistribution of electrons between the one-electron reduced product superoxide ($O_2^{\tau}$) and the divalently reduced hydrogen peroxide:

$$O_2^{\tau} + H_2O_2 \rightarrow O_2 + OH^- + OH^{\cdot}$$

This reaction is commonly referred to as the Haber-Weiss reaction, and has been shown to require the participation of a transition metal catalyst, usually iron. The reaction may be catalyzed extracellularly by the iron-containing protein transferrin, and intracellularly by iron-adenosine diphosphate chelates. The free radical product of the Haber-Weiss reaction, the hydroxyl radical, is a much more potent oxidant than either superoxide or hydrogen peroxide. It should be obvious from the above reactions that, in the absence of scavengers, the production of the superoxide radical can give rise to all of the intermediate reduction states of oxygen shown in Table 1.

The term "active oxygen" is sometimes used to include singlet oxygen, an electronically excited state of oxygen. It is isoelectronic with molecular oxygen, but much more reactive due to the elimination of a spin restriction imposed by the unusual occurrence of two unpaired electrons in ground state oxygen. There is some evidence that suggests that singlet oxygen may be a product of the Haber-Weiss reaction.

## WHAT ARE THE PHYSIOLOGICAL SOURCES OF FREE RADICALS?

### Mitochondria

Certain autoxidizable metabolites such as hydroquinones or reduced flavins may react with molecular oxygen by transferring one electron at a time to the oxygen, generating superoxide. In a normal mitochondrion approximately 1% of the electrons that pass down the electron-transport chain "leak off" to molecular oxygen by just such a reaction at coenzyme Q. When tissues are exposed to hyperoxia, the rate of this leakage goes up in direct proportion to the partial pressure of molecular oxygen at the level of the mitochondrion. Thus, when an animal is exposed to 100% oxygen, the mitochondria, in the pneumocyte at least, may produce five times the normal flux of superoxide. Much evidence (2) suggests that most of the toxic effects that result from hyperoxic exposure are due to increased rates of production of superoxide and hydrogen peroxide.

### Leukocytes

*A major pathological source of superoxide is from metabolically stimulated phagocytes, especially polymorphonuclear leukocytes* (see Chapter 13). As is frequently the case, nature has learned to make something useful from something bad. The major task of these cells is to engulf and kill invading microorganisms. To do so, the phagocyte intentionally produces cytotoxic species, which would normally be very undesirable products; chief among these is superoxide. *Not only does superoxide participate in the killing of these ingested microbes, but it also serves to activate a chemotactic "beacon," enabling other phagocytes to find and assist those which are actively involved in the killing of microbes.* It is by preventing the activation of this superoxide-dependent chemoattractant that superoxide dismutase exerts its antiinflammatory effect (7).

### Ischemia, Reperfusion, and Xanthine Oxidase Activity

More recently, we have found yet another pathological source of superoxide. *The radical appears to be produced in great abundance when ischemic tissues are reperfused*, and, hence, reoxygenated (5,6). The phenomenon occurs in all tissues with the probable exception of skeletal muscle, and is the result of several coincidental metabolic events (8). Certain of these events are well known and well documented; others are currently under study and are not yet understood in great detail. The sequence of events is represented schematically in Fig. 1. It begins with the loss of high-energy phosphates in the substrate- and oxygen-starved ischemic tissue, manifested in a decrease in adenosine triphosphate (ATP) concentration within the cell. As adenosine monophosphate (AMP) content rises, the nucleotide is catabolized to adenosine, inosine, and finally the free purine base hypoxanthine. As the energy level of the cell drops, the cation pumps can no longer keep calcium ions pumped out of the cytosol. The influx of calcium results in the activation of a calcium-dependent (and possibly calmodulin-regulated) protease in the cytosol. This protease attacks a normally innocuous enzyme, xanthine dehydrogenase, which catalyzes the reaction:

$$\text{hypoxanthine} + \text{NAD}^+ + \text{H}_2\text{O} \rightarrow \text{xanthine} + \text{NADH} + \text{H}^+$$

converting it to a new enzyme activity, xanthine oxidase, which can no longer reduce $\text{NAD}^+$ (nicotinamide adenine-dinucleotide) but rather can reduce molecular oxygen to produce the superoxide radical:

$$\text{hypoxanthine} + 2\text{O}_2 + \text{H}_2\text{O} \rightarrow \text{xanthine} + 2\text{O}_2^- + 2\text{H}^+$$

This proteolytic conversion of the dehydrogenase to the oxidase has been well studied *in vitro*, but was only recently shown to occur *in vivo*.

*At this stage in the ischemic tissue two important things have occurred: a new enzyme activity has appeared and, coincidentally, one of its two required substrates, hypoxanthine, has accumulated.* When the tissue is reperfused and reoxygenated, the second required substrate, molecular oxygen, is supplied. *The reaction then proceeds with a burst of free radical production and consequent destruction of the tissue.* In the feline intestinal ischemia model we have found (6) dramatic protection of the tissue if the animal is treated at some point prior to reperfusion with agents that either scavenge superoxide (superoxide dismutase) or prevent its production (allopurinol).

A question of obvious importance was to determine whether the mechanism put forth in Fig. 1 was unique to the intestine or common to all tissues, especially the

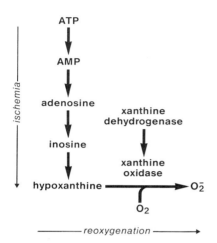

**FIG. 1.** Events Occurring During Ischemia and Reperfusion. Pathways for the degradation of adenine nucleotide, the interconversion between xanthine dehydrogenase and xanthine oxidase, and the formation of superoxide.

myocardium? Table 2 shows that the mechanism is a common one; all tissues examined contained xanthine dehydrogenase and only in skeletal muscle did it fail to convert to the oxidase upon nonperfusion. Furthermore, although the content of xanthine dehydrogenase as well as the rate at which it is converted to the oxidase varied considerably from tissue to tissue, there was a definite correlation between these factors and the clinically observable sensitivity of the tissue to ischemic injury. That is, the mucosal lining of the intestine is extremely susceptible to ischemic injury; skeletal muscle, on the other hand, is very resistant to such injury.

## IS SUPEROXIDE A MAJOR CULPRIT IN MYOCARDIAL ISCHEMIC INJURY?

The studies performed to date may be too preliminary to provide a definitive answer to this important question, but *they strongly suggest that the generation of superoxide does indeed make a major contribution to the genesis of ischemic injury.* One justification for making such speculation on the basis of preliminary data is the specificity of the probes that have been utilized in the experiments. Superoxide dismutase has been studied intensively for 15 years, and its specificity for super-

TABLE 2. *Xanthine oxidase content of various tissues of the rat*

| Tissue | Units/g protein | Half-time for conversion |
|--------|-----------------|--------------------------|
| Intestine | 10 | 4 s |
| Heart | 0.82 | 5 min |
| Liver | 0.78 | 30 min |
| Kidney | 0.40 | 30 min |
| Lung | 1.15 | 30 min |
| Spleen | 0.91 | 30 min |

oxide remains unquestioned. It is, therefore, a reasonably safe assumption that any effect of superoxide dismutase is due to the elimination of superoxide free radicals. As drugs go, allopurinol, too, has a high degree of specificity, although it is not absolute. The drug was specifically developed to be a potent inhibitor of xanthine oxidase; it was not simply empirically discovered to have that activity.

It is encouraging to note that superoxide dismutase, alone or in combination with catalase, has provided protection against the deleterious effects of ischemia in a variety of models, both *in vivo* and *in vitro*, as well as in several species (dog, cat, rat). Furthermore, the indices upon which injury has been assessed have ranged from measurements of necrosis (1,6) to more subtle measurements of physiological function (postreperfusion ventricular pressure development, maximal ventricular dP/dt, etc.) (10).

## RELATIONSHIP BETWEEN FREE RADICAL- AND CALCIUM-INDUCED INJURY

An influx of calcium has been linked to the initiation of free radical production by at least two lines of evidence. We have demonstrated that rats pretreated with stelazine (trifluoperazine—a calmodulin inhibitor) showed a significantly slowed rate of conversion of dehydrogenase to oxidase in the nonperfused gut (8). Additionally, the so-called "calcium paradox" seen with the isolated perfused working rat heart model was shown to initiate dehydrogenase-to-oxidase conversion in the absence of either low oxygen or low flow (9). That is, the mechanism by which ischemia triggers free radical production appears to depend on the elevation of cytosolic calcium, as described earlier. *Another way of viewing this is that much of what is commonly referred to as calcium-induced damage may, in fact, be free-radical-mediated damage.* It is, however, clear that the calcium paradox results in substantial damage to the myocardium even under complete anoxia; that portion of the damage cannot be attributed to oxygen-derived free radicals.

Perhaps the point is too obvious to make, but those who are not biochemically inclined should keep in mind that it *is not sufficient to say "the cells died due to an influx of calcium." This is not a biochemical explanation of the phenomenon.* The calcium may activate proteases, which activate free radical production, or the calcium may activate calmodulin-regulated phospholipases which promptly degrade cell membranes, or it may physically disrupt mitochondrial structure by precipitating as calcium phosphate, or it may act by all of the above plus many additional mechanisms not yet considered. *But calcium is only the trigger, it is not the gun.*

## EXTENT OF FREE RADICAL PRODUCTION IN ISCHEMIA, HYPOXIA, REPERFUSION, AND REOXYGENATION

In attempting to assess the quantitative or qualitative clinical importance of free radicals as mediators of injury during both oxygen deprivation and oxygen repletion, it is necessary to ask if frequently used experimental models (such as total anoxia followed by reoxygenation) might not be so severe as to inadequately reflect the clinical situation? Because many models rely on the sudden and complete deprivation of flow or oxygenation (or whichever variable is being studied) followed by the sudden and complete restoration of flow or oxygen, the validity of such models is sometimes questioned. Arising from this are other questions, including: How can superoxide production be important during ischemia or hypoxia where oxygen availability is reduced? Can superoxide or other toxic radicals be produced under conditions of total anoxia where there is little or no available oxygen? Does the method of oxygen deprivation, or restoration, influence the extent of formation or cytotoxicity of free radicals, i.e., is there a difference between ischemia (with a reduced flow but normoxia) and hypoxia with normal flow?

### Can Superoxide Be Produced During Ischemia or Hypoxia?

If the enzyme xanthine oxidase is considered to be the primary source of ischemia-induced superoxide production, and much evidence suggests that this is the case, the answer to the question should be provided by examining the enzyme's $K_m$ for molecular oxygen. This however is not a simple matter. The enzyme can deal with oxygen in two distinct ways: It can add two electrons simultaneously to produce a molecule of hydrogen peroxide, or it can add one electron to produce a superoxide radical. The former predominates at lower concentrations of oxygen, with an apparent $K_m$ of 27 micromolar oxygen (or a partial pressure of 20 mm), while the latter mode of reduction becomes dominant at higher concentrations of oxygen ($K_m = 800$ micromolar oxygen, or 600 mm) (4). What this unusual behavior means is that under hypoxic conditions it is to be expected that the newly formed xanthine oxidase will be functioning, but at only a fraction of its maximal velocity. The predominant product will be hydrogen peroxide. As tissue $P_{O_2}$ rises back toward normal, or even beyond, due to reactive hyperemia, the turnover rate of the enzyme may increase in an almost linear relationship, but with a slightly larger fraction of the product now consisting of superoxide. In fact, over the entire range of physiologically attainable oxygen concentrations, there should be a nearly linear relationship between tissue $P_{O_2}$ and the rate of superoxide production by xanthine oxidase, once that activity is created.

In the intestinal model which led to the hypothesis outlined in Fig. 1, the ischemia was partial (20% of normal flow and a tissue $P_{O_2}$ of 3 mm or less) and reperfusion was complete (100% of normal flow and a tissue $P_{O_2}$ of about 15 mm) (5,6). Hence, during ischemia the increase in xanthine oxidase activity was roughly offset by a corresponding decrease in the concentration of available oxygen, and there was little net change in superoxide production. During reperfusion, however, there would have been at least a fivefold increase in superoxide production, relative to the normal.

If the ischemia were complete (no flow) and the tissue were completely anoxic, it should be obvious that no superoxide could be made under these conditions. Varying degrees of hypoxia will result in varying rates of superoxide production, ranging from less than normal to greater than normal, depending on the tissue $P_{O_2}$

and the extent of conversion of xanthine dehydrogenase to xanthine oxidase. Complete restoration of oxygen concentration will necessarily result in elevated rates of superoxide production, assuming that some conversion of dehydrogenase to oxidase has occurred.

In the intestinal model (5,6) where complete ischemia was followed by reperfusion, superoxide dismutase and allopurinol were much less effective at preventing the injury; apparently overriding factors enter the picture under these circumstances. It is not surprising that tissues totally deprived of blood flow will eventually suffer irreversible damage that is not free radical-dependent. The heart, however, appears to be protected by superoxide dismutase and catalase even after 2 hr of complete global ischemia (10), so there may be significant differences among the tissues.

In clinical myocardial ischemia, regions of total ischemia may be very unusual; in fact they may never occur due to the collateralization of the heart. Varying degrees of partial ischemia and tissue hypoxia may be the most commonly encountered situation. In studies in the dog *in vivo*, complete ligation of the left anterior descending coronary artery for 1 hr produced a region of necrosis after 4 hr of reperfusion that was markedly reduced in animals treated with superoxide dismutase or allopurinol (1).

Is reperfusion required if the ischemia is partial? This question has not been adequately addressed experimentally as yet. Most of the models which have been used are reperfusion models. It is certainly conceivable that in a certain range of hypoxia the events in Fig. 1 could be triggered (i.e., catabolism of ATP and conversion of the dehydrogenase to the oxidase) at partial pressures of oxygen which are adequate to support the production of superoxide by the xanthine oxidase. If this proves to be the case, chronically ischemic tissues may be subjected to continuous free radical insult of various degrees.

## Perfusion Versus Oxygenation

It appears that the most important factor in determining the rate of radical production is likely to be tissue $P_{O_2}$, and that enhanced radical production may be possible even under hypoxic conditions. Perfusion, however, may also affect rates of radical production by at least two mechanisms. Nonperfused tissues become acidotic, and, all other factors being equal, xanthine oxidase makes more hydrogen peroxide and less superoxide at lower pH values. On the other hand, during nonperfusion, hypoxanthine accumulates in the tissue. Hypoxanthine is, of course, the driving force behind the production of superoxide by xanthine oxidase. The greater the perfusion, the less accumulation of hypoxanthine. In practice, this "washout" of hypoxanthine may not be so important because the concentrations of hypoxanthine which can accumulate in ischemic tissues may exceed the enzyme's $K_m$ by two orders of magnitude. That is, oxygen, not hypoxanthine, is likely to be the limiting substrate.

The superoxide and hydroxyl free radicals have lifetimes measured in fractions of a second under these conditions. For this reason, direct washout of the radicals themselves is not possible by perfusion of the tissue.

### Validity of Models

Good models are absolutely vital to the progress of medical research, yet they are inevitably the focal points of criticism and controversy. Clinicians argue that the model creates conditions never seen in clinical practice, and the basic scientist occasionally loses sight of the fact that a model, by definition, must represent something that exists, and not simply something that is convenient to study. Most real situations involve multiple contributing factors, each of which may exist in many "shades of gray." Ideally, a good model should be able to isolate one or more of the multiple variables individually, and to vary them independently of one another. Furthermore, it may be important (for practical reasons) to maximize the effect of any given variable beyond the magnitude of its natural occurrence. These features do not necessarily invalidate a model. If, for example, it appears that total global ischemia in an isolated heart does not bring into play any new factors not seen in partial regional ischemia, but rather simply amplifies the end-result, then the model may be accepted, with some caution, as useful and valid.

From a consideration of free radical metabolism, a potentially serious difference between the commonly used isolated organ models and their real counterparts is perfusion with oxygenated salt solutions rather than with whole blood. Not only are there substantial differences in $Po_2$ (the model is much higher) and capacity (much lower), but whole blood has substantial ability to scavenge superoxide and hydrogen peroxide, as well as the ability to catalyze their reaction to produce the hydroxyl radical. These factors could conceivably account for dramatic differences in response to an ischemic insult.

## WHAT CAN WE DO TO COMBAT FREE RADICALS?

Two significant sources of superoxide radical have been identified in the ischemically injured myocardium: the major source appears to be the enzyme xanthine oxidase; the other source appears to be metabolically activated polymorphonuclear leukocytes. We are probably very fortunate in that a potent inhibitor with a high degree of specificity already exists for the enzyme xanthine oxidase. That inhibitor, allopurinol, is a drug widely used in the treatment of gout. (The problem in gout, of course, is high serum levels of uric acid, the purine end-product of the enzyme's action on hypoxanthine. Allopurinol inhibits both uric acid production and superoxide production.) It may not be the ideal drug; it is given orally and is rather slow-acting. It might be desirable to have a fast-acting injectable xanthine oxidase inhibitor available in cases of sudden-onset, severe ischemia. In cases of chronically recurring ischemic episodes or where distinct reperfusion is brought about by clinical intervention, however, it makes very good biochemical sense to prophylactically inhibit xanthine oxidase with allopurinol. Other approaches, such as the injection of the scavenger enzymes, superoxide dismutase and catalase, have been invaluable as laboratory tools to elucidate the biochemical mechanisms involved, but have a number of practical problems which may limit their clinical utility for the foreseeable future.

The inflammatory component of ischemic injury involves superoxide in the same capacity as any other neutrophil-mediated event (7). A potent and specific inhibitor of the NADPH oxidase responsible for neutrophil-generated superoxide would, without doubt, be a powerful and useful new antiinflammatory drug. No such drug has as yet been identified.

## CONCLUDING COMMENTS

It is now clear that oxygen-derived radicals play important roles in several pathophysiological processes and among these is ischemic injury. The primary source of superoxide in reperfused tissues is the enzyme xanthine oxidase, created during ischemia by a calcium-triggered proteolytic attack on xanthine dehydrogenase. Reperfused tissues are protected in a variety of laboratory models by scavengers of superoxide radicals or hydroxyl radicals, or by allopurinol, an inhibitor of xanthine oxidase. Free radical-induced injury may be a major component of calcium-induced injury, as well as neutrophil-mediated inflammation. I believe that each of these processes has its role in human heart disease, and as our understanding of each process increases we may expect to see the clinical implementation of rational new approaches to the management of heart disease.

## REFERENCES

1. Chambers, D. E., Parks, D. A., Patterson, G., Yoshida, S., Burton, K., Parmley, L. F., McCord, J. M., and Downey, J. M. (1983): Role of oxygen derived radicals in myocardial ischemia. *Fed. Proc.*, 42:1093.
2. Freeman, B. A., Young, S. L., and Crapo, J. D. (1983): Liposome-mediated augmentation of superoxide dismutase in endothelial cells prevents oxygen injury. *J. Biol. Chem.*, 258:12534–12542.
3. Fridovich, I. (1983): Superoxide radical: an endogenous toxicant. *Annu. Rev. Pharmacol. Toxicol.*, 23:239–257.
4. Fridovich, I., and Handler, P. (1962): Xanthine oxidase. V. Differential inhibition of the reduction of various electron acceptors. *J. Biol. Chem.*, 237:916–921.
5. Granger, D. N., Rutili, G., and McCord, J. M. (1981): Superoxide radicals in feline intestinal ischemia. *Gastroenterology*, 81:22–29.
6. Parks, D. A., Bulkley, G. B., Granger, D. N., Hamilton, S. R., and McCord, J. M. (1982): Ischemic injury in the cat small intestine: role of superoxide radicals. *Gastroenterology*, 82:9–15.
7. Petrone, W. F., English, D. K., Wong, K., and McCord, J. M. (1980): Free radicals and inflammation: superoxide-dependent activation of a neutrophil chemotactic factor in plasma. *Proc. Natl. Acad. Sci. USA*, 77:1159–1163.
8. Roy, R. S., and McCord, J. M. (1983): Superoxide and ischemia: conversion of xanthine dehydrogenase to xanthine oxidase. In: *Oxy Radicals and Their Scavenger Systems*, Vol. II, edited by R. Greenwald and G. Cohen, pp. 145–153. Elsevier, New York.
9. Schaffer, S. W., Roy, R. S., and McCord, J. M. (1984): Possible role for calmodulin in calcium paradox-induced heart failure. *Eur. Heart J. (in press)*.
10. Shlafer, M., Kane, P. F., Wiggins, V. Y., and Kirsh, M. M. (1982): Possible role for cytotoxic oxygen metabolites in the pathogenesis of cardiac ischemic injury. *Circulation*, 66(Suppl.I):85–92.

*Therapeutic Approaches to Myocardial Infarct
Size Limitation*, edited by D. J. Hearse and
D. M. Yellon. Raven Press, New York © 1984.

13

# Do Leukocytes Influence Infarct Size?

*Benedict R. Lucchesi, **Joseph L. Romson, and †Stanley R. Jolly

*Department of Pharmacology, University of Michigan Medical School, Ann Arbor,
Michigan 48109; **Department of Surgery, Division of Cardiothoracic Surgery, University
of Washington, Seattle, Washington 98195; and †Department of Pharmacology, Medical
College of Georgia, Augusta, Georgia 30912

Three important observations have given impetus to the development of pharmacologic means of limiting the extent of irreversible myocardial injury resulting from an acute ischemic insult or from ischemia followed by reperfusion. First, the number of deaths attributable to ischemic heart disease in the United States is staggering, accounting for nearly two-thirds of the 980,000 annual deaths of cardiovascular origin (69). The manifestations of ischemic heart disease, in particular, acute myocardial infarction, account for one-third of *all* deaths occurring in the United States each year (60).

Second, the short- as well as long-term prognosis of patients presenting with acute myocardial infarction is in direct correlation with the extent of myocardial injury resulting from the ischemic insult. Of those patients surviving long enough to be admitted to the coronary care unit, most deaths from myocardial infarction are due to the loss of ventricular function secondary to extensive *de novo* infarction or reinfarction (15). Sobel et al. (65) have shown that when the size of the infarct is estimated by serial measurement of plasma creatine phosphokinase (CK), those patients with smaller myocardial infarcts had a considerably better prognosis than those patients with larger infarcts. *These data clearly indicate the importance of minimizing the extent of irreversible myocardial injury resulting from an acute ischemic event.*

The third pertinent observation deals with the temporal sequence of events beginning with the onset of regional myocardial ischemia and culminating in the infarct attaining its ultimate size. Although complex biochemical changes that occur during regional ischemia are not understood completely, it is apparent that the transformation of myocardial cells from the reversibly to the irreversibly injured state is a gradual process occurring over the course of several hours. In experimental models of acute myocardial infarction, irreversible injury occurs after 40 min of regional ischemia. Without reperfusion, infarct extension continues up to 6 hr after the start of the ischemic insult (53). Cell death is not instantaneous, but, instead, the deterioration occurs over a period of time that makes efforts to salvage jeopardized (reversibly injured) myocardium a realistic endeavor (15). Most recently, there has been an increasing emphasis placed on efforts to establish reperfusion of the once ischemic myocardium with the intended goal of salvaging myocardial tissue before it becomes irreversibly damaged. Therefore, patients with evolving myocardial infarctions may be subjected to coronary artery angioplasty and/or thrombolytic therapy with the hope of reestablishing regional coronary artery blood flow and restoring regional contractility of the once jeopardized and functionally compromised myocardial segment. There is concern that reperfusion may lead to cellular processes that extend the area of cell necrosis beyond that which could be attributed solely to the mechanisms associated with ischemia.

## APPROACHES TO LIMIT INFARCT SIZE

In 1971, Maroko et al. (43) demonstrated that the extent of irreversible myocardial injury is worsened by factors that increase myocardial oxygen consumption. Conversely, factors that decrease myocardial oxygen demand were shown to lessen myocardial injury during ischemia. Ensuing efforts to limit the extent of ischemia-induced myocardial injury focused on pharmacologic means of correcting the imbalance between myocardial oxygen supply and demand during an ischemic episode. Altering the major determinants of myocardial oxygen consumption (such as heart rate, myocardial contractility, and ventricular wall tension) by pharmacologic agents were evaluated in animal models of myocardial ischemia and infarction. Several laboratories have observed that the β-adrenergic receptor antagonist, propranolol, favorably alters indices of ischemic myocardial injury and report that this beneficial effect is due, at least in part, to the ability of the drug to reduce myocardial oxygen consumption (see Chapter 11 and review in ref. 31).

### Alteration of Myocardial Oxygen Supply and Demand

Efforts to increase oxygen delivery to the ischemic myocardium have focused primarily on enhancing myocardial blood flow to ischemic tissue by surgical (coronary artery bypass), mechanical (intraaortic balloon counterpulsation) or pharmacologic (coronary vasodilators) means (31). Thus, increasing oxygen and nutrient supply to ischemic tissue by pharmacologic and/or mechanical interventions appears to be a feasible approach to limiting ultimate myocardial infarct size.

*Implicit in previous efforts to salvage ischemic myocardium by altering myocardial oxygen supply or demand is the assumption that myocardial tissue injury results from the inability of the coronary vasculature to deliver necessary oxygen and nutrients to maintain myocyte viability. However, we believe that other pathophysiologic processes are contributing to the ultimate extent of irreversible myocardial injury resulting from an acute ischemic insult.*

### Recent Alternative Approaches: A Role for Leukocytes?

In the past few years, a number of cardioprotective compounds have been developed that do not appear to alter myocardial oxygen supply or demand. The efficacy of these compounds in animal models of myocardial ischemia has prompted expansion of the conceptual framework that forms the basis of efforts to pharmacologically limit infarct size. *One promising avenue of current research is the investigation of the role of leukocytes in the pathophysiology of myocardial ischemia and infarction. The demonstrated efficacy of certain antiinflammatory agents in protecting the ischemic myocardium implicates the inflammatory response as one source of tissue injury in the hypoperfused and, in particular, the reperfused myocardium.* The role of the polymorphonuclear neutrophils has been investigated for they are the first leukocytic elements to be mobilized subsequent to the ischemic insult. The importance of the neutrophils in the pathophysiology of acute myocardial infarction, and various pharmacologic approaches to modifying neutrophil function during ischemic myocardial injury and/or reperfusion is the major subject of our discussion.

### INFARCT SIZE LIMITATION BY NEUTROPHIL INHIBITION

Between 1977 and 1979, several reports appeared in the literature indicating that the nonsteroidal, antiinflammatory agent, ibuprofen, provided cardioprotection in animal models of myocardial infarction (28,37,39,40,54,55) (Fig. 1). However, Jugdutt et al. (28) and Romson et al. (55) reported that ibuprofen did not alter

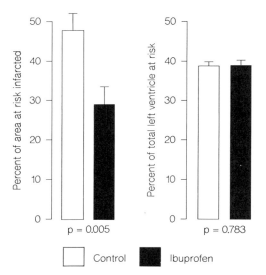

**FIG. 1.** Reduction in Ultimate Infarct Size by Ibuprofen. Effect of ibuprofen on the extent of irreversible myocardial injury after 60 min of left circumflex occlusion followed by reperfusion ($n = 14$ in control group, $n = 13$ in ibuprofen group). Myocardial infarct size *(left)* is expressed as a percent of the area at risk. Oral ibuprofen (12.5 mg/kg, q 4 hr) reduced the extent of myocardial infarction by 35% based on the area at risk. The percent of the total left ventricle occupied by the area at risk was not different in the two groups of dogs *(right)*. (From ref. 55., with permission.)

distribution of regional myocardial blood flow (Fig. 2) or reduce myocardial oxygen consumption during acute myocardial ischemia.

## Mechanisms of Ibuprofen Action

The balance between myocardial oxygen supply and demand has been postulated to be a critical factor in determining the ultimate extent of myocardial injury. It then stands to reason that an intervention that reduces myocardial oxygen demand might prove beneficial during regional myocardial ischemia. Ibuprofen, however, does not appear to exert its cardioprotective effects in this fashion. The product of heart rate and mean arterial pressure, the rate-pressure product, has become an established approximation of myocardial oxygen consumption. In our canine model of regional ischemia, ibuprofen had no significant effect on myocardial oxygen consumption, as indicated by the rate-pressure product data. The isolated, blood-perfused cat heart was used as an experimental model in which ibuprofen's direct myocardial effects could be assessed apart from the hemodynamic and autonomic influences that occur in an intact animal. Under carefully controlled conditions, ibuprofen did not reduce myocardial oxygen consumption in the nonischemic, isolated, blood-perfused cat heart (55). Ibuprofen did not alter the intrinsic heart rate, left ventricular peak pressure (LVPP), or dP/dt (indices of myocardial contractility) of nonischemic cat isolated hearts. The data rule out the possibility that ibuprofen aids the ischemic myocardium by reducing myocardial oxygen consumption or by redistributing myocardial blood flow to ischemic tissue. Redistribution of myocardial blood flow and reduction of myocardial oxygen consumption are but two mechanisms by which a compound may salvage ischemic myocardium.

Several authors have speculated on other possible mechanisms by which ibuprofen exerts its cardioprotective effects. Lefer and associates (1,36,37) postulated that ibuprofen salvages ischemic myocardium by inhibiting prostaglandin synthesis, inhibiting platelet aggregation, causing coronary vasodilation, and preventing release of lysosomal enzymes. Jugdutt et al. (28) suggested that the beneficial effects of ibuprofen resulted from the inhibition of platelet aggregation in the border zone of the ischemic myocardium, inhibition of lysosomal enzyme release, and inhibition of prostaglandin synthesis. *Ibuprofen's capacity to reduce the extent of irreversible myocardial injury in experimental models of myocardial infarction was clear; on the other hand, the mechanism by which ibuprofen produced its salutory effect was very much in doubt.*

### Role of Antiinflammatory Reactions

In 1982, Romson et al. (57) studied the effect of ibuprofen on the accumulation of platelets and leukocytes in ischemic and infarcted myocardium in the dog. It was known that ibuprofen possessed both platelet inhibitory (44,47) and antiinflammatory (29) properties. This study was designed to determine whether ibuprofen's cardioprotective action could be attributed to the inhibition of platelet and/or polymorphonuclear neutrophil (PMN) accumulation in infarcted canine myocardium. Briefly, the experimental protocol consisted of administering indium-111-

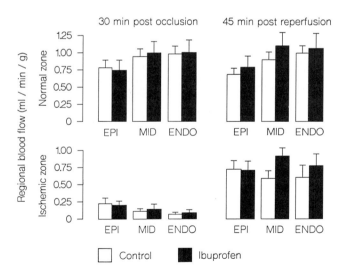

**FIG. 2.** Regional Myocardial Blood Flow. Effects of ibuprofen (12.5 mg/kg, q 4 hr) on regional myocardial blood flow during left circumflex coronary artery occlusion and reperfusion. Regional myocardial blood flows were measured using the radioactive microsphere technique. Subepicardial (EPI), midmyocardial (MID), and subendocardial (ENDO) tissue samples from the normal and ischemic zones were obtained. Ibuprofen or drug vehicle was administered orally beginning 1 hr prior to occlusion. No statistical differences in regional myocardial blood flow were observed between control and ibuprofen-treated dogs. (From ref. 55., with permission.)

labeled platelets or polymorphonuclear leukocytes to open chest, anesthetized dogs subjected to 60 min of left circumflex (LCX) coronary artery occlusion followed by 24 hr of reperfusion. The animals were sacrificed after 24 hr and the extent of irreversible myocardial injury resulting from the temporary ischemic insult was determined by an *ex vivo* staining technique using the histochemical reagent, triphenyltetrazolium. The technique identifies the area at risk of infarction and, within this area, distinguishes viable from irreversibly injured and/or infarcted myocardium. Myocardial tissue samples from the area at risk, containing both infarcted and viable myocardium, and tissue samples from the nonischemic region were taken to determine the extent of radiolabeled platelet or leukocyte accumulation (Fig. 3). The results of these experiments indicated that treating the animals with ibuprofen (12.5 mg/kg i.v. every 4 hr beginning 30 min before LCX coronary artery occlusion) resulted in a 40% reduction in the extent of myocardial infarction [48 ± 4% of the area at risk infarcted in control animals ($n = 14$) versus 29 ± 4% in ibuprofen-treated animals ($n = 13$); $p < 0.005$, $\bar{X} \pm$ SEM]. Ibuprofen did not

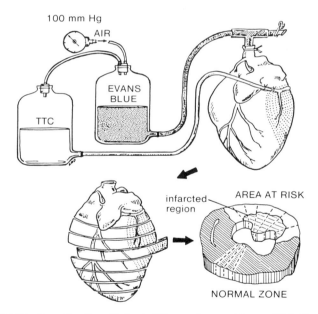

**FIG. 3.**   Method for Quantification of Infarcted Myocardium and Area at Risk. The left circumflex vascular bed is perfused with 1.5% triphenyltetrazolium (TTC) and the aorta is perfused in a retrograde manner with 0.5% Evans blue. The Evans blue delineates the nonrisk region, and the TTC distinguishes viable myocardium from infarcted tissue within the area at risk. Both the TTC and Evans blue reservoirs are maintained at a constant pressure of 100 mm Hg. Tissue sampling for determination of indium-111 radioactivity in infarcted and nonischemic myocardium was done by gamma spectrometry. Transmural sections are taken from the area at risk and normal zone. Each tissue section from the area at risk is carefully traced onto clear sheets, noting the regions of infarcted myocardium.

influence the accumulation of indium-111-labeled platelets in the infarcted myocardium, but had a significant effect on leukocyte accumulation. In myocardial samples with 0.41 to 0.61-g-infarct, there was a 67% reduction of leukocyte accumulation in tissue obtained from ibuprofen-treated animals as compared to control dogs. The infarcted/normal tissue ratio of leukocyte radioactivity was $12 \pm 2$ in control dogs and $4 \pm 1$ in ibuprofen-treated dogs (Fig. 4).

That ibuprofen significantly limits indium-111-labeled leukocyte accumulation in infarcted myocardium is a most noteworthy observation. Autoradiography of transverse myocardial tissue sections indicated that indium-111-labeled leukocyte accumulation occurred primarily within the boundaries of infarcted myocardium (Fig. 5). Gamma spectrometry of myocardial tissue sections permitted quantification of indium-111-labeled leukocyte radioactivity and the calculation of leukocyte accumulation ratios. Ibuprofen lessened the accumulation of leukocytes in infarcted myocardium. While the leukocyte accumulation ratios for control dogs were $3.6 \pm 0.3$ (0.01–0.20-g-infarct interval) to $17.9 \pm 3.0$ (1.01 + g-infarct interval), ibuprofen-treated dogs had averaged leukocyte accumulation ratios of $3.7 \pm 0.6$ (0.01–0.20-

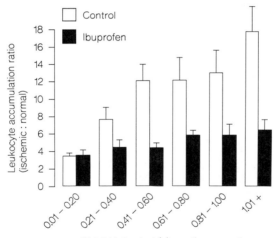

**FIG. 4.** Distribution of Indium-111-Labeled Leukocytes in Nonischemic Myocardium. Effect of ibuprofen (12 mg/kg, q 4 hr, i.v.) on the accumulation of indium-111-labeled leukocytes in infarcted myocardium ($n = 9$ in control group, $n = 7$ in drug group). Quantitative assessment of the accumulation of indium-111-labeled leukocytes was accomplished by calculating the leukocyte accumulation ratio, defined as the increase in radioactivity present in infarcted myocardium compared with the indium-111 activity present in nonischemic tissue. The leukocyte accumulation ratio was calculated for each transmural myocardial tissue section taken from the area at risk. These values were then grouped according to the number of grams of infarcted tissue in each transmural section. In control dogs, leukocyte accumulation ratio increased substantially with greater amounts of infarcted tissue in each section. Treating the dogs with ibuprofen markedly suppressed leukocyte accumulation in infarcted myocardium. The 1.01 + g-infarct division includes tissue samples with more than 1.0 g but less than 1.4 g of infarcted tissue.

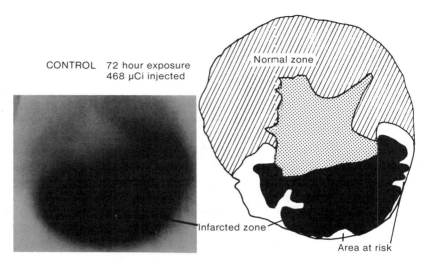

CONTROL    72 hour exposure
468 µCi injected

Normal zone

Infarcted zone

Area at risk

**FIG. 5.** Autoradiograph of Indium-111 Accumulation in Infarcted Myocardium. An autoradiograph indicating the accumulation of indium-111-labeled leukocytes in a transverse myocardial section from a control animal. The transverse myocardial section indicating the boundaries of the differentially stained myocardial regions is drawn from a trace of the tissue section made prior to the start of autoradiography. On the *left* is a photograph of the autoradiograph indicating specific regions of intense exposure of the film. The borders of the area of intense radioactivity always exactly match the regions of infarcted myocardium. The length of the film exposure and the total amount of indium-111 activity administered to the animal are presented.

g-infarct interval) to $6.5 \pm 1.2$ ($1.01 +$ g-infarct interval). Averaged over all six g-infarct intervals, ibuprofen treatment reduced leukocyte accumulation ratios by 46% compared with control dogs.

## Neutrophils and Superoxide Production

*With the growing understanding of the involvement of leukocytes in the "reparative" process of transforming necrotic myocardium into scar tissue has come the realization that massive accumulation of inflammatory cells may actually injure viable myocardium.* Stimulated neutrophils transform molecular oxygen into highly reactive and cytotoxic free radical superoxide anion (Chapter 12), hydroxyl radical, hydrogen peroxide, and, perhaps, singlet oxygen. When not limited to phagocytic vacuoles, these oxygen radicals degrade extracellular macromolecules, attack membrane phospholipids, and promote cell injury or death. In addition, the release of the enzymatic contents of neutrophil granules into the extracellular space may result in proteolytic attack on viable tissue. *It is our belief that the influx of leukocytes into regions of myocardial cell damage, in numbers far greater than necessary for the repair and resolution of injured myocardium, may exacerbate the ischemic insult. Thus, the antiinflammatory properties of ibuprofen may be an important mechanism by which the drug exerts its cardioprotective effects during myocardial ischemia and especially in those instances where reperfusion occurs after a period of regional ischemia (Fig. 6).*

## ROLE OF NEUTROPHILS IN ISCHEMIC INJURY

The hypothesis that the antiinflammatory properties of ibuprofen accounted for its cardioprotective effect and the postulated deleterious effects of neutrophil accumulation in ischemic myocardium (57) suggested a series of experiments which investigated the role of circulating neutrophils in mediating ischemic myocardial injury. The protocol called for selective depletion of dog polymorphonuclear leukocytes by the administration of antiserum to canine neutrophils.

### Neutrophil Depletion Studies

#### *Brief Ischemia*

In an initial set of experiments in our laboratory (56), open chest, anesthetized dogs were assigned randomly to three treatment groups: saline controls ($n = 8$), those treated with neutrophil antiserum ($n = 8$) and those receiving nonimmune serum ($n = 7$). Each dog was subjected to 90 min of left circumflex coronary artery occlusion, followed by 6 hr of reperfusion. The animals were sacrificed and the extent of myocardial injury assessed utilizing the *ex vivo* histochemical staining method shown in Fig. 3. Myocardial tissue samples from the area at risk were taken for histopathologic assessment of leukocyte infiltration by light microscopy. The administration of canine neutrophil antiserum reduced the circulating neutrophil count by an average of $77 \pm 2\%$ ($\bar{X} \pm$ SEM) over the course of the experiment. The effect of neutrophil depletion on the extent of irreversible myocardial injury is summarized in Table 1. Dogs treated with neutrophil antiserum developed myo-

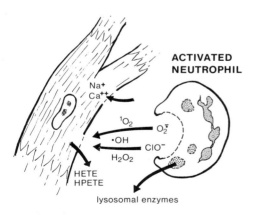

lysosomal enzymes

**FIG. 6.** Potential Role of the Leukocyte as a Mediator of Myocardial Cell Injury. The leukocyte is attracted to the site of ischemic myocardial cell injury perhaps by a noncomplement-derived substance (HETE and/or HPETE) which is chemotactic for neutrophils. The stimulated neutrophil develops an incomplete phagocytic vacuole, undergoes degranulation and the production of toxic products of oxygen metabolism ($^1O_2$, singlet oxygen; $O_2^-$, superoxide anion; $\cdot$OH, hydroxyl radical; lysosomal enzymes). The inability of the activated neutrophil to engulf the injured cell leads to the release of the contents of the vacuole into the extracellular space. The lack of specific protective enzymes (superoxide dismutase, glutathione peroxidase) in the extracellular space allows the released toxic oxygen products to mediate cell injury (influx of sodium and calcium ions) beyond that attributable to the ischemic process alone. The events are exaggerated in those instances where reperfusion occurs after a period of ischemia.

TABLE 1. *Infarct size data from saline, nonimmune serum, and neutrophil antiserum groups*

| Group | n | Left ventricle wt. (g) | Infarct size as a % of | | Area at risk as a % of left ventricle |
|---|---|---|---|---|---|
| | | | Area at risk | Left ventricle | |
| Saline | 8 | 88.9 ± 8.0 | 48.0 ± 4.7 | 20.3 ± 1.9 | 42.9 ± 1.3 |
| Nonimmune serum | 7 | 78.0 ± 6.2 | 47.1 ± 7.5 | 20.1 ± 3.5 | 42.6 ± 3.0 |
| Neutrophil antiserum | 8 | 86.1 ± 6.2 | 27.0 ± 4.5[a] | 9.6 ± 1.6[a] | 37.0 ± 1.6 |

Data were analyzed using analysis of variance followed by Bonferroni's method for multiple comparisons. Values are mean ± SEM.
[a] $p < 0.05$ vs nonimmune serum and saline groups.

cardial infarcts that were 43% smaller than those in dogs treated with nonimmune serum ($27 ± 4.5\%$ versus $47.1 ± 7.5\%$ of the area at risk, respectively; $p < 0.05$). In the saline-treated control group, infarct size was $48.0 ± 4.7\%$ of the area at risk, a value not significantly different from that in the group which received nonimmune serum, but significantly larger than that of the neutrophil antiserum group ($p < 0.05$). Figure 7 presents the results of the histopathologic examination of the myocardial tissue samples taken from each animal. Infarcted myocardium from dogs treated with saline or nonimmune serum had a substantial neutrophilic infiltrate, while PMN infiltrate was virtually absent in infarcted tissue from dogs treated with neutrophil antiserum. *Thus, neutrophil depletion reduced the extent of the leukocytic infiltrate in infarcted myocardium and was associated with a 43% reduction in the extent of irreversible myocardial injury.*

## Extended Ischemia

The above study was extended by another series of experiments in which circulating neutrophils in the dog were depleted by the administration of antiserum to canine neutrophils and the extent of irreversible myocardial injury assessed 24 hr after the ischemic insult. Similar methods were used as in the previous study (56) and equivalent neutrophil depletion was obtained, approximately 85% depletion, over the first 10 hr. However, neutrophil counts had recovered by 24 hr to 60% of the initial control value. The effects of neutrophil depletion on infarct size at 24 hr were similar to the previous results (56). Neutropenic animals had significantly smaller infarcts compared to those which received nonimmune serum ($27 ± 4\%$ versus $41 ± 4\%$ of the area at risk; $p < 0.05$). Again, the extent of myocardial infarction in animals which received nonimmune serum was not different from that observed in hearts from the saline-treated group. Histopathologic examination suggested reduced tissue neutrophil counts, but there was significant overlap with controls, which was probably attributable to the late recovery of circulating neutrophils. In addition to confirming the results of the initial study (56), *these results suggest that allowing the return of neutrophils after the initial ischemic event does not cause a resumption of tissue injury and infarct progression.* Since the neutrophil may play an integral role in the organization and healing of myocardial infarcts, this facet of the problem deserves further study.

These results indicate the importance of circulating neutrophils in the pathophysiology of acute myocardial infarction. In a recent study using a canine model of myocardial infarction consisting of 60 min of left anterior descending coronary artery occlusion followed by 5 hr of reperfusion, Mullane et al. *(personal communication)* reported that in animals in which leukopenia was induced by 5 daily injections of hydroxyurea, there was a 67% reduction in the percent of the area at risk infarcted as compared to controls ($16.5 \pm 3.4\%$ versus $50.1 \pm 0.2\%$; $p < 0.001$). These observations have been extended recently in the report by Ksiezycka et al. (33) who noted that neutrophil depletion resulted in a reduction in ultimate infarct size in the canine heart subjected to permanent coronary artery occlusion.

*Recognition of the release of cytotoxic products by stimulated neutrophils has led to the suggestion that neutrophil infiltration into infarcted myocardium may exacerbate ischemic injury by the destruction of otherwise viable tissue. The results of our experiments as well as those of others are in accord with that suggestion and emphasize the importance of the acute inflammatory response in the pathophysiology of myocardial infarction.*

The major advantages of inducing neutropenia by using neutrophil antiserum as opposed to chemical means, such as mechlorethamine hydrochloride or hydrox-

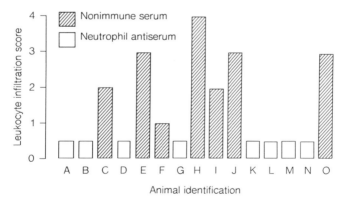

**FIG. 7.** Effect of Leukocyte Depletion upon the Inflammatory Response in Infarcted Myocardium. Results of the histopathologic assessment of leukocyte infiltrate into infarcted myocardium for dogs given nonimmune serum and those given neutrophil antiserum. Each coded tissue specimen was ranked for the extent of leukocytic infiltrate associated with infarcted myocardium on a scale ranging from 0 (no white cells) to +4 (assigned to the specimen with the most extensive accumulation of leukocytes). The score for each dog is presented in the order in which the coded samples were evaluated. Each dog treated with neutrophil antiserum received a score of 0, representing the rare presence of interstitial leukocytes. Dogs treated with nonimmune serum had scores ranging from +1 to +4, indicating substantial neutrophil accumulation in the infarcted myocardium. Samples from dogs given saline exhibited leukocytic infiltration comparable to that in the nonimmune serum group (data not shown).

yurea, include specificity of cell depletion and minimal side-effects. The most noticeable side-effect associated with the administration of neutrophil antiserum was a transient vasodepressor response, but mean arterial blood pressure returned to baseline values within 30 to 45 min.

In contrast to the marked reduction in circulating neutrophils in dogs that received neutrophil antiserum, dogs given nonimmune serum or saline had substantially higher neutrophil counts. The elevation in the circulating neutrophil count was not attributable to nonimmune serum, since similar increases in neutrophil counts were observed in the saline-treated group. Furthermore, the extent of irreversible myocardial injury averaged 47.1 ± 7.5% of the area at risk in the group treated with nonimmune serum, compared with 48.0 ± 4.7% in the saline group. The increase in circulating neutrophil counts was probably related to surgical trauma associated with the experimental induction of ischemic myocardial injury.

## Possible Mechanisms of Protection

### Hemodynamic Effects?

Reduction of circulating neutrophil counts was associated with a reduction in the extent of irreversible myocardial injury when expressed as a percentage of either the area at risk or as a percentage of the left ventricle (Table 1). The hemodynamic data indicated that no substantial differences were seen among dogs treated with saline, nonimmune serum, or neutrophil antiserum. The only noticeable difference was a reduction in the average left ventricular end-diastolic pressure after 6 hr of reperfusion, probably a result of the smaller amount of infarcted myocardium observed in the dogs which received neutrophil antiserum. Thus, the significant reduction in the extent of irreversible myocardial injury in the dogs treated with neutrophil antiserum cannot be attributed to an alteration in hemodynamics that reduced myocardial oxygen consumption during regional ischemia.

### Coronary Flow Effects?

Any explanation of the mechanism by which an intervention could reduce infarct size must consider possible alterations in the distribution of myocardial blood flow and myocardial contractility. Whereas we did not study regional myocardial blood flow or assess regional myocardial contractility, such changes, if they did occur, would have to be attributed to the presence of the antibody, because the nonimmune serum dogs and the saline-treated dogs had similar degrees of irreversible myocardial injury. In future studies of antineutrophil serum, alterations in regional coronary blood flow and myocardial contractility should be considered as possible mechanisms by which the depletion of circulating neutrophils might reduce the extent of ischemic myocardial cell injury. Leukocytes, because of their ability to adhere to impaired vascular endothelium, lead to capillary obstruction, which may further impair reperfusion to the jeopardized myocardial region. Plasma proteins, erythrocytes, and granulocytes have been observed in capillaries and venules, in the extracellular space, as well as adhering to damaged myocardial cells. Neutrophil depletion might prevent the influence of such a mechanism, particularly upon reperfusion, therefore resulting in the further salvage of jeopardized myocardial tissue.

## Extent of Leukocyte Infiltration?

Histopathologic examination of myocardial tissue revealed a striking difference in the extent of leukocytic infiltrate in infarcted myocardium from dogs treated with neutrophil antiserum compared with tissue from dogs receiving nonimmune serum. Although changes in myocardial cells characteristic of irreversible injury were present in all groups of dogs, neutrophilic infiltrate was virtually absent in infarcted myocardium from dogs receiving neutrophil antiserum. The semiquantitative assessment of leukocyte infiltrate clearly demonstrated the pronounced differences between the two groups of dogs receiving serum. The dogs receiving neutrophil antiserum consistently were found to have virtually no neutrophilic infiltrate, whereas dogs treated with nonimmune serum had a significant degree of neutrophil accumulation in infarcted tissue. In short, the two treatment groups did not overlap with respect to the semiquantitative assessment of leukocyte infiltrate. Although these data do not prove that neutrophil depletion spares ischemic myocardium, *there is certainly a strong association between the lack of neutrophilic infiltrate in infarcted myocardium and the reduction in the extent of ischemia-induced myocardial injury.*

It has been established that migration of polymorphonuclear neutrophils into recently infarcted myocardium represents an initial phase in a complex process which includes demolition and subsequent organization of injured tissue and culminates in the replacement of necrotic myocardium with fibrous scar tissue (35,41). Infiltration of neutrophils into irreversibly injured myocardium facilitates the breakdown of necrotic tissue which, in turn, promotes reabsorption or phagocytosis by tissue macrophages. After the removal of tissue debris, capillaries and fibroblasts invade the infarcted area, ultimately leading to the formation of collagen-rich scar tissue that replaces the necrotic area (35).

*During the initial stages of an acute inflammatory response, polymorphonuclear neutrophils undergo a complex series of functional and biochemical alterations that promote tissue lysis. Although these events are ultimately of importance to the repair process, they may also result in the destruction of potentially viable tissue elements.* Stimulated neutrophils release highly reactive and cytotoxic activated oxygen species, which promote cell injury or death (9,12,67). In addition, activated neutrophils release lysosomal enzymes capable of proteolytic disruption and liquefaction of viable as well as irreversibly injured tissue (72). Finally, stimulated neutrophils trigger membrane phospholipids to release arachidonic acid which is converted by specific lipoxygenases to potent chemotactic hydroxy-eicosatetraenoic acids (HETEs), hydroperoxy-eicosatetraenoic acid (HPETEs), and leukotriene $B_4$ (LTB$_4$) (4,64). The chemoattractant, LTB$_4$, promotes the further recruitment of neutrophils as well as monocytes into the acutely inflamed region at the site of ischemic tissue injury. The monocytes, in contrast to the polymorphonuclear neutrophils, have the capacity to generate leukotriene $C_4$ and $D_4$ which, in addition to producing coronary artery vasoconstriction, also enhance vascular permeability, thereby increasing the extent of ischemic injury. *In short, the migration and accumulation of neutrophils at the site of tissue injury may exacerbate the extent of tissue destruction by cellular mechanisms considered essential for the ultimate organization and repair of the injured tissue.*

## ROLE OF FREE RADICALS IN ISCHEMIC INJURY

It has been known for some time that *under the appropriate stimulus, polymorphonuclear leukocytes and other granulocytes reduce molecular oxygen to superoxide anion free radical (Chapter 12) and hydrogen peroxide (3) which are released into the extracellular space (58).* These reduced oxygen species are thought to be generated by a membrane-associated nicotinamide adenine dinucleotide oxidase enzyme system (10). Other highly reactive oxygen-derived free radicals produced by stimulated phagocytic cells include the hydroxyl radical, singlet oxygen, and hypochlorous acid. *There is little doubt that these oxygen metabolites are capable of producing significant cellular and tissue injury by altering cellular proteins, nucleic acids, membrane lipids, cytosolic molecules, and extracellular matrix constituents (11).* In addition to the cellular damage caused by activated granulocytes, Meerson et al. (45) suggested that incomplete reduction of oxygen within the phospholipid matrix serves as an additional source of lipid peroxidation of myocyte membranes during myocardial ischemia leading to further membrane injury.

### Natural Protection Against Free Radicals

Over the course of evolution, cells have developed a number of protective mechanisms to adapt to the constant challenge of free radical formation, which is a normal consequence of existence in an oxidizing environment. Some of these mechanisms include production of free radical scavengers such as vitamin E, vitamin C, and glutathione, or development of enzymatic systems such as catalases, peroxidases, and superoxide dismutases (11). All of these "free radical" scavengers protect the cell from reduced oxygen species generated from normal cellular metabolism. Evidence suggests that cellular protective systems are injured by myocardial ischemia. *Tissue activities of myocardial superoxide dismutase (16,45) and glutathione peroxidase (16,45,52) are depleted after experimental myocardial ischemia. When the myocardium is rendered ischemic, toxic oxygen species generated either within the plasma membrane, the mitochondria, the cytosol, or by stimulated granulocytes infiltrating the ischemic area, overwhelm the capacity of these protective cellular mechanisms.*

### Free Radical Scavengers and Infarct Size

To test the above hypothesis superoxide dismutase (SOD) plus catalase (CAT) were administered by intraatrial infusion to dogs undergoing experimental myocardial infarction (5). *Animals receiving the free radical protective enzymes showed an overall reduction in ultimate infarct size* of approximately 50% (19.4 ± 5.0 versus 43.6 ± 3.5% of the area at risk; $p < 0.05$) compared to controls. The percent of left ventricle at risk did not differ between groups. *The beneficial effects of SOD plus CAT could not be explained on the basis of hemodynamic differences.*

Our studies employing SOD and CAT demonstrated that reperfusion of the once ischemic myocardium is associated with an extension of the region of myocardial cellular injury and necrosis. As illustrated schematically in Fig. 8, total occlusion of the left circumflex coronary artery in the canine heart for 24 hr is associated with a degree of myocardial necrosis involving 75% of the area at risk. On the other hand, occlusion of the circumflex coronary artery for a period of 90 min followed by reperfusion for 24 hr results in 45% of the area at risk undergoing infarction, thereby leading one to assume that reperfusion after 90 min of regional ischemia salvages approximately 30% of the myocardium within the area at risk. There is no doubt that, in the absence of reperfusion, the ultimate extent of necrosis would have been much greater. However, if one assumes that the act of reperfusion

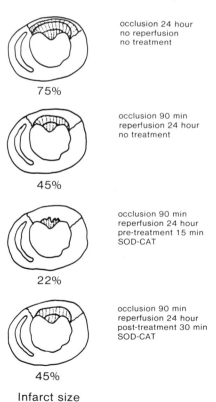

occlusion 24 hour
no reperfusion
no treatment

75%

occlusion 90 min
reperfusion 24 hour
no treatment

45%

occlusion 90 min
reperfusion 24 hour
pre-treatment 15 min
SOD-CAT

22%

occlusion 90 min
reperfusion 24 hour
post-treatment 30 min
SOD-CAT

45%

$$\frac{\text{Infarct size}}{\text{Area at risk}} \%$$

**FIG. 8.** Extent of Injury Associated with Reperfusion of the Ischemic Heart. Schematic summary of data supporting the observation that reperfusion of the heart after a 90-min period of regional ischemia is accompanied by an extension of the ultimate region of the infarction beyond that which could be attributed solely to the ischemic insult. Reperfusion injury was prevented by the administration of superoxide dismutase (SOD) plus catalase (CAT) 15 min before coronary blood flow was restored. Delaying the introduction of the SOD and CAT until a time after reperfusion had been established did not result in myocardial salvage.

in itself is capable of inducing cell damage *via* the reintroduction of molecular oxygen and leukocytes, leading to the formation of oxygen free radicals, then *the possibility arises that oxygen radical scavengers may exert a protective effect upon the heart being subjected to reperfusion for the purpose of preserving myocardial tissue.* As illustrated in Fig. 8, occlusion of the circumflex coronary artery for 90 min with the systemic administration of SOD plus CAT being instituted 15 min before initiating reperfusion and continuing for a total of 1 hr resulted in 22% of the area at risk undergoing necrosis when examined at 24 hr. The same enzyme treatment commencing 45 min after the start of reperfusion did not afford any protection over that observed in the control group undergoing 90 min of occlusion followed by reperfusion.

*These results support the theory that the toxic effects of oxygen free radicals and/or hydrogen peroxide contribute to ischemic injury (16,45) and suggest that therapies directed against reactive oxygen species could salvage jeopardized myocardium.* Similar results have been obtained recently by Chambers and co-workers (7). *Thus, it is conceivable that the damage to ischemic myocardium by free radicals or lipid peroxidation may be minimized by the exogenous administration of a free radical scavenger such as superoxide dismutase. This is particularly true when the source of free radicals is extracellular as would be the case where leukocytes are migrating into an area of injury, a phenomenon which certainly would be enhanced with reperfusion of the once ischemic region.*

## ROLE OF LYSOSOMAL ENZYMES IN ISCHEMIC INJURY

In 1975, Wildenthal (70) postulated that cellular biochemical changes occurring during ischemia resulted in enhanced membrane permeability that allowed lysosome contents to gain access to the cytosol of the cell, an argument that became known as the "lysosomal hypothesis." Wildenthal theorized that abnormal hydrolysis of cellular macromolecules by these lysosomal enzymes could contribute to myocardial cell injury and, if severe enough, would result in cell death. There is compelling evidence to indicate that myocardial cell lysosomes become permeable after 30 min of ischemia (71) with increasing amounts of lysosomal enzyme marker, cathepsin D, appearing in the cytosol over a 2-hr time span. *While there is little doubt that the contents of myocardial cell lysosomes gain access to the cytoplasm after prolonged ischemia, the extent of cell injury caused by leakage of these proteolytic enzymes is not clear.* The lysosomal hypothesis, if truly a factor in the pathophysiology of myocardial infarction, has important implications in the treatment of acute ischemia, since drugs are available which have been shown to stabilize lysosomal membranes and prevent protease release.

### Lysosomes, Granulocytes, Free Radicals, and Ischemic Injury

*The lysosomal hypothesis can be extended to consider the degranulation of activated granulocytes as another source of enzymes capable of proteolytic attack on ischemic myocardial cells.* The involvement of granulocyte lysosomal enzymes in the pathogenesis of inflammatory arthritis has been documented (21). It is conceivable that an acute ischemic insult may trigger an inflammatory response which provides a similar proteolytic attack on myocardial cell membranes and connective tissue. *In short, inflammation may contribute to the extension of irreversible myocardial cell injury by increasing the production of oxygen-derived free radicals produced by activated granulocytes, and through the release of leukocyte lysosomal enzymes into the extracellular space.* The recognition of these deleterious effects of the inflammatory response prompted efforts to protect ischemic myocardium by the administration of antiinflammatory agents in experimental models of myocardial infarction.

### Membrane and Lysosome "Stabilizers" and Infarct Size

Previous attempts using glucocorticoids to inhibit the inflammatory response after an acute ischemic insult led to somewhat mixed results with some investigators reporting a beneficial effect on myocardial infarct size while other authors observed no effect (reviewed in ref. 31). Kloner et al. (32) demonstrated that high doses of methylprednisolone inhibited the inflammatory response to myocardial injury and slowed the removal of necrotic myocytes, resulting in impaired healing in an experimental model of myocardial infarction. However, the potential deleterious effects of methylprednisolone might be more directly attributable to the inhibitory effects of glucocorticoids on protein synthesis and tissue healing; these events are independent of neutrophil function. *Thus, it appears that any pharmacologic attempt to protect ischemic myocardium by modulating neutrophil function may prevent nonspecific neutrophil-mediated injury of viable tissue, but not interfere with the necessary resolution and repair of injured myocardium.*

More recently, efforts to inhibit the inflammatory response while minimizing the unwanted side-effects of glucocorticoid administration have led to the evaluation of newer nonsteroidal antiinflammatory agents in animal models of myocardial ischemia and infarction. One such compound, ibuprofen, was discussed earlier and shown to reduce the extent of irreversible myocardial injury presumably through its antiinflammatory properties. Other investigators have postulated that ibuprofen (1) and naproxen (63) protect ischemic myocardium by stabilizing cardiac lysosomal and cellular membranes. Clearly, these nonsteroidal antiinflammatory agents have the potential to provide cardioprotection in a number of different ways. It remains to be seen which drug effects prove to be the most beneficial during regional myocardial ischemia with or without reperfusion.

### INHIBITION OF LEUKOCYTE CHEMOTAXIS

*Chemotaxis of leukocytes is a cornerstone of the inflammatory response for it is through this directional migration that granulocytes accumulate at the site of tissue injury and carry out their function of resolution and repair. As previously described, this is also true in ischemic myocardium where neutrophils begin to accumulate soon after the start of irreversible myocardial injury.* Leukocyte chemotaxis is a complex physiologic phenomenon and may be stimulated by a wide variety of substances (62,64).

For the sake of discussion, we have simplified the classification scheme for chemotactic factors involved in myocardial ischemia and infarction, and divided them into two categories: complement factors and factors originating from the arachidonic acid cascade.

*This section will focus on efforts to inhibit the production of chemotactic substances so as to prevent the accumulation of leukocytes at the site of ischemic myocardial injury. It should be apparent that the goal of this approach is not to suppress completely the inflammatory response but, instead, to modulate it in such a way as to limit leukocyte infiltration without preventing the resolution and repair of irreversibly injured myocardium.*

## Role of Complement Activation

In 1971, Hill and Ward (19) reported that a tissue protease found in myocardium was released during "nonspecific" ischemic injury induced by coronary artery ligation in the rat. A tissue protease was shown to cleave the third component of the complement system ($C_3$) into fragments possessing chemotactic activity. After treating the rats with fractionated cobra venom factor which depletes serum $C_3$, no $C_3$ fragments were detected after the ischemic insult and neutrophil infiltration into the injured myocardium was reduced.

### Complement Depletion and Infarct Size Limitation

Maroko et al. (42) attempted to reduce the extent of myocardial necrosis resulting from left anterior descending coronary artery ligation by the administration of purified cobra venom factor 30 min after the start of the ischemic insult. The extent of myocardial injury resulting from 24 hr of coronary artery occlusion was evaluated by correlating epicardial electrograms with CK activity and histologic assessment of myocardial tissue samples. For any given degree of epicardial ST-segment elevation there was less loss of CK activity in tissue samples from animals treated with cobra venom factor as compared to samples taken from control animals. In addition, less neutrophilic infiltrate was observed in myocardial tissue biopsies from animals treated with cobra venom factor than in nontreated control animals.

In a similar study, Pinckard and associates (51) evaluated the effect of $C_3$ depletion by cobra venom factor administration in an experimental model of myocardial infarction in the anesthetized baboon. These investigators reported significantly more CK activity per milligram protein in infarcted and "intermediate" ischemic sites (defined by epicardial ECG mapping) 24 hr after the onset of ischemia in those animals treated with cobra venom factor, as compared to the CK activity in comparable tissue samples from control animals. Direct immunofluorescence revealed uniform $C_3$ distribution in those sites classified as "infarcted" and heterogeneous distribution of $C_3$ at those sites considered "intermediate" in samples taken from the control group of baboons. In contrast, there was a failure to localize $C_3$ in any of the tissue samples taken from animals treated with cobra venom factor.

The results of experiments evaluating the effect of $C_3$ depletion on regional myocardial ischemia serve to *emphasize the importance of the complement cascade in the pathophysiology of acute myocardial infarction.*

## *Possible Mechanisms of Injury and Protection*

The mechanism by which $C_3$ depletion provides cardioprotection during regional myocardial ischemia has not been determined completely. *One straightforward explanation could be that by inhibiting the formation of chemotactic complement fragments ($C_3$ and $C_5$) there is a decrease in the leukocytic infiltrate which, in turn, reduces the degree of "nonspecific" myocardial injury from products released by activated granulocytes.*

Jacob (22) has suggested that complement activation may promote the aggregation of granulocytes in the microvasculature of the ischemic myocardium, thus exacerbating the ischemic injury. In this light, perhaps microvascular "sludging" of granulocytes may be prevented by the administration of cobra venom factor or other interventions that modify leukocyte reactivity. Little is known about the possible direct cytotoxic effect of complement localization on ischemic myocytes. Whatever the mechanism of action, it remains to be seen whether the information gained from these studies can be utilized to develop a therapeutic approach to the management of regional myocardial ischemia by manipulation of the complement cascade.

*One can only speculate on the mechanism by which the complement-mediated injury is brought about in the ischemic myocardium.* The subject has been reviewed recently by Fantone and Ward (10). Thus, injured myocardial tissue is believed to release a protease capable of cleaving $C_3$ into leukotactic fragments resulting in the accumulation of neutrophils in the injured myocardial tissue and the regions bordering the ischemic and jeopardized heart muscle. *It is possible that the local product of the oxygen metabolites (hydrogen peroxide, and superoxide, and hydroxyl radicals) by the sequestered leukocytes leads to vascular endothelial and myocardial cell injury. Furthermore, the leukocyte-generated free radicals may augment the inflammatory responses by the enhanced production of a chemotactic lipid resulting from the metabolism of arachidonic acid by the lipoxygenase pathway. Therefore, the leukocyte-derived oxygen metabolites may serve as a positive feedback mechanism that potentiates the local inflammatory response through the generation of chemotactic factors.* Our recent demonstration (5) that continuous infusion of SOD and CAT to the anesthetized dog could reduce the extent of regional myocardial ischemic injury in response to occlusion/reperfusion of the circumflex coronary artery supports this concept.

Based on our previous observations, we suggest that neutrophil accumulation in ischemic myocardial tissue is an important determinant of the ultimate extent of tissue necrosis due to myocardial ischemia. The duration of our studies was intentionally limited, and our studies do not provide any information about the potential long-term benefits of reducing the circulating neutrophil count. It would be valuable to know whether a return of the neutrophil count, after its initial reduction, could result in a resumption of the cellular destructive processes and the ultimate extention of the infarct, or whether neutrophil depletion only delays the development of cellular changes leading to necrosis. *These questions are extremely important and should be of interest to those who seek to limit infarct size experimentally or clinically.*

The present observations are even more significant in view of two recent reports describing the infarct size-sparing effects of BW755C (27,46), a dual inhibitor of lipoxygenase and cyclooxygenase. The beneficial effects of the drug may be related to an effect on leukocytes, either to prevent their migration or to inhibit their function by inhibiting the lipoxygenase-mediated metabolism of arachidonic acid. The production by leukocytes of products of arachidonic acid metabolism, which are known chemotactic agents (49), and the leukotrienes, which can cause coronary artery vasoconstriction (38), along with free radical formation (10), can enhance the degree of myocardial cell injury. *Thus, myocardial cell damage in response to ischemia may, in part, be mediated by the cells that migrate into the ischemic region and the immediate surrounding regions (area of extension).* Therefore, the proposed role of the leukocyte as a mediator of myocardial cell injury offers an opportunity to examine pharmacologic interventions that act to prevent or modify the actions of the leukocytes in response to tissue injury.

Additional studies are needed to define more completely the role of the leukocyte and modification of its function in attempts to limit ischemic myocardial injury.

## Role of Arachidonic Acid Metabolites

*The metabolism of arachidonic acid by prostaglandin synthetase and/or lipoxygenase leads to the production of both pro- and antiinflammatory eicosanoids.* Actions of prostaglandins in inflammation (34) and in myocardial ischemia (20) have been reviewed elsewhere. In this discussion we will focus on products of arachidonic acid metabolism by the lipoxygenase pathway (61). Granulocytes possess 5-lipoxygenase activity and produce lipoxygenase products. Production of $LTB_4$ by polymorphonuclear neutrophils is of particular interest (61). $LTB_4$ is an extremely potent chemotactic substance (48) which may interact with complement fragments to promote leukocytic infiltration in ischemically injured myocardial cells. Other lipoxygenase products such as leukotrienes $C_4$ ($LTC_4$) and $D_4$ ($LTD_4$) have been shown to produce coronary vasoconstriction and to decrease myocardial contractility (50,68). Pharmacologic studies with BW755C, which inhibits the cyclooxygenase and lipoxygenase pathways of arachidonic acid metabolism, suggest that endogenous leukotrienes contribute to myocardial ischemia. Mullane et al. (46) have demonstrated that BW755C reduces myocardial infarct size. Independent studies from our group reached similar conclusions (27). Animals treated with

BW755C (3 or 10 mg/kg) developed smaller infarcts than control animals which received saline (Fig. 9). The high dose of BW755C (10 mg/kg) did not impair the ability of platelets to aggregate *ex vivo* in response to appropriate stimuli. This suggests that lipoxygenase inhibition was the most likely mechanism by which BW755C exerted its beneficial action (27). *Further work with lipoxygenase inhibitors or leukotriene antagonists may lead to useful therapeutic approaches for protecting the ischemic myocardium especially when it is subjected to reperfusion.*

## PATHOPHYSIOLOGY OF ISCHEMIC AND REPERFUSION INJURY AND THE ROLE OF NEUTROPHILS

To summarize the concepts covered in this chapter, a brief description of the pathophysiology of myocardial infarction (see Chapter 3) and reperfusion injury, *with a focus on leukocyte involvement,* is given. Figure 10 is a representation of some of the pathologic processes contributing to a decline in myocyte membrane integrity and, ultimately, cell death. Also noted are sites at which various pharmacologic agents may act to minimize the disruption of the myocardial cell membrane.

### Ischemia-Induced Cellular Changes

The reduction in regional myocardial blood flow may be precipitated by a variety of pathologic processes including atherosclerosis, coronary artery spasm, and coronary artery thrombosis. All that is required is reduction of coronary blood flow to a point where the amount of oxygen and nutrients delivered to the myocardium is inadequate to meet its metabolic demands. Shortly after becoming ischemic, the previously functional myocardium undergoes a rapid decline in contractile activity and concomitantly ceases aerobic metabolism. This shift in metabolism to anaerobic glycolysis results in a decrease in creatine phosphate, followed by a reduction in

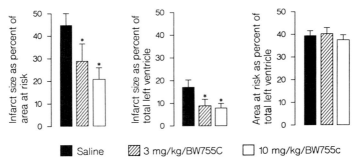

**FIG. 9.** Reduction in Ultimate Infarct Size by BW755C. Effects of BW755C on 24-hr myocardial infarct size. Shows infarct zone normalized as a percent of area at risk, or as a percent of total left ventricle and area at risk as a percent of total left ventricle. Three groups were studied: saline treatment ($n = 16$); low dose BW755C (3 mg/kg, $n = 7$); high dose BW755C (10 mg/kg, $n = 8$). *Asterisks* indicate significant differences compared to the saline control group by one-way analysis of variance followed by Duncan's multiple range test. No differences in area at risk between groups were observed.

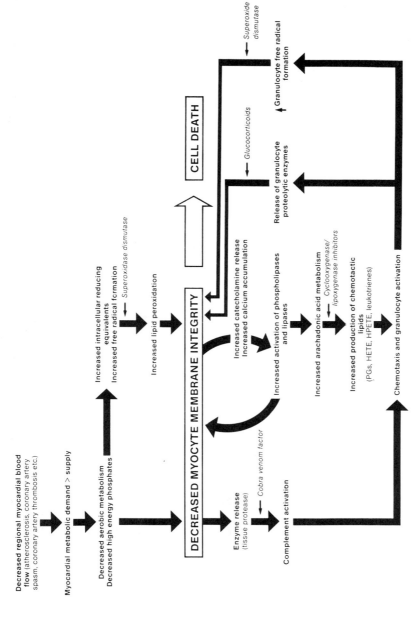

**FIG. 10.** Schematic Representation of the Pathologic Processes Involved in Acute Myocardial Infarction. The diagram indicates the importance of myocardial myocyte membrane integrity in events leading to ischemia induced cell death (see text for details). Also noted are sites at which pharmacologic interventions described in the text are thought to act.

the cellular ATP concentration, production of excess lactate, a decline in myocardial pH, and accumulation of reducing equivalents (NADH) within the cell (8). These derangements in normal cellular metabolism indirectly lead to disruption of myocyte membrane integrity which, in turn, activates other deleterious pathologic processes. For example, with the decline in intracellular ATP, the sodium pump ($Na^+/K^+$, ATPase) is impaired resulting in the loss of $Na^+/K^+$ ion regulation, the loss of cell volume control, and eventual cell swelling. Although early cell swelling is considered a reversible change, the inability to regulate cell volume results in membrane permeability changes which herald the start of a decline in membrane integrity. Once the myocyte membrane becomes permeable to intracellular constituents, two major pathologic mechanisms are activated. First, cellular enzymes released due to a decline in membrane integrity lead to complement activation by tissue proteases thus producing chemotactic $C_3$ fragments (19).

Second, a decrease in membrane integrity and the enhanced sympathetic activity resulting from the "stress" of the ischemic insult combine to increase local catecholamine and $Ca^{2+}$ ion concentrations at the plasma membrane. *These conditions stimulate the activation of membrane phospholipases and lipases which serve to further disrupt membrane integrity (45) and increase the release of chemotactic products from enhanced arachidonic acid metabolism.*

### *Inflammatory Response and Activation of the Complement System*

*The acute inflammatory response is accompanied by activation of the alternative complement pathway with the production of $C_{3a}$ and $C_{5a}$. The cleavage fragments possess anaphylotoxic properties which result in vasoconstriction, vasodilation, and histamine release.* Furthermore, through the action of a naturally occurring plasma carboxypeptidase, $C_{5a}$ undergoes cleavage of the COOH-terminal arginine to give rise to $C_{5a}$-desarg. The latter is a chemotactic factor which recruits additional granulocytes to the area of injury. *The importance of these events is illustrated by previous studies (22,51) in which myocardial infarction was associated with activation of the complement system and in which ultimate infarct size could be reduced by procedures which resulted in modifying the alternative complement pathway.*

The presence of $C_{5a}$-desarg appears to be essential for the margination of leukocytes along the endothelial surface of the vascular bed leading to both functional and morphologic damage that is dependent on the close adhesion of the leukocyte to the endothelial cell. The release of oxygen radicals by the activated and adherent leukocyte causes disruption of intracellular junctions between adjacent endothelial cells, and enhanced vascular permeability, along with migration of inflammatory cells into the immediate extracellular environment, whereby the continued production of cytotoxic oxygen species and vasoactive products cause further extension of the tissue injury. The evidence to date suggests that the systemic activation of the complement system during the initial phase of tissue injury facilitates the adhesion of leukocytes to the vascular endothelial cells. The initial event may be specific for attracting polymorphonuclear leukocytes which, in turn, can be stimulated to produce $LTB_4$, a chemoattractant for neutrophils and monocytes, thereby accounting for the observation that polymorphonuclear leukocyte migration precedes mononuclear cell infiltration to an area of injury.

The mononuclear cell, in addition to being a source of superoxide anion, is capable of producing metabolites of arachidonic acid, including products of both the cyclooxygenase and lipoxygenase pathways. The products of arachidonic acid metabolism have immediate effects on the vasculature, especially $LTC_4$ and $LTD_4$, which cause intense, but short-lived, constriction of arterioles and extravasation of macromolecules from postcapillary venules.

*The combination of the production of chemotactic complement fragments and arachidonic acid metabolites provides potent stimuli for the migration of activated granulocytes to the site of ischemic injury.* Further injury to potentially viable myocytes is thought to result from the activated granulocytes which release oxygen-derived free radicals and proteolytic enzymes in the adjacent extracellular space. Meerson et al. (45) have suggested that the shift to anaerobic metabolism in the ischemic myocardium indirectly contributes to membrane disruption. Anaerobic metabolism leads to the accumulation of reducing equivalents in the form of NADH due to the inhibition of the electron transport chain of aerobic mitochondrial respiration. The accumulation of NADH is thought to contribute to the decline in membrane function by participating in the endogenous generation of oxygen radicals thus leading to further lipid peroxidation and membrane injury. Thus, all of these pathophysiologic processes impinge on the myocardial cell membranes which, when sufficiently damaged, lead inevitably to cell death.

## Reperfusion-Induced Cellular Changes

The deleterious effects of myocardial ischemia, whether regional or global, have been recognized and studied in great detail. Despite extensive investigative efforts, there is still disagreement as to the exact time when the ischemic process progresses to the point of irreversible cell injury. It has been stated that 40 min of regional ischemia in the working heart leads to irreversible myocardial cell damage characterized by well defined ultrastructural changes (23) which become progressive with time. Periods of ischemia less than 40 min followed by reperfusion produce no evidence of ischemia-induced cell death (24). Part of the uncertainty about the point at which ischemic myocardial cells become irreversibly injured stems from the fact that the reintroduction of oxygenated blood, after a period of regional or global ischemia in excess of 40 min, is associated with the phenomenon of "reperfusion injury" characterized by a major extension of cell damage (13,17,18,25), an event that can be reduced or even prevented by cold cardioplegic techniques that decrease myocardial energy demands.

Thus, we are confronted with a paradox—whereas the ischemic myocardium will undergo progressive cellular injury as the ischemic period continues, the restitution of coronary blood flow itself is capable of extending the area of injury. It is thus made essential that we understand those separate cellular destructive mechanisms associated with ischemia as opposed to those resulting from the return of blood flow to the once ischemic myocardial tissue. *Our current thinking is that the reintroduction of leukocytes upon the restitution of coronary blood flow is, in part, responsible for the extensive injury associated with reperfusion.*

## Leukocytes and Reperfusion Injury

The polymorphonuclear leukocyte, monocyte, and tissue macrophage become activated as a result of the ischemic process (2,19). The leukocyte-mediated release of oxygen free radicals and other reduced products of oxygen result in an alteration in vascular permeability to macromolecules, the migration of leukocytes to the extravascular space and their close approximation to injured and viable myocytes. *The process of leukocyte accumulation and the development of an acute inflammatory response are aided by the formation of chemotactic factors as discussed earlier and enhanced by the act of reperfusion.*

The continued production of oxygen radicals by the inflammatory cells causes an accumulation of superoxide anion and hydrogen peroxide because of the low extracellular concentrations of SOD and CAT. The lack of SOD in the extracellular space permits the superoxide anion to generate reduced metal chelates resulting in the formation of the highly destructive hydroxyl radical. It is important to note that hydrogen peroxide is a substrate for myeloperoxidase which leads to the formation of additional oxidative products such as hypochlorite and perhaps singlet oxygen (30,59), both of which can cause extensive tissue injury. These reactions can be mediated by the neutrophil and constitute the process whereby the polymorphonuclear leukocyte exerts an effective bacteriocidal action (2). The important point to note is that the reactive products of oxygen are not specific and will destroy structural molecules such as hyaluronic acid and cause peroxidation of lipid membranes. Thus, the leukocyte, a cell necessary for host defense mechanisms, also may be capable of doing harm.

There are now sufficient data to suggest that some, if not most, of the actions of stimulated neutrophils may be related to the metabolism of arachidonic acid. Special attention must be given to the oxidized derivatives of arachidonic acid which result from the lipoxygenase pathway. The HETEs are synthesized by activated neutrophils and serve to amplify the chemotactic response to the original perturbation (ischemia) of the myocardial cell. Furthermore, the lipoxygenase-produced products of arachidonic acid metabolism may enhance permeability of the leukocyte membrane to the calcium ion. The increase in calcium ion influx would produce a further activation of phospholipase $A_2$ and release of additional arachidonic acid. The essential role of calcium in the activation of the leukocyte suggests a possible site at which selective pharmacologic antagonism may be applied effectively in an effort to modulate the intensity of the inflammatory response. To date, there are no data to suggest that inhibitors of the slow calcium channel are capable of modifying leukocyte function. It is known, however, that several inhibitors of the slow calcium channel are effective in protecting the ischemic heart *in vivo* (6). In this connection, the editors of this book and their colleagues (73) have recently discussed the possibility that slow calcium channel blocking drugs may exert their protective properties, in part, by an inhibition of free radical formation, possibly by influencing the calcium-calmodulin controlled protease reactions. This, in turn, might act to limit free radical production.

### Approaches to Myocardial Protection

There exists a complex relationship between the production of free radicals and other active species of oxygen and the synthesis of eicosonoids by activated leukocytes. The data are convincing that the ability to modulate the reactions of the leukocyte in response to ischemic myocardial injury may serve as an important means by which one could limit the ultimate extent of irreversible cellular injury. More importantly, *attempts to reperfuse ischemic myocardium may be improved by recognition of the role of the leukocyte as a mediator in reperfusion injury.* Several recent reports (14,26,66) have demonstrated the protective effects of free-radical scavengers, superoxide dismutase and catalase, upon the globally and regionally reperfused myocardium. These encouraging results indicate *the need for a better appreciation of the interrelationships that exist between the release of oxygen-free radicals from inflammatory cells, the activation of the complement system, and the other biochemical events which comprise the inflammatory response seen in the ischemic heart or in heart muscle which has been subjected to a period of ischemia followed by reperfusion.* Progress in this area could have important clinical significance in efforts directed toward the salvage of jeopardized, but recoverable, ischemic myocardial tissue. *The evidence at hand suggests that increased attention must be directed at the leukocytes as potential mediators of myocardial cell injury under those circumstances where reperfusion of the ischemic myocardium is employed in an effort to protect the heart against irreversible cellular injury.*

### CONCLUDING COMMENTS

There have been numerous attempts directed at the salvage of ischemic myocardial tissue through the use of a wide variety of pharmacologic agents in both experimental animal studies and in patients with an evolving myocardial infarction. The therapeutic approaches have focused on interventions whereby myocardial oxygen demand would be reduced or in which regional myocardial blood flow would be improved, in either case restoring the balance between oxygen supply and demand. Although the application of this concept has resulted in some success in experimental animals, more recent studies have shown that several nonsteroidal antiinflammatory agents provided protection to the ischemic/reperfused heart without altering the balance between myocardial oxygen supply and demand. Attempts to identify the underlying mechanism for the salutory effects of the nonsteroidal antiinflammatory drugs has led to a consideration of the role of the inflammatory response in mediating myocardial cellular injury associated with ischemia and/or reperfusion. The data support the concept that oxygen derivatives, primarily the superoxide anion radical, hydrogen peroxide, and the hydroxyl radical are important participants in the acute inflammatory response associated with myocardial ischemic injury and/or reperfusion damage. Recent evidence has implicated the polymorphonuclear leukocyte as an important source of reactive oxygen species. Modulation of neutrophil function or the depletion of circulation neutrophils has resulted in protection against the injury associated with ischemia and reperfusion. The administration of the free radical scavenging agents, superoxide dismutase plus catalase, just before the initiation of myocardial reperfusion, reduced the ultimate extent of irreversible myocardial injury. The data support the concept that the reactive *oxygen species derived from extracellular sources* are responsible, in part, for the phenomenon of reperfusion injury, and that myocardial protection can be achieved by modulating the function of the circulating neutrophils and/or by scavenging the reduced species of oxygen produced from this extracellular source. The data are supportive of the notion that reperfusion of the once ischemic myocardium results in cellular injury which extends beyond that which can be attributed to the ischemic process alone, and that *efforts directed at limiting the cytotoxic actions of the leukocyte can lead to an enhancement of myocardial salvage afforded by reperfusion of the previously ischemic heart.*

## REFERENCES

1. Araki, H., and Lefer, A. (1980): Lysosomal stabilizing effect of two nonsteroidal antiinflammatory agents in the hypoxic liver. *Naunyn Schmiederbergs Arch. Pharmacol.*, 311:79–84.
2. Babior, B. (1978): Oxygen-dependent billing of phagocytes. *N. Engl. J. Med.*, 298:659–668.
3. Babior, B., Kipnes, R., and Curnutte, J. (1973): Biological defense mechanisms. The production of leukocytes of superoxide, a potential bacteriocidal agent. *J. Clin. Invest.*, 52:741–744.
4. Bach, M. (1982): Mediators of anaphylaxis and inflammation. *Annu. Rev. Microbiol.*, 36:371–413.
5. Bailie, M., Jolly, S., and Lucchesi, B. R. (1982): Reduction of myocardial ischemic injury by superoxide dismutase plus catalase. *Fed. Proc.*, 41:1736 (abstract).
6. Bush, L. R., Romson, J. L., Ash, J. L., and Lucchesi, B. R. (1982): Effect of diltiazem on the extent of ultimate myocardial injury resulting from temporary coronary artery occlusion in dogs. *J. Cardiovasc. Pharmacol.*, 4:285–296.
7. Chambers, D., Parks, D., Patterson, G., Yoshida, S., Burton, K., Parmley, L., McCord, J., and Downey, J. (1983): Role of oxygen derived radicals in myocardial ischemia. *Fed. Proc.*, 42:1093 (abstract).
8. DeJung, J. (1979): Biochemistry of acutely ischemic myocardium. In: *The Pathophysiology of Myocardial Perfusion*, edited by W. Schaper, pp. 719–750. Elsevier/North-Holland, Amsterdam.
9. Del Maestro, R., Thaw, H., Bjork, J., Planer, M., and Arfors, K. (1980): Free radicals as mediators of tissue injury. *Acta Physiol. Scand. (Suppl.)*, 492:43–57.
10. Fantone, J., and Ward, P. (1982): Role of oxygen derived free radicals and metabolites in leukocyte-dependent inflammatory reactions. *Am. J. Pathol.*, 107:397–418.
11. Freeman, B., and Crapo, J. (1982): Biology of disease. Free radicals and tissue injury. *Lab. Invest.*, 47:412–426.
12. Fridovich, I. (1978): The biology of oxygen radicals. *Science*, 201:875–880.
13. Ganote, C., Seabra-Gomez, R., Nayler, W., and Jennings, R. (1975): Irreversible myocardial injury in anoxic perfused rat hearts. *Am. J. Pathol.*, 80:419–450.
14. Gardner, T., Stewart, J., Casale, A., Downey, J., and Chambers, D. (1983): Reduction of myocardial ischemic injury with oxygen-derived free radical scavengers. *Surgery*, 94:423–427.
15. Gillespie, T., and Sobel, B. (1977): A rationale for therapy of acute myocardial infarction: Limitation of infarct size. *Adv. Intern. Med.*, 22:319–353.

16. Guarnieri, C., Flamingi, F., and Caldarera, C. M. (1980): Role of oxygen in the cellular damage induced by reoxygenation of hypoxic heart. *J. Mol. Cell. Cardiol.*, 12:797–808.
17. Hearse, D. J., Humphrey, S. M., and Chain, E. B. (1973): Abrupt reoxygenation of the anoxic potassium arrested perfused rat heart: A study of myocardial enzyme release. *J. Mol. Cell. Cardiol.*, 5:395–407.
18. Hearse, D. J., Humphrey, S. M., Nayler, W., Slade, A., and Border, D. (1975): Ultrastructural damage associated with reoxygenation of the anoxic myocardium. *J. Mol. Cell. Cardiol.*, 7:315–324.
19. Hill, J., and Ward, P. (1971): The phlogistic role of $C_3$ leukotactic fragments in myocardial infarcts in rats. *J. Exp. Med.*, 133:885–900.
20. Hirsh, P., Campbell, W., Willerson, J., and Hillis, L. (1981): Prostaglandins and ischemic heart disease. *Am. J. Med.*, 71:1009–1026.
21. Honig, S., Hoffstein, S., and Weissman, G. (1978): Leukocyte lysosomes and infiltration: The example of arthritis. *Pathobiol. Ann.*, 8:315–331.
22. Jacob, H. (1981): The role of activated complement and granulocytes in shock states and myocardial infarction. *J. Lab. Clin. Med.*, 98:645–653.
23. Jennings, R., and Ganote, C. (1974): Structural changes in myocardium during acute ischemia. *Circ. Res.*, 34,35 (Suppl. III):156–172.
24. Jennings, R., and Reimer, K. (1979): Biology of experimental, acute myocardial ischemia and infarction. In: *Enzymes in Cardiology: Diagnosis and Research*, edited by D. J. Hearse and J. de Leiris, pp. 21–57. John Wiley, Chichester.
25. Jennings, R., Sommers, H., Smyth, G., Flack, H., and Linn, H. (1960): Myocardial necrosis induced by temporary occlusion of a coronary artery in the dog. *Arch. Pathol.*, 70:68–78.
26. Jolly, S., Kane, W., Bailie, M., Abrams, G., and Lucchesi, B. (1983): Reduction of reperfusion injury after canine myocardial ischemia by superoxide dismutase plus catalase. *Circulation*, 68:III–185 (abstract).
27. Jolly, S., and Lucchesi, B. (1983): Effect of BW755C in an occlusion-reperfusion model of ischemic myocardial injury. *Am. Heart J.*, 106:8–13.
28. Jugdutt, B., Hutchins, G., Bulkley, B., and Becker, L. (1980): Salvage of ischemic myocardium by ibuprofen during infarction in the conscious dog. *Am. J. Cardiol.*, 46:74–82.
29. Kantor, T. (1979): Ibuprofen. *Ann. Int. Med.*, 91:877–882.
30. Klebanoff, S. (1975): Antimicrobial systems of the polymorphonuclear leukocyte. In: *The Phagocytic Cell in Host Resistance*, edited by J. A. Bellanti and D. H. Dayton. Raven Press, New York.
31. Kloner, R., and Braunwald, E. (1980): Observations on experimental myocardial ischemia. *Cardiovasc. Res.*, 14:371–395.
32. Kloner, R., Fishbein, M., Lew, H., Maroko, P., and Braunwald, E. (1978): Mummification of the infarcted myocardium by high doses of corticosteroids. *Circulation*, 57:56–63.
33. Ksiezycka, E., Hastie, R., and Maroko, P. R. (1983): Reduction in myocardial damage after experimental coronary artery occlusion by two techniques which deplete neutrophils. *Circulation*, 68:III-185 (abstract).
34. Kuehl, F., and Egan, R. (1980): Prostaglandins, arachidonic acid and inflammation. *Science*, 210:978–984.
35. Lautsch, E. (1979): Morphologic factors of clinical significance in myocardial infarction—A review. *Tex. Rep. Biol. Med.*, 39:371–386.
36. Lefer, A., and Crossley, K. (1980): Mechanisms of the optimal protective effects of ibuprofen in acute myocardial ischemia. *Adv. Shock Res.*, 3:133–141.
37. Lefer, A., and Polansky, E. (1979): Beneficial effects of ibuprofen in acute myocardial ischemia. *Cardiology*, 64:265–279.
38. Letts, L. G., and Piper, P. J. (1982): The actions of leukotrienes $C_4$ and $D_4$ on guinea-pig isolated hearts. *Br. J. Pharmacol.*, 76:169–176.
39. MacLean, D., Fishbein, M. C., Braunwald, E., and Maroko, P. R. (1978): Long-term preservation of ischemic myocardium after experimental coronary artery occlusion. *J. Clin. Invest.*, 61:541–551.
40. MacLean, D., Fishbein, M., Maroko, P., and Braunwald, E. (1979): Long-term salvage of ischemic myocardium by depleting catecholamines and inhibiting inflammation. *Clin. Res.*, 25:455A (abstract).
41. Mallory, G., White, P., and Salcedo-Salger, J. (1939): The speed of healing of myocardial infarction. A study of the pathologic anatomy in seventy-two cases. *Am. Heart J.*, 18:647–671.

42. Maroko, P., Carpenter, C., Chiariello, M., Fishbein, M., Radvany, P., Knostman, J., and Hale, S. (1978): Reduction by cobra venom factor of myocardial necrosis after coronary artery occlusion. *J. Clin. Invest.*, 61:661–670.
43. Maroko, P., Kjekshus, J., Sobel, B., Watanabe, T., Covell, J., Ross, J., and Braunwald, E. (1971): Factors influencing infarct size following experimental coronary artery occlusion. *Circulation*, 43:67–83.
44. McIntyre, B., and Philip, R. (1977): Effect of three nonsteroidal anti-inflammatory agents on platelet function and prostaglandin synthesis *in vitro*. *Thromb. Res.*, 12:67–77.
45. Meerson, F., Kagan, V., Kozlov, Y., Belkina, L., and Arkhippenko, Y. (1982): The role of lipid peroxidation in pathogenesis of ischemic damage and the anti-oxidant protection of the heart. *Basic Res. Cardiol.*, 77:465–485.
46. Mullane, K., and Moncada, S. (1982): The salvage of ischemic myocardium by BW755C in anesthetized dogs. *Prostaglandins*, 24:255–266.
47. O'Brien, J. (1968): Effect of antiinflammatory agents on platelets. *Lancet*, 1:894–895.
48. Palmblad, J., Malmetin, C., Uden, O., Radmark, O., Engstedt, L., and Sammuelsson, B. (1981): Leukotriene B$_4$ is a potent and stereo-specific stimulator of neutrophil chemotaxis and adherence. *Blood*, 58:658–661.
49. Palmer, R. M. J., Stepney, R. J., Higgs, G. A., and Eakins, K. E. (1980): Chemokinetic activity of arachidonic acid lipoxygenase products of leukocytes of different species. *Prostaglandins*, 20:411–418.
50. Panzenbeck, M., and Kalaz, G. (1983): Leukotriene D$_4$ reduces coronary blood flow in the anesthetized dog. *Prostaglandins*, 25:661–670.
51. Pinckard, R., O'Rourke, R., Crawford, M., Grover, F., McManus, L., Ghidoni, J., Storrs, S., and Olson, M. (1980): Complement localization and mediation of ischemic injury in baboon myocardium. *J. Clin. Invest.*, 66:1050–1056.
52. Rao, P. S., and Mueller, H. S. (1982): Lipid peroxide production and glutathione peroxidase depletion in rat myocardium after acute infarction. *Clin. Chem.*, 27:1027 (abstract).
53. Reimer, K., and Jennings, R. (1979): The "wavefront phenomenon" of myocardial ischemic cell death. II. Transmural progression of necrosis within the framework of ischemic bed size (myocardium at risk) and collateral flow. *Lab. Invest.*, 40:633–644.
54. Ribeiro, L., Yasuda, T., Lowenstein, E., Braunwald, E., and Maroko, P. (1979): Comparative effects of anatomic infarct size of verapamil, ibuprofen and morphine chlorpromazine combination. *Am. J. Cardiol.*, 43:398 (abstract).
55. Romson, J., Bush, L., Jolly, S., and Lucchesi, B. (1982): Cardioprotective effects of ibuprofen in experimental regional and global myocardial ischemia. *J. Cardiovasc. Pharmacol.*, 4:187–196.
56. Romson, J., Hook, B., Kunkel, S., Abrams, G., Schork, A., and Lucchesi, B. (1983): Reduction in the extent of ischemic myocardial injury by neutrophil depletion in the dog. *Circulation*, 67:1016–1023.
57. Romson, J., Hook, B., Rigot, V., Schork, A., Swanson, D., and Lucchesi, B. (1982): The effect of ibuprofen on accumulation of Indium-111 labelled platelets and leukocytes in experimental myocardial infarction. *Circulation*, 66:1002–1011.
58. Root, R., and Metcalf, J. (1977): H$_2$O$_2$ release from human granulocytes during phagocytosis: Relationship to superoxide anion formation and cellular catabolism of H$_2$O$_2$: Studies with normal and cytochalasin B-treated cells. *J. Clin. Invest.*, 60:1266–1279.
59. Rosen, H., and Klebanoff, S. (1979): Bacteriocidal activity of a superoxide anion-generating system: A model for the polymorphonuclear leukocyte. *J. Exp. Med.*, 149:27–39.
60. Rosenberg, H., and Klebba, A. (1979): Trends in cardiovascular mortality with a focus on ischemic heart disease: United States, 1950–1976. In: *Proceedings: Conference on Decline in Coronary Heart Disease Mortality*, edited by R. Havlik and M. Fienleib, pp. 11–39. Department of Health, Education and Welfare, National Institutes of Health, Washington, D.C.
61. Sammuelsson, B., Hammerstrom, S., Murphy, R., and Borgeat, P. (1980): Leukotrienes and slow reacting substance of anaphylaxis. *Allergy*, 35:375–381.
62. Schifferman, E. (1982): Leukocyte chemotaxis. *Annu. Rev. Physiol.*, 44:553–568.
63. Smith, E., and Lefer, A. (1981): Stabilization of cardiac lysosomal and cellular membranes in protection of ischemic myocardium due to coronary occlusion: Efficacy of the nonsteroidal antiinflammatory agent, naproxen. *Am. Heart J.*, 101:394–402.
64. Synderman, R., and Goetzl, E. (1981): Molecular and cellular mechanisms of leukocyte chemotaxis. *Science*, 213:830–837.

65. Sobel, B., Bresnahan, G., Shell, W., and Yoder, R. (1972): Estimation of infarct size in man and its relation to prognosis. *Circulation*, 46:640–648.
66. Stewart, J., Blackwell, W., Crute, S., Loughlin, V., Greenfield, L., and Hess, M. (1983): Inhibition of surgically-induced ischemia/reperfusion injury by oxygen free radical scavengers. *J. Thorac. Cardiovasc. Surg.*, 86:262–272.
67. Snyderman, R., and Goetzle, E. (1981): Molecular and cellular mechanisms of leukocyte chemotaxis. *Science*, 213:830–839.
68. Terashita, Z., Fukui, H., Hirata, M., Terao, A., Olikama, S., Nishikawa, K., and Kikuchi, S. (1981): Coronary vasoconstriction and $PGI_2$ release by leukotrienes in isolated guinea pig hearts. *Eur. J. Pharmacol.*, 73:357–361.
69. Thom, T., and Kannel, W. (1981): Downward trend in cardiovascular mortality. *Annu. Rev. Med.*, 32:427–434.
70. Wildenthal, K. (1975): Lysosomes and lysosomal enzymes in the heart. In: *Lysosomes in Biology and Pathology*, Vol. 4, edited by J. T. Dingle and R. T. Dean, pp. 167–190. North-Holland, Amsterdam.
71. Wildenthal, K. (1978): Lysosomal alterations in ischemic myocardium: Result or cause of myocellular damage? *J. Mol. Cell. Cardiol.*, 10:595–603.
72. Weissmann, G., Smolen, J., and Korchak, H. (1980): Release of inflammatory mediators from stimulated neutrophils. *N. Engl. J. Med.*, 303:27–34.
73. Yellon, D. M., Downey, J. M., and Hearse, D. J. (1984): Myocardial infarct size limitation: principles, problems and possibilities. *Ital. J. Cardiol. (in press)*.

# Subject Index

## DATE DUE

| AG  6 '97 | | | |
|---|---|---|---|
| | | | |
| | | | |
| | | | |
| | | | |
| | | | |
| | | | |
| | | | |
| | | | |
| | | | |
| | | | |
| | | | |
| | | | |
| | | | |
| | | | |
| | | | |
| | | | |
| | | | |
| | | | |